3D Printing in Bone Surgery

Carmine Zoccali
Pietro Ruggieri • Francesco Benazzo
Editors

3D Printing in Bone Surgery

Springer

Editors
Carmine Zoccali
Department of Anatomical, Histological
Forensic Medicine and Orthopaedic
Science
Sapienza University of Rome
Rome, Italy

Pietro Ruggieri
Department of Orthopedics and
Orthopedic Oncology
University of Padova
Padova, Italy

Francesco Benazzo
Sezione di Chirurgia Protesica ad
Indirizzo Robotico - Unità di
Traumatologia dello Sport
U.O. Ortopedia e Traumatologia
Fondazione Poliambulanza
Brescia, Italy

ISBN 978-3-030-91899-6 ISBN 978-3-030-91900-9 (eBook)
https://doi.org/10.1007/978-3-030-91900-9

This Springer imprint is published by the registered company Springer Nature Switzerland AG
The registered company address is: Gewerbestrasse 11, 6330 Cham, Switzerland

Foreword

Progress in 3D technology (imaging, printing, and modeling) is changing our approach to surgery.

Three-dimensional CT scan and MRI increased consistently our knowledge about anatomy, both normal and pathological. But they actually give us a 3D simulation on a computer screen (with ultimate expression as virtual reality) and it may be sometimes hard to incorporate all the information available in real surgery.

Computer-assisted and robot-assisted systems of surgery are two of the philosophies that, at the present day, are trying to fill this gap. But they need a significant investment in terms of resources, training, and time to become effective in daily practice.

A completely different approach is to create a three-dimensional life-sized model of a normal or abnormal anatomical structure.

This model can offer us a multisensory interaction to a pathological condition or to plain anatomy, based both on binocular vision and touch, with a consistent improvement in spatial conceptualization: this term stands for complex subject of planning and the related practical activities (to define surgical strategy, create surgical guides, project and make custom implants, provide tangible references during surgical procedures).

Besides the surgical applications, almost unlimited possibilities may arise from the use of individual anatomy models: for educational purpose in teaching programs, for patient information in consent collection to mention just two of them.

In Orthopedic Surgery, a three-dimensional model seems to significantly improve the understanding of complex anatomic situation as often encountered in complex primary joint reconstruction (post-traumatic arthritis, congenital or acquired joint or segmental dysplasia, tarsal and carpal avascular necrosis, adaptive changing in near bone or joint structures) or where a severe bone loss has to be managed as in Revision Joint Surgery or in primitive and secondary bone and soft tissue neoplastic lesions.

This "touch and see" process to comprehend anatomy is not limited to bone and may include vascular structures and soft tissues.

Moreover, these models allow creating custom implants that match individual anatomy and restore biomechanics, giving a simpler and time-saving procedure during reconstructive steps.

It becomes evident especially when a 3D model of the custom implant is available to the surgeon in the preoperative phase, giving the opportunity to become familiar with its reciprocal relationship with anatomic resin model and where, besides the main prosthetic device manufacturing, additional details have been accurately planned and simulated (i.e., type, length, and screws positioning; choice of modularity, if available).

"Additive" techniques and advancement in trabecular metal technologies dramatically improve primary stability and osteointegration of these implants, together with the potential perfect match to patient anatomy.

In Trauma Surgery, a three-dimensional depiction of segmental or joint injuries gives the opportunity to surgeons to outline key point in anatomical reduction, hardware type and placement, even to predict screws length and their optimal positioning (because the model is life-sized).

Finally, in all body areas bone loss after both traumatic and neoplastic pathologies (i.e., in oro-maxillary surgery, craniofacial surgery, both for skull and spine loss, in some aspects of thoracic surgery) can be successfully addressed with custom prosthetic implants, and resin models are frequently used to improve preoperative plan and surgeon skills to reduce operative times.

Undoubtedly technological improvements significantly reduced time and costs of manufacturing, both for plastic models and final implants, contributing to push forward practical applications: the possibility to share real-time imaging files with manufacturers and the option to remotely control 3D printers for resin modeling open the way to a daily use of this technology for clinical and educational purpose.

It is my opinion that this volume will represent an excellent guideline in the comprehension of the possible applications of this technology, supporting those willing to approach the use of this not only for planning purpose but also for reconstructive issues taking advantages of their choice of the experiences reported by different authors of the volume.

Francesco Falez
Department of Orthopaedics, ASL Roma 1
Rome, Italy

Ospedale San Filippo Neri
Rome, Italy

Sapienza University of Rome
Rome, Italy

Preface

In the last decades, there has been an important increase in the global survival of patients affected by musculoskeletal tumors. This improvement has given way to the research of new reconstructive techniques to assure better function and higher quality of life for the patient.

The idea to produce "spare parts" specifically for the patient originates with surgery; actually, the first prostheses, although rudimentary, were produced based on the patient's specific anatomic characteristics.

Later, the development of modular prostheses made the first custom-made prostheses obsolete, also because they were characterized by high costs and a long production time.

The development of additive manufacturing and its application to medicine, specifically to bone reconstruction, has made custom-made prosthesis affordable for everyone.

We are currently witnessing a fundamental change also in materials: the present is titanium, the immediate future is composite materials whereas the future is biological materials and the production of "original spare parts."

Research goes on, society evolves, and one who hesitates is lost.

This book aims at taking stock of the situation regarding additive manufacturing applied to bone reconstruction in the different segments and at giving new inspiration for the future.

The authors evaluated the application of custom-made reconstruction, proposed their experience, and underlined related problems and possible solutions for all segments.

Rome, Italy — Carmine Zoccali
Padova, Italy — Pietro Ruggieri
Brescia, Italy — Francesco Benazzo

Contents

Indications: Didactical Use of 3D Printing, Surgical Didactical Use, Surgical Planning, Patient Information, Custom-Made Prosthesis, Spacer and Template, External Prosthesis, Cast

1

Michele Boffano, Alessandro Aprato, and Raimondo Piana

Introduced in the last decade, the use of 3D printing in the field of orthopedics is relatively new. It helps in understanding anatomy, teaching, research, surgical planning, and manufacturing customized implants. This innovative technology is growing fast in the orthopedic markets [1, 2].

1.1 3D Model Development

Rapid Prototyping (RP), whether CT or MRI based, allows to create quickly and precisely 3D devices that help orthopedic surgeons to study the shape of the fracture, the bone or joint involved, or the neoplasms and tailor surgical solutions. A CT scan with slice thickness of 1 mm is requested to create an accurate bone model. Angio-CT or angio-MRI sequences are requested to add vessels to the model. MRI also adds information to study muscles and other soft tissues. The combination of CT and MRI can better visualize the pelvic organs and the shape and margins of a neoplasm [1–4].

An intraoperative alternative to computer navigation is Patient-Specific Instrument (PSI). Following the previous use for total knee and hip arthroplasty, for pedicle screw insertion and for corrective osteotomy, PSI has recently also been adapted to bone tumor surgery. The PSI is a customized tool, designed to have bone-specific contact surfaces aiming to guide a saw or a drill into the desired resection planes or positions. These cutting guides are designed on the basis of patient 3D reconstructed images and Computer-Aided Design (CAD) softwares, allowing surgeons to plan surgeries based on the patient's unique anatomy. The blocks of the PSI consist of three components: (1) a surface of contact, that conforms to the footprints contour predetermined by the surgeons, so that the blocks could be positioned consistently near the site of the planned resections without translation; (2) three-planar cutting slot in the blocks, based on the unique orientation of the resection planes defined during virtual simulation in the software; (3) cylindrical guides for the insertion of Kirschner wires to fix the PSI to pelvic bone after correctly positioning the PSI (Fig. 1.1). In addition, PSI provides calibration marks to control over the cutting depth to prevent

M. Boffano (✉) · R. Piana
Oncologic Orthopaedic Surgery Department, CTO Hospital, AOU Città della Salute e della Scienza di Torino, Torino, Italy
e-mail: mboffano@cittadellasalute.to.it

A. Aprato
Orthopaedic and Traumatology 1 Department, CTO Hospital, AOU Città della Salute e della Scienza di Torino, Torino, Italy

C. Zoccali et al. (eds.), *3D Printing in Bone Surgery*, https://doi.org/10.1007/978-3-030-91900-9_1

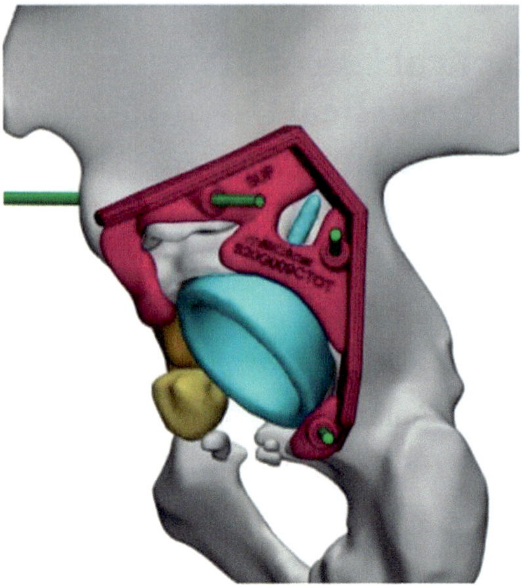

Fig. 1.1 PSI model for chondrosarcoma pelvic resection with adequate margins

a soft tissue tear by the saw. These marks represent the distance along the associated direction line measured between the outer edge of the PSI and the deepest bone structure to be cut. Following surgeons' indications about the surgical approach or exposure, the nearby soft tissues, the defined position and the direction for the placement of PSI, the engineers combine the different components of PSI and create a unique contact interface between the PSI and the host bone [1, 5–7].

Orthopedic surgeons could also practice and familiarize with the proper placement of the PSI on bone models, fabricated on a 3D printing machine, before approving the final design. The final product is made of a thermoplastic material, with high chemical resistance and high tensile strength, stable to temperatures up to 130 °C and thus sterilizable for the use in the operating theater [1, 7, 8].

Intraoperatively, surgeons can generally use a standard surgical approach and soft tissue dissection. A possible limit to the technique might be the need for an adequate exposure of the bone surface to optimally fit to it without interfering with soft tissues (ligaments, muscles insertions, etc.) or noble structures (nerves and vessels) [8, 9]. However, Gouin et al. [6] showed that PSI requires only a limited extra bone exposure (less than 10 mm).

1.2 Didactical Use and Patient Information

The complexity of orthopedic surgical techniques is increasing. Often it is difficult to correctly explain the surgery to the patients. Sometimes the surgeon should plan in advance if to realize patient-specific instrumentation (PSI), which is the proper implant or the relationships with major vessels or intrapelvic organs. A case study can be prepared using CT and/or MRI to develop a 3D model either on an interactive pdf file or even printed [1].

On the other hand, Computer Navigation is a passive system of image-guided techniques that provides a real-time, interactive, 3D digital map of a patient's anatomy. A process called "registration" allows to associate the patient's imaging information and anatomical landmarks using an intraoperative navigated device. This procedure increases spatial accuracy during dissection, surgical resection and instrumentation through a continuous control of images by the surgeon on a video monitor.

The first interesting results in orthopedic oncology were obtained by Cartiaux and al., with simulation on plastic pelvic models [11]. They affirmed that the probability for an experienced surgeon to obtain a 10-mm surgical resection margin with a 5-mm tolerance above or below was only 52% (95% CI 37–67). Also, the degree of host–graft contact for reconstruction was found to be poor. This group went on to demonstrate in another experimental study that cutting accuracy was significantly improved with computer navigation guidance [11]. In a simulated sawbone model, the error of navigated cutting was only 2.8 mm, whereas that of the non-navigated group was 5.2 mm [1, 8, 10, 11].

While Computer Navigation is an operative instrument to deal orthopedic surgery with high precision, 3D modeling and 3D printing are excellent instruments to plan surgery in advance and prevent theoretical complications. 3D modeling and printing are also an important supplementary learning and teaching resource in undergraduate anatomy education and postgraduate surgical training. Unexperienced surgeons can simulate the surgical procedure without fear and with lower costs than a cadaver lab. The experienced surgeon can show and simulate the surgery to his/her fellows to explain the main steps and obtain a better collaboration in operating room [12].

An interactive pdf file containing a 3D model is a simple way to explain surgery to the patient and his/her relatives showing the starting point, the expected results, and the difficulties of the surgery. Furthermore, it is a demonstration of the accurate case study performed and the attention dedicated to the patient's medical problem.

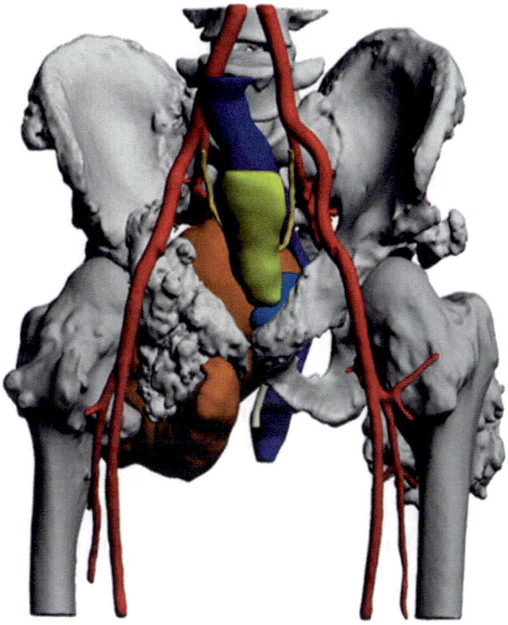

Fig. 1.2 3D model of pelvic chondrosarcoma in close proximity to iliac and femoral vessels, rectum, bladder, and prostate

1.3 Surgical Planning

Custom pelvic prostheses are used to reconstruct the bone defect following complex pelvic bone tumor resection. CAOS allows the engineers to design and tailor-made an implant that matches exactly to the anticipated bone loss after tumor resection. However, the degree of fitting of the custom implant greatly depends on the ability of the surgeons to reproduce intraoperatively the resection as planned. Pelvic tumor surgery is challenging because of the complex bony anatomy and the close proximity to pelvic organs and neurovascular structures. Accurate resections with wide margins are the most important prognostic factor in managing pelvic bone tumors [1, 5].

Thanks to the use of different colors in the 3D model, oncology surgeons can obtain a better mental picture of the tumor location and accurately define the surgical resection planes with specific orientation on the virtual patient image (Fig. 1.2). Preoperative planning also consists in selecting the best surgical approach and defining the location of the noble structures to detect and protect during surgery.

A local recurrence rate of up to 70% is observed after a marginal resection, and 92% after an intralesional resection [5]. To date, three modalities are possible to perform free margin resections and the closest to preoperative planning: free-hand resections, 3D computer navigation and patient-specific Instrument (PSI). Free-hand resections are certainly the least accurate, despite the surgeon can train on plastic three-dimensional models printed on patient image data. In recent years, intraoperative 3D navigation and PSI guides have been described with good results. Comparing free-hand cutting of pelvic bone tumors with PSI cutting, a significant difference was demonstrated [1, 13]. In fact, free-hand cutting is not accurate enough to ensure wide margins: the errors on the desired safe margin averaged 5.3 mm, with a standard deviation ranging from 2.7 to 5.3 mm among the experienced surgeons, and two resections out of 12 were intralesional. Instead, PSI enables the surgeon to intraoperatively replicate the planned resections with a very good cutting accuracy. Wong et al. [7] reported a millimetric accuracy during a PSI-assisted bone tumor resection of the femur. Khan et al. [8] also investigated bone-cutting accuracy and reported a 2-mm location accuracy during a PSI-assisted multiplanar resection on a cadaveric femur. The observed level of accuracy suggests that a 5-mm safe margin should be sufficient to obtain clear surgical margins when using PSI. This decrease in the level of desired safe margins allows to perform resections closer to the tumor boundary, offering the possibility to preserve for example the sacroiliac or the hip joint, a specific portion of a supporting bone, muscle insertions, or nerve roots. Similarly, a recent cadaveric study compares navigation-assisted and PSI techniques in simulated pelvic bone resections [9]. The mean average deviation error from the planned resection was not different for the navigation and the PSI groups: in both techniques it was less than 2 mm. The mean time required for the bone resection in the navigation group, instead, was significantly greater than that in the PSI group. In fact, Cartiaux [10] showed a similar trend. In this study, the time required for a pelvic resection was 49 min for navigation assistance versus 6.9 min with PSI assistance. The increased operative time in the navigation group can be due to the time required for the placement of patient's tracker, system calibration and image-to-patient registration prior to the navigated bone resections. In addition, surgeons have to manually control the direction of the sawblade for the resection under visual guidance on the navigation display, as the existing navigation system does not support a navigated saw. The greatest risk of PSI is the wrong positioning of its components on the bone surface that leads to a complete lack of precision during the bone-cuts. Further studies are needed to investigate how much bone contact surface is necessary for an accurate placement of the PSI. According to the actual results, the PSI can be performed safely and provides a good cutting accuracy. The intraoperative use of the PSI appeared to be quick and easy-to-handle and to require minimal operative setup. The next step is designing the reconstructive planning after tumor resection. Based on precise 3D resection planning and preoperative CT images, a prosthetic or an allograft reconstruction are possible.

Thanks to the advances in technology that allow 3D preoperative plan and models, it is possible to ensure a better execution of surgical procedures in trauma, hip preserving surgery, and arthroplasty. Virtual joints model can be applied in Femoro-Acetabular Impingement (FAI), Developmental Dysplasia of the Hip (DDH), pelvic or femoral osteotomies, complex arthroplasties [4, 14]. A virtual 3D model gives to the surgeon many information about bone deformities and joint biomechanics but sometimes a real model is mandatory. Furthermore, 3D technologies may also helpful in trauma settings: they help in planning the fracture reduction techniques, in the choice of type and allocation of devices and also in customizing plates before surgery.

The Rapid Prototyping (RP) can be the answer: it is defined as a set of techniques to achieve physical models useful for features verification of a model. The target is to create a prototype of the bone component to be corrected which faithfully reproduces the size and shape and which is possible to handle. RP is a procedure composed by three fundamentals steps: the creation of a "Standard Triangulation Language to Layer" file (STL), the STL file verification and preparation before the actual construction of the prototype, and the construction of the prototype layer by layer. The deposition of material can occur by different ways; one of these is the "Fused Deposition Modeling" (FDM) [4, 14]. As described by Ratnadurai et al. [15] FDM is a rapid method to obtain a real model that can be sterilized by gamma radiation and can be handled by the surgeon in the operating room.

1.4 Custom-Made Prosthesis

Tailored solutions are not a novelty in orthopedic surgery, although not involving 3D. During pioneer years, THA have been built following silicone molds with disastrous results [1, 16]. Nevertheless, custom-made implants have been extensively used in hip, knee, or humerus showing good outcomes. Oncologic surgery soon made the most with 3D printing, starting with maxillofacial surgery and neurosurgery, but involving just later most of the other surgical specialties [17–20]. Orthopedic oncology has an historical background of custom-made implants; in fact, the first custom-made implant for limb salvage procedure had been implanted in Wien in 1975 [21]. From the early 1990s, the use of custom-made prostheses began to be commonly accepted [22]. Orthopedic oncology received many benefits from 3D technologies, especially in pelvic surgery where the increasing use of 3D printing gave the possibility to build custom-made implants in an easier and (theoretically) less expensive way. In literature, several case reports and small series are reported [23]. Clavicular, scapular, vertebral, knee, and pelvic implants have been described [24]. Virtually any kind of anatomical site could be reconstructed with 3D custom implants for bone or soft tissue tumors, but pelvic is the elective one. Custom-made implants in orthopedic oncology are nowadays a reality in surgical reconstruction of massive periacetabular defects. As previously described, pelvis has a complex 3D anatomy and very important close neurovascular structures. Moreover, being the fulcrum of high forces, implants with the highest probability of ingrowth are the most suitable for long term survival. 3D printing permits easily to add pins, to fit short stems in case of poor bone quality, to guide screw holes, till to foresee screws length. All these features allow, in selected cases, to merge ideal qualities of bespoke shape with high-tech surfaces, in order to minimize the limb loss of function. Nevertheless, custom-made implants are a small part of global reconstructions. Still highly expensive, they need to be implanted in super-specialized centers, with a solid environment of clinicians, surgeons, engineers, and manufacturers. Postoperative care as well needs to be tailored on the patient. When a custom-made component is planned and implanted in an oncologic patient, it is the result of a strong cooperation and a solid workflow [1, 4, 25].

Choosing a custom-made implant presents several benefits that may lead to relevant advantages for the surgeon and subsequently for the patient.

1. *Surgical margins.* The choice of a custom-made implant in orthopedic oncology permits to clarify preoperatively surgical resections, magnifying the chance to obtain adequate surgical margins.
2. *Surgical time.* Preoperative planning, with predetermined screw length, permits an easy-to-fix implant. Custom-made cutting guides or navigation add further advantages. The combination of these two techniques potentially shortens surgical timings, preventing infections and improving general clinical conditions in high complexity patients. A shorter surgical time means frequently lower blood loss and a better recovery for the patient. In addition, a shorter surgical time reduces the cost of surgery.
3. *Reconstruction quality.* 3D printing technique permits highly congruent implants that improve significantly bone–metal interface, creating a wider surface to promote integration. Recent studies described the functional improvement and the lower revision rate in comparison to older techniques for 3D custom implants. Moreover, finite element analysis have been used to evaluate the different behavior of implants, in order to identify more stressed zones and to use the more technically efficient design [23, 26].

A biomechanically efficient design of 3D-printed components can obviate to those situations where muscular forces are modified due to extensive resections. A shorter surgical time, wider margins with lower recurrence rate, lower revision rate, and a faster recovery can improve the Quality of Life (QoL) of the patient and determine less expensive global costs counterpointed to an expensive implant [1, 3].

On the other side, there are many problems that may affect significantly the use of 3D implants and they are mainly related to orthopedic oncology.

1. *Learning curve.* Resection of pelvic tumors is highly demanding from a surgical point of view. Few centers treat a sufficient number of cases to train skilled young surgeons. The importance to be precise and safe is even more requested in pelvic surgery. Moreover, computer-assisted resections need further skills that are partially independent from specific oncologic surgical abilities [1, 4, 27]. Nevertheless, this problem affects globally

pelvic oncologic surgery and not specifically 3D-assisted surgery.

2. *Intraoperative resection changes.* This is the main topic to explore when using a custom implant. In fact custom implants works properly to fill a predefined bone loss. Some problems may emerge if a wider resection is needed. If preoperative Imaging is done as closer as possible to the interventions, very few intraoperative changes are expected. In most of the cases intraoperative changes are probably due to a lack of accuracy in the preoperative planning more than an effective problem with 3D-printed implants. In some cases, the implant could be adapted without compromising the final result. In extreme cases, it would be better to convert the reconstructive procedure to "traditional" solutions (hip transposition, allograft, reconstruction cages). A two-steps procedure (resection first, production and reconstruction with custom-made implant in a second surgery) has recently been described in some centers [1, 27, 28].
3. *Routine use.* It is important to keep in mind that the use of custom 3D-printed implants it is not an every-day solution. One problem is the effective time needed to properly plan resection, design, print, and sterilize the implant. In rapidly growing, poor responding masses, like in some cases of malignant soft tissue tumors involving the bone, a custom-made implant could not be the best option. In fact, during the whole design and manufacturing time, tumor may grow putting at risk not only the effectiveness of the implant but the feasibility of limb salvage as well. In some other cases (i.e., fractured metastatic patients) the patient may not have a real QoL improvement from a custom implant. Life expectancy, pain control, and residual function have to be carefully evaluated to choose the best treatment option. Case centralization in highly specialized center is the best way to control and use in the proper way all the existing techniques [1, 3, 26].
4. *Costs.* A 3D implant requires a huge organization. 3D printing, although its enormous expansion during these years, is still expensive. The entire organization, from Computer Assisted Drafting (CAD) till physical manufacturing of the definitive implant, involves many people. Sometimes cutting guides are printed with selective laser sintering (SLS) or FDM, while electron beam melting (EBM) printers are used for the implant. Additional intraoperative navigation increases the costs. Nevertheless, no cost-effectiveness [29] studies are available to support one option against the others.

Like many other innovations, 3D printing implants seems to be very promising and they could make a radical difference in complex reconstructive cases. 3D-printed implants and global planning could substantially help the surgeon. Like many others, these technologies have some limitations too.

1. *Presence of previous metal implants:* metal implants lead to artifacts. Either if diamagnetic steel, titanium or CrCoMo, all metal implants are quite incompatible with 3D-printing implants. Advanced MRI and CT scanners, even if with metal signaling suppression, do not have the sufficient detecting power to avoid completely the scattering phenomenon [6]. Nevertheless, 3D-printed specimens could be used to preoperatively evaluate and to explain to the patient some difficult situations, such as complications after a previous surgery (heterotopic ossifications, failed synthesis, etc.) [1, 30]. New radiotransparent implant (PEEK, composite carbon fibers-PEEK) are recently available. Their potential interference with navigation systems or 3D planning softwares has yet to be studied [31, 32].
2. *Technical feasibility:* to allow good quality of all procedures, good quality images are mandatory. If neither narrow slice CT scan nor MRI could be performed due to technical problems, no 3D reconstruction/planning could be hypothesized [1, 4].
3. *Potential metal allergies:* to our knowledge, there are no reported cases of allergic reac-

tions to custom-made metal implants in literature. These implants, being usually printed in titanium alloys, have very low allergenic potential; titanium is commonly used in metal allergic patients. Nevertheless, in highly reactive patients with documented allergy (i.e., patch tests), the use of a metal-printed implant has to be carefully assessed [1, 30].

Total Hip Arthroplasty (THA) is well defined in most cases and described principles should be followed to obtain the expected functional results and for long term implant survival [25, 33]. To restore a correct hip biomechanics sometimes also a primary THA may be complex: anatomical deformities may represent an issue for the surgeon. Coxavara, leg length discrepancy, acetabular dysplasia, Legg-Calve-Perthes disease, epiphysiolysis, heterotopic ossifications, avascular necrosis of femoral head, trauma in acetabular traumatic fractures are the most common ones. Bone dystrophies (Paget's disease, osteoporosis, osteopetrosis, irradiated bone) may also complicate the surgical steps. 3D customized implants may be useful in those severe deformities [25].

In the last decade, introduction of modularity has been as an alternative to monoblock femoral stems. Large use of modular implants has been made in primary complex arthroplasty. As widely proved in literature and by experience, it shows remarkable advantages. The claimed advantage of this type of prosthesis is the possibility of choosing intraoperatively neck version and neck length independently of the stem size. With modular neck, restoration of hip biomechanics including femoral offset and soft tissue tensioning and abductor muscle imbalances, is easier, mostly in complex hip replacement [34–36]. However, an increasing number of recently published reports and studies describe failures of modular femoral neck prostheses. The addition of an interface is associated with complications such as corrosion or stem-neck disassociation [37, 38]. Another option for complex hip arthroplasty is the implant of short stem. Short stems may be used in selected morphological anomalies of proximal femur in younger patient with a good bone quality. Unfortunately, only a little rate of complex arthroplasty may be safely performed using short femoral stems, for example, coxavara and high dysplastic femoral neck antetorsion are known contraindications [39, 40].

Several surgical techniques have been also proposed to improve implant positioning and stability in complex arthroplasty. Classic shelf augmentation, cotyloplasty, medial protrusion technique, and a controlled fracture of the medial wall are the most known. Osteotomy of the iliac ala with distal sliding of the detached fragment, proximal positioning of the acetabular component, proximal femoral shortening osteotomy, sub-trochanteric shortening and/or derotation osteotomy have also been widely used [25, 33, 41, 42]. All of them are still considered as reliable in specific group of patient but 3D technology may decrease their popularity.

- Cup Customizing

In severe acetabular deformities, cup placement may be technically difficult. Standard anatomic landmarks may not be identified therefore choosing cup size, inclination, anteversion, and coverage may be complex. Several techniques have been proposed to solve this issue [42–46]. These techniques use standard acetabular cup or, in more complex cases, of revision cups. Indication for custom-made cup in primary THA is rare but it should be considered in extreme cases: major alterations of acetabular anatomy, very small or very large dimensions of the acetabular cavity.

- Femoral Customizing

Literature reports several studies about custom-made femoral implants for femoral deformities. Each patient with major deformity of proximal femur is a unique case. The complex femoral anatomy in combination with soft tissue and leg length discrepancy precludes the implantation of classical stem in several situations. Use of modular stem or cone type stems can solve most of the cases. When excessive rotational deformity, coxavara and cortical thinning are present and no anatomical fitting could be achieved with standard stems, a custom femoral implant should be considered. A custom design may improve strain distribution and help to reconstruct hip biomechanics. Abnormal helitorsion of proximal femur is treated creating an asymmetrical proximal part of the stem and neck geometry may be corrected in a triplanar way. The main purpose is to follow canal morphology by varying the implant surface in contact with the bone. This approach is named "fill and fit." It consists in the physiological distribution of stress to the femoral shaft. Stems are normally designed with circular cross section and stem tip has hemispheric shape in order to facilitate the implantation to the femoral canal and avoiding localized stress shields. All reported custom-made femoral stems are made of titanium alloy. Bone integration is helped by surface settings: specific roughness and hydroxyapatite coatings. In the majority of custom-made femoral stem, the hydroxyapatite coating is applied to the proximal part of the implant although, some authors used a fully hydroxyapatite coated stem [47–50]. Furthermore, custom stems present all the advantages of monoblock design: no stress concentrations at the neck and stem junction and a low rate of aseptic loosening. The main disadvantages of custom-made femoral stems are the long production time and the high cost. Production times can take up to 3 months. The work flow includes the selection of images from CT scans and the production of a prototype that has to be sent to the surgeon, who can approve or modify it. This process can be repeated several times before achieving a perfect stem. Costs increase two or three times if compared to the production of a standard stem. In cases of severe dysplasia, custom-made stems may simplify surgical procedure, avoiding in several cases trochanteric osteotomy, which may increase complication rates. The femoral cut height and direction is either preoperatively decided by CAD measurements, or obtained by creating custom-made cutting guides. Preparation of femoral canal is done with one or two custom-made broaches, usually 1 mm smaller than definitive stem. Broaches have the same shape as the custom stem. Femoral anteversion, varus/valgus correction, lateral offset are defined in preoperative planning. In those complex cases, custom-made implants may increase life expectancy of stem and reduce revision rate. Literature showed high rates of stem survival prosthesis (from 93% to 100% in a range from 6 to 14 years follow up). All studies demonstrated a significant improvement in postoperative clinical score compared to preoperative situation. No studies reported major complications after custom-made femoral stem implantation. Considering the available huge variability of solution (i.e., modularity, short-neck stems) an expert surgeon does not need custom-made prostheses for the standard first total hip arthroplasty. On the other hand, in severe deformities, custom-made femoral stems are a valid choice. According to our point of view, custom-made stems should be used when an accurate preoperative planning shows the impossibility to get a correct anatomic reconstruction and a good fitting. In those cases, the custom implant form is chosen in order to get an excellent stability, to achieve a better distribution of loads and a better reconstruction of hip biomechanics [25].

Revision hip arthroplasty, especially in case of multiple revisions, is one of the most complex topic in orthopedic surgery. The custom 3D-printed acetabular implant is indicated in complex cases with a multiple revision history associated with poor bone stock (Fig. 1.3a, b). It can be a viable option either in Paprosky III A/B cases or in pelvic discontinuity [4, 51–54], and according to reported data in various arthroplasty registers, with ageing populations and trends for total hip replacements in younger patients it is likely that the demand for these implants will increase [55–57].

The goal of this kind of implants is to allow a restoration of the acetabular anatomy, filling the periacetabular bone defects and restoring hip biomechanics, with a stable fixation of the implant to the host bone implant stability is ensured by screws introduced through prepared holes in three flanges spreading from the component and laying on ilium, ischium, and pubis. Presence of these flanges, in the beginnings, gave the name to this kind of solutions, known as triflanged cup. The implant can be tailored with

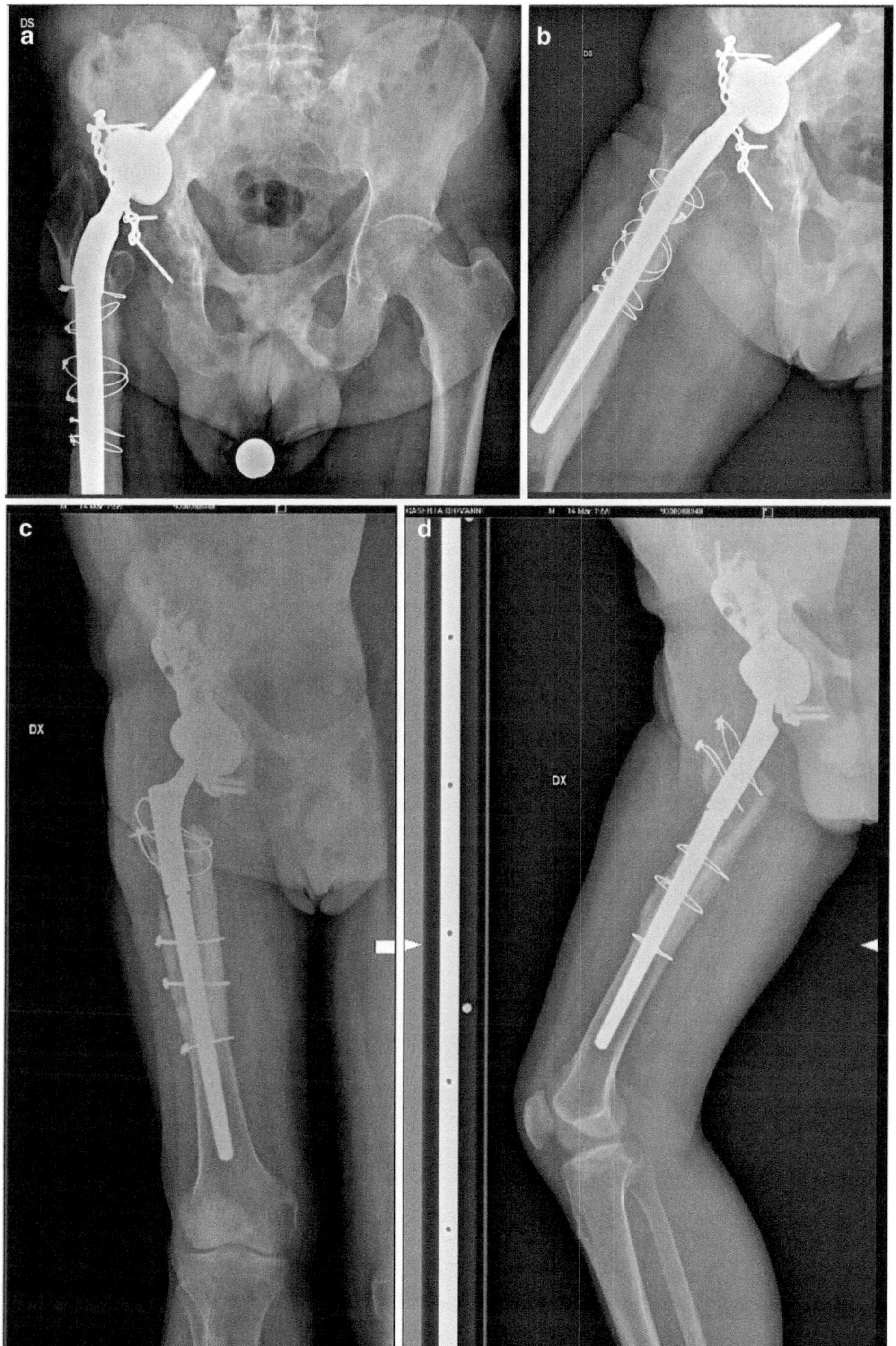

Fig. 1.3 (**a**, **b**) Preoperative anteroposterior and lateral views of acetabular loosening in a 65 years old male who underwent the fourth hip revision. (**c**, **d**) Postoperative anteroposterior and lateral views of the sixth revision with a custom-made cup and a long revision stem

different zones depending on specific mechanical and biological problem to address. Porous surfaces are used to promote bone on-growth while smooth surfaces can diminish potential irritation of soft tissues. Depending on the CT scan data, locking screw trajectory and length can be planned to maximize fixation, to obtain the most efficient purchase in host bone and to minimize vascular risk. Previous implants removal has to be performed being careful not to further compromise the residual bone. Then periacetabular bone has to be prepared to receive the customized implant as planned. The aim is to achieve a good amount of contact surface between component and vital bone, without removing too much tissue. The precision-fit of the implant to the remaining patient's bone stock minimizes the need for more bone resection to fit a standard acetabular revision component [4, 57]. At this point 3D-printed trial models of the involved hemipelvis and of the customized implant, suitably sterilized so that can be handled by members of the surgical team, provide visual and tactile reproduction of the deficient pelvic bony anatomy and of the mutual relationship with the component. This, besides the mentioned help in the preoperative planning, enables and improves understanding of the anatomy during surgery, facilitating intraoperative decisions.

Depending on the patient's specific anatomy and the resulting chosen solution, the main cavity is reamed until the diameter planned and also the nearby defects can be minimally reamed with smaller dedicated instrumentation to even out any roughness and to allow better fitting of any eventual bumps of the custom implant. Component is fixed to the hemipelvis by the porous metal back surface through a press fit concept, and usually by some locking screws going into ilium, ischium, and pubis. Screws can be inserted from holes eventually present inside the cup, or from holes on flanges of the component (Fig. 1.3c, d). Then a liner is introduced inside the metal back either with or without cementation, depending on the implant concept design. Also regarding the femoral side, in the last few years, custom-made implants have been proposed for patients undergoing revision hip surgery, with the goals of promoting axial stability and preserving proximal bone stock. Custom-made femoral stems have been developed usually for younger patients with the objective to attain contact all around medial and lateral stem in the metaphysis and diaphysis of the femur. These solutions are built custom-fitted to patient's anatomy, obtained from CT reconstruction of the femur, to allow a broad stress distribution and best possible fit between bone and stem surface. However nowadays, long-stemmed standard implants or modular distal stems are more cost-effective than custom devices in revision surgery. For this reason, their use is not frequently seen [4, 52, 56].

1.5 Conclusions

3D printing is an innovative and expanding field in orthopedic surgery. Preoperative study, surgical planning for didactical use, specific instruments for resection, and custom-made implants are nowadays viable options to treat more complex cases.

References

1. Boffano M, Pellegrino P, Ratto N, Piana R. Chapter 8. 3D customizing in oncologic hip and pelvic surgery. In: Aprato A, editor. 3D applications in hip surgery. Hauppauge, NY: Nova Science; 2015. ISBN: 978–1–53612-308-1.
2. Wong K-C, Kumta S-M. Use of computer navigation in orthopedic oncology. Curr Surg Rep. 2014;2:47.
3. Aprato A, Greco V, Massè A. Total hip arthroplasty: anything new? Lo Scalpello. 2019;33:178–80. https://doi.org/10.1007/s11639-019-00312-4.
4. Aprato A, D'Amelio A, Marra F, Favuto MM, Mellano D, Massè A. Chapter 7. 3D customizing in revision hip replacement. In: Aprato A, editor. 3D applications in hip surgery. Hauppauge, NY: Nova Science; 2015. ISBN: 978–1–53612-308-1.
5. Jeys L, Matharu GS, Nandra RS, Grimer RJ. Can computer navigation-assisted surgery reduce the risk of an intralesional margin and reduce the rate of local recurrence in patients with a tumour of the pelvis or sacrum? Bone Jt J. 2013;95-B(10):1417–24.
6. Gouin F, Paul L, Odri GA, Cartiaux O. Computer-assisted planning and patient-specific instruments for bone tumor resection within the pelvis: a series of 11 patients. Sarcoma. 2014;2014:842709.

7. Wong KC, Kumta SM, Sze KY, Wong CM. Use of a patient-specific CAD/CAM surgical jig in extremity bone tumor resection and custom prosthetic reconstruction. Comput Aided Surg. 2012;17(6):284–93.
8. Khan FA, Lipman JD, Pearle AD, Boland PJ, Healey JH. Surgical technique: computer-generated custom jigs improve accuracy of wide resection of bone tumors. Clin Orthop. 2013;471(6):2007–16.
9. Wong K-C, Sze K-Y, Wong IO-L, Wong C-M, Kumta S-M. Patient-specific instrument can achieve same accuracy with less resection time than navigation assistance in periacetabular pelvic tumor surgery: a cadaveric study. Int J Comput Assist Radiol Surg. 2016;11(2):307–16.
10. Cartiaux O, Paul L, Francq BG, Banse X, Docquier P-L. Improved accuracy with 3D planning and patient-specific instruments during simulated pelvic bone tumor surgery. Ann Biomed Eng. 2014;42(1):205–13.
11. Cartiaux O, Banse X, Paul L, Francq BG, Aubin C-É, Docquier P-L. Computer-assisted planning and navigation improves cutting accuracy during simulated bone tumor surgery of the pelvis. Comput Aided Surg. 2013;18(1–2):19–26.
12. Li K, Kui C, Lee E, Ho C, Wong S, Wu W, Voll J, Li G, Liu T, Yan B, Chan J, Tse G, Keenan I. The role of 3D printing in anatomy education and surgical training: a narrative review. MedEdPublish. 2017;6(2):31. https://doi.org/10.15694/mep.2017.000092.
13. Cartiaux O, Docquier P-L, Paul L, Francq BG, Cornu OH, Delloye C, et al. Surgical inaccuracy of tumor resection and reconstruction within the pelvis: an experimental study. Acta Orthop. 2008;79(5):695–702.
14. Di Benedetto P, Buttironi MM, Causero A. Chapter 4. A virtual model in hip preserving surgery. In: Aprato A, editor. 3D applications in hip surgery. Hauppauge, NY: Nova Science; 2015. ISBN: 978-1-53612-308-1.
15. Ratnadurai DYN. FDM models and FEA in dysplastic hip. Rapid Prototyp J. 2012;18(3):215–21.
16. Salvi V. Identifit: a silicone mould used to intraoperatively construct a cementless femoral stem. Chir Organi Mov. 1992;77(4):443–5.
17. Al-Khateeb H, Kwok IHY, Hanna SA, Sewell MD, Hashemi-Nejad A. Custom cementless THA in patients with Legg-calve-Perthes disease. J Arthroplasty. 2014;29(4):792–6.
18. Batta V, Coathup MJ, Parratt MT, Pollock RC, Aston WJ, Cannon SR, et al. Uncemented, custom-made, hydroxyapatite-coated collared distal femoral endoprostheses: up to 18 years' follow-up. Bone Jt J. 2014;96-B(2):263–9.
19. McGrath A, Sewell MD, Hanna SA, Pollock RC, Skinner JA, Cannon SR, et al. Custom endoprosthetic reconstruction for malignant bone disease in the humeral diaphysis. Acta Orthop Belg. 2011;77(2):171–9.
20. Malik HH, Darwood ARJ, Shaunak S, Kulatilake P, El-Hilly AA, Mulki O, et al. Three-dimensional printing in surgery: a review of current surgical applications. J Surg Res. 2015;199(2):512–22.
21. Kotz RI. Progress in musculoskeletal oncology from 1922–2012. Int Orthop. 2014;38(5):1113–22.
22. Schindler OS, Cannon SR, Briggs TW, Blunn GW. Stanmore custom-made extendible distal femoral replacements. Clinical experience in children with primary malignant bone tumours. J Bone Joint Surg Br. 1997;79(6):927–37.
23. Wong KC, Kumta SM, Geel NV, Demol J. One-step reconstruction with a 3D-printed, biomechanically evaluated custom implant after complex pelvic tumor resection. Comput Aided Surg. 2015;20(1):14–23.
24. Fan H, Fu J, Li X, Pei Y, Li X, Pei G, et al. Implantation of customized 3-D printed titanium prosthesis in limb salvage surgery: a case series and review of the literature. World J Surg Oncol. 2015;13(1):308. http://www.wjso.com/content/13/1/308. Accessed 20 Jan 2017 Jan 20.
25. Aprato A, De Vivo S, Marra F, Nicodemo A, Bistolfi A, Massè A. Chapter 6: 3D customizing in complex primary hip replacement. In: Aprato A, editor. 3D applications in hip surgery. Hauppauge, NY: Nova Science; 2015. ISBN: 978–1–53612-308-1.
26. Danışman M, Mermerkaya MU, Bekmez Ş, Ayvaz M, Atilla B, Tokgözoğlu AM. Reconstruction of periacetabular tumours with saddle prosthesis or custom-made prosthesis, functional results and complications. Hip Int J Clin Exp Res Hip Pathol Ther. 2016;26(2):e14–8.
27. Farfalli GL, Albergo JI, Ritacco LE, Ayerza MA, Milano FE, Aponte-Tinao LA. What is the expected learning curve in computer-assisted navigation for bone tumor resection? Clin Orthop Relat Res. 2017;475(3):668–75.
28. Aprato A, Olivero M, BrancaVergano L, Massè A. Outcome of cages in revision arthroplasty of the acetabulum: a systematic review. Acta Bio Medica Atenei Parmensis. 90(1S):24–31.
29. Tack P, Victor J, Gemmel P, Annemans L. 3D-printing techniques in a medical setting: a systematic literature review. Biomed Eng Online. 2016;15(1):115.
30. Aprato A, Governale G, Stucchi A, Deregibus M, MassèA. Biomaterials in bearing surface for total hip arthroplasty: state of the art. Recent patents on. Biomed Eng. 2010;3(2):75–85.
31. Koff MF, Shah P, Koch KM, Potter HG. Quantifying image distortion of orthopedic materials in magnetic resonance imaging. J Magn Reson Imaging. 2013;38(3):610–8.
32. Zimel MN, Hwang S, Riedel ER, Healey JH. Carbon fiber intramedullary nails reduce artifact in postoperative advanced imaging. Skeletal Radiol. 2015;44(9):1317–25.
33. Boisgard S, Descamps S, Bouillet B. Complex primary total hip arthroplasty. Orthop Traumatol Surg Res. 2013;99(1 Suppl):S34–42.
34. Bobyn JD, Tanzer M, Krygier JJ, Dujovne AR, Brooks CE. Concerns with modularity in total hip arthroplasty. Clin Orthop Relat Res. 1994;298:27–36.
35. Blaha JD. The modular neck: keystone to functional restoration. Orthopedics. 2006;29:804–5.

36. Aprato A, Massè A, Stucchi A, Governale G. Femoral stem's designs: review of the literature. In: Colombo DF, Rossi GS, editors. Prostheses: design, types and complications. Hauppauge, NY: Nova Science; 2012.
37. Fokter SK, Moličnik A, Kavalar R, Pelicon P, Rudolf R, Gubeljak N. Why do some titanium-alloy total hip arthroplasty modular necks fail? J Mech Behav Biomed Mater. 2017;69:107–14.
38. Wodecki P, Sabbah D, Kermarrec G, Semaan I. New type of hip arthroplasty failure related to modular femoral components: breakage at the neck-stem junction. Orthop Traumatol Surg Res. 2013;99:741–4.
39. Wittenberg RH, Steffen R, Windhagen H, Bucking P, Winkle A. Five-year results of a cementless short-hip-stem prosthesis. Orthop Rev (Pavia). 2013;5(1):e4.
40. Gruner A, Heller KD. Patient selection for shorter femoral stems. Orthopedics. 2015;38(3 Suppl):S27–32.
41. Park MS, Kim KH, Jeong WC. Transverse subtrochanteric shortening osteotomy in primary total hip arthroplasty for patients with severe hip developmental dysplasia. J Arthroplasty. 2007;22(7):1031–106.
42. Aprato A, Nardi M, Favuto M, Cominetti G, Zoccola K, Masse A. Chapter 5. Hip dislocation: types, causes and treatments. In: Duncan LT, editor. Advances in health and disease, vol. 3. Hauppauge, NY: Nova Science. ISBN:978–1–53613-020-1.
43. Russotti GM, Harris WH. Proximal placement of the acetabular component in total hip arthroplasty. A long-term follow-up study. J Bone Joint Surg Am. 1991;73(4):587–92.
44. Hartofilakidis G, Stamos K, Karachalios T. Treatment of high dislocation of the hip in adults with total hip arthroplasty. Operative technique and long-term clinical results. J Bone Joint Surg Am. 1998;80:510–7.
45. Haddad FS, Masri BA, Garbuz DS, Duncan CP. Primary total replacement of the dysplastic hip. Instr Course Lect. 2000;49:23–39.
46. Bicanic G, Barbaric K, Bohacek I, Aljinovic A, Delimar D. Current concept in dysplastic hip arthroplasty: techniques for acetabular and femoral reconstruction. World J Orthop. 2014;5(4):412–24.
47. Tsiampas DT, Pakos EE, Georgiadis GC, Xenakis TA. Custom-made femoral implants in total hip arthroplasty due to congenital disease of the hip: a review. Hip Int. 2016;26(3):209–14.
48. Koulouvaris P, Stafylas K, Sculco T, Xenakis T. Custom designed implants for severe distorted proximal anatomy of the femur in young adults followed for 4–8 years. Acta Orthop. 2008;79(2):203–10.
49. Hartofilakidis G, Karachalios T. Total hip arthroplasty for congenital hip disease. J Bone Joint Surg Am. 2004;86-A(2):242–50.
50. Yang S, Cui Q. Total hip arthroplasty in developmental dysplasia of the hip: review of anatomy, techniques and outcomes. World J Orthop. 2012;3(5):42–8.
51. Aprato A, Giachino M, Bedino P, Mellano D, Piana R, Masse A. Management of Paprosky type 3b acetabular defects by custom made components: early results. Int Orthop. 2019;43:117–22. https://doi.org/10.1007/s00264-018-4203-5.
52. Christie MJ, Barrington SA, Brinson MF, et al. Bridging massive acetabular defects with the triflange cup: 2- to 9-year results. Clin Orthop Relat Res. 2001;393:216–27.
53. Holt GE, Dennis DA. Use of custom triflanged acetabular components in revision total hip arthroplasty. Clin Orthop Relat Res. 2004;429:209–14.
54. Taunton MJ, Fehring TK, Edwards P, et al. Pelvic discontinuity treated with custom triflange component: a reliable option. Clin Orthop Relat Res. 2012;470(2):428–34.
55. Wyatt MC. Custom 3D-printed acetabular implants in hip surgery—innovative breakthrough or expensive bespoke upgrade? Hip Int. 2015;25(4):375–9.
56. Massè A, Aprato A, Turchetto L, Rizzi L, Lasagna G, Arrigoni C, Ganz R. Reconstruction with rib graft for acetabular revision in pelvic discontinuity: an extreme solution? Tech Orthop. 2015;30:269–74.
57. Artiaco S, Fusini F, Colzani G, Aprato A, Zoccola K, Masse A. Long-term results of Zweymüller SLL femoral stem in revision hip arthroplasty for stage II and IIIA femoral bone defect: a 9–15-year follow-up study. Musculoskelet Surg. 2020;104(3):273–8. [Epubahead of print]. https://doi.org/10.1007/s12306-019-00617-y.

The Rationale of 3D Printing in Oncological Orthopaedics

2

Rodolfo Capanna and Lorenzo Andreani

2.1 Introduction

Orthopaedic oncological surgery, unlike traditional orthopaedic surgery, is by definition invasive and often requires wide resections of bone, soft tissue or both. For a long time, the classical treatments for patients with large malignant tumours of the limbs was demolitive surgery. In the last decades, because of the availability of more accurate modalities for imaging, the use of neoadjuvant chemotherapy, improved resection techniques and prosthetic devices, the majority of cases have been treated with the so-called *limb-salvage surgery*. The diffusion of reconstructive procedures led to a reduction of functional and psychological disability for the oncological patient [1–4]. Methods for skeletal reconstruction include massive osteoarticular allograft, endoprosthetic reconstruction and prosthetic–allograft composites. Inter alia, the advent of metallic prostheses allowed a functional recovery nearly 80% of the normal function and, in the follow-up, only 16% of the patients goes towards definitive failure and/or secondary amputation [4]. The reconstruction is of primary importance and is actually the most challenging act for the orthopaedic surgeon.

Technological development significantly contributed to surgical advance in the last years and if we are able to implant 3D prostheses today, it is thanks to Charles W. Hull, a well-known engineer who invented 3D printing in the late 1980s. He was the inventor of the so-called stereolithography, an adding manufacturing process that produces objects by hitting photosensitive liquid resin with ultraviolet light; the resin photochemically polymerize adding layers that make up the body of a solid object. Following evolutions of the technique enabled its expansion to a multitude of sectors. In the medical field stereolithographic models are actually used to aid diagnosis, preoperative planning and reconstruction devices. The modern printers are based on the traditional additive manufacturing technique by adding the use of specific software for computer aided design or computer aided manufacturing (CAD/CAM).

These software are able to acquire patients' data from CT, MRI or other scan and to translate them into a format suitable for stereolithography, through a process called segmentation. Accurate 3D models of a specific anatomic region can be produced using this technique. The modern 3D printers that are so-called powder based have a further evolution: instead of the liquid resin, a powder bed interacts with the moving head of the printer that releases a laser beam or a binding material; the parts touched by the laser or the glue fuse together creating the desired model. The use of specific metallic powders allows the creation of customized products in stainless steel,

R. Capanna · L. Andreani (✉)
University of Pisa, Pisa, Tuscany, Italy

C. Zoccali et al. (eds.), *3D Printing in Bone Surgery*, https://doi.org/10.1007/978-3-030-91900-9_2

titanium, ceramic, high performance plastic [5, 6]. To remove debris and powder excess a post-processing stage is necessary, in order to obtain biocompatible and sterile products ready to be implanted in human body. According to the type of fusion technique, material and porosity, the post-processing can be complex, leading to increased time of fabrication and costs. Particularly, the removal of unfused powder from porous implant micro-channels and holes is an arduous issue. Usually it requires a blasting phase or abrasive jet machining with rotate and vibrate system, followed by washing steps with distilled water and other solutions such as ethanol or aceton [7]. Moreover, some implants surface is coated with hydroxyapatite or other material to improve osteointegration and fit.

The success of 3D printing application in orthopaedic oncological surgery relies exactly in the customization of the products. Soft tissue and bone malignant tumours are rare and often develop in unusual patterns, requiring often personalized treatments. Moreover because of the histologic variability and the local aggressiveness, a case-specific approach is mandatory.

In orthopaedic oncological surgery, 3D printing technique finds application in the following major fields:

(a) Preoperative planning and training (3D-models);
(b) Intraoperative support for precise bone cutting (guiding jigs);
(c) Method for reconstruction (3D prostheses or scaffold).

2.1.1 3D Models

(a) The **creation of models**, reproducing the lesion within its anatomical region, for preoperative training enables the surgeon to improve his/her technique and self-confidence becoming more expert; this eventually leads to a reduction of surgical times, intraoperative bleeding, X-rays exposure, risk of nerve or vascular damage and also a better aesthetic result [8]. Moreover, the same models can be used as part of medical students training but also for an educational purpose towards the patient in order to explain the effects of the disease and its surgical treatment obtaining an informed consent as clear as possible [9–11].

2.1.2 Guiding JIGS

(b) 3D print is also commonly used to produce **surgical cutting guides** for bone resection. These are devices that, positioned intraoperatively to given landmarks, guide the surgeon throughout the osteotomy. Despite their cost, they offer more precise resection, with minimal sacrifice of noble structures and healthy tissue. Patients treated with intraoperative use of surgical guides seem to report better functional outcomes with higher MSTS (Musculoskeletal Tumour Society Score); moreover, patients with joint involvement, seem to develop less mechanical complications during follow up [12, 13]. Surgical cutting guides can help preparing the osteoarticular allograft too: a precise and personalized osteotomy on the donor bone improves allograft fit with patient's bone, with a far better result compared to freehand saw (Fig. 2.1).

Beyond the benefits regarding the application of 3D-printed cutting guides, there are a few disadvantages to keep in mind. The costs, the surgical times often related to the confidence of the surgeon, the need of a wide surgical exposure to point out the anatomical landmarks are all aspects that should be taken into consideration [11, 13].

Sometimes, the presence of soft tissues on the bone surface does not allow a perfect match of the cutting guide on the bone surface preventing its correct use. Furthermore, in order to have a good stability and to recognize the right positioning, the cutting guide must have a large support area and it requires a large stripping of the muscles in the areas of osteotomies. Moreover, there are some dangerous areas for the application of cutting guides as sacroiliac joint, sciatic notch, anterior groin region, where there is the passage of neuro-vascular bundle or the major branches (i.e. gluteal and hypogastric arteries).

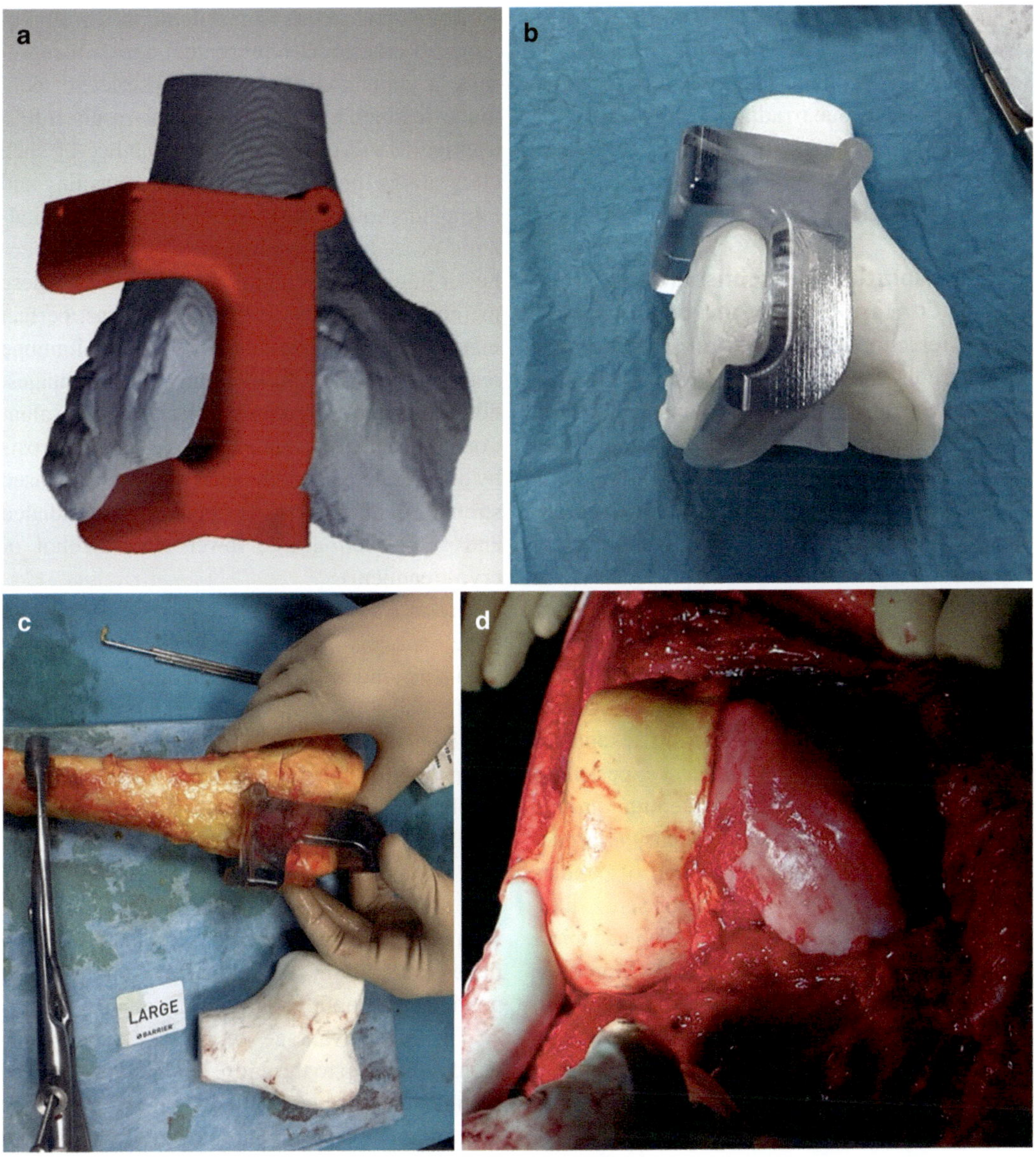

Fig. 2.1 Grade I chondrosarcoma of the lateral femoral condyle with indication to condyle surgical resection and reconstruction. A surgical cutting guide was produced through the acquisition of preoperative CT, MRI and PET scan. 3D-CAD model and the cutting guide (**a**, **b**). The guide was used both for tumour resection and to obtain the allograft from the donor, achieving a high congruency of the surfaces (**c**, **d**). The excellent functional scores at follow-up (MSTS and KSS) confirmed the success

Finally, the cut must be done throw a slotted guide not throw a sliding surface. Moreover, the guide should be thick enough to avoid oblique cut caused by bending of the saw or should have a thick surface for sliding cut of the saw. These solutions require a bulky toll.

2.1.3 3D Prostheses

(c) In orthopaedic oncological surgery massive demolition is mandatory to achieve free-of-disease margins and therefore decrease the rate of local recurrence of malignant tumours. The restoration of the resulting defects can be addressed with various approaches and materials depending on several factors including the site and width of the resection, local tissue irradiation, previous site of biopsy or intervention, diagnosis and grade of tumour, patient age, comorbidities and life expectation [14–16].

2.1.3.1 Evolution of Reconstruction Concept and Technology

Among resections, those performed in the pelvic region are the most challenging to face to for its three-dimensional anatomy and the closeness to vulnerable structures. A few decades ago most pelvic tumours were treated with hindquarter amputation. Later on simple **biological reconstruction** were introduced periacetabular resections involving ileo and ischio-pubic branches (II + III Type of Duhann-Enneking Classification) were reconstructed by ileo-femoral coaptation or ileo-femoral arthrodesis [2]. The construct was simple and resulted in a stable and painless limb, but the usual evolution was in a stiff pseudoarthrosis or in arthrodesis. Patients experienced restricted motion and limb shortening (around 4–5 cm). On the other hand, a primary arthrodesis was successful in less than a half of patients due to limited contact, thin area for screw fixation, impaired blood supply and biomechanical disadvantage for the long lever arm. Moreover, even if ileo-femoral fusion was achieved with excellent stability, patient satisfaction was low for the lack of motion, spine pain and difficulty to reach the sitting position.

In periacetabular resection involving the ileum (I + II type of pelvic resection), ischiofemoral arthrodesis was performed with screws or wiring. The first procedure was particularly successful in children due to frequent ischiofemoral union rate, hip motion hinging in pubic symphysis associated with limited shortening and acceptable function. The wiring, instead, particularly in adult patients, usually failed ending in a flail hip, shortening and instability, with poor functional results.

All these difficulties associate to unsatisfactory functional outcomes led orthopaedic surgeons to search alternative limb sparing techniques.

Bone transplants from a donor (allografts) or recycled autografts represented, and still represent, a valid and effective reconstructive technique leading to good functional results (70% average MSTS). Moreover, availability of such allografts is limited. In alternative, recycling and reimplantation of the resected bone after devitalizing procedures (irradiation, autoclaving, alcohol or liquid nitrogen bath) could be done. These methods have many advantages such as: perfect matching of the cut surfaces and no immune reaction. But they also have many disadvantages: not applicable for osteolytic lesions, no evaluation of surgical specimen and induced necrosis by preoperative neoadjuvant treatment, decreased strength of the grafts, particularly for irradiated and autoclaved grafts, lower after alcohol or cryo-treatment).

Fresh frozen, sterile allografts, taken from bone bank and chosen by a computer according with site and size are commonly used today. Grafts must be treated with rifampicin before application to prevent infections [17].

In periacetabular pelvic resection with involvement of ilium (type I + II), the graft can be fixed with cannulated screws both to the sacrum and pelvic ramus. In periacetabular reconstruction after type II + III resection (periacetabular with pelvic ramus) the graft can be fixed with two plates to the ilium, while fixation to the anterior pelvic arch is optional and not mandatory.

The main advantages of graft are the possibility to replace up to the entire hemipelvis and to be moulded in the operative field to better fit to bone gap, compensating any intraoperative unexpected variations of the resection margins. While their versatility is evident, still it's hard to obtain perfect interface contact to the native bone considering both three-dimensional aspect of pelvis and freehand osteotomy.

Both allografts and autografts expose to a certain risk of major post-operative complications like deep infections, non-unions or fractures, hip dislocations and nervous palsy (sciatic or femoral nerve) [18–20]. High is the revision rate of these implants [21].

Infection is a major complication (~ 20%). It is a predictable event, considering closeness to viscera (rectum, bladder, urethra), long operative times and the low immune defences of oncological patients [19, 22–26].

In order to decrease the infective risk an antibiotic bath is suggested before implantation. Infection often requires allograft removal and two stage revision with the implantation of a moulded cemented antibiotic loaded spacer.

The high risk of non-union in sacral or iliac interface should be considered especially when an irradiated or autoclaved graft is implanted (around 50% of cases) [27]. The rate of non-union for cryopreserved allograft is rare. More frequent is non-union in particularly of the anterior arch bones but it is clinically irrelevant. Non-union risk factors can be local (especially due to narrow bone anchorage and to mismatch between native bone and graft interface) or systemic (including poor vascularization, diabetes, infections or chronic use of corticosteroids) [19, 28]. The risk of non-union is very low when the proximal osteotomy is transverse, oblique or V-shaped through the iliac bone and solid osteosynthesis with one or two plates is performed. A posterior plate following the ideal projection of sacroiliac joint and crossing the osteotomy is recommended. In this way, the screws have a solid grip in the thick bone of the sacroiliac area. However, in total hemipelvis resection when the proximal osteotomy is vertically drawn through the sacroiliac joint or the sacral wing, important shear stress are present at the interface with increased risk of pseudoarthrosis or screw fatigue failures. When cannulated screws are inserted through the allograft into the sacrum, these should have an oblique direction (postero-anterior) and reach the anterior part of S1 and S2 body (thicker bone) avoiding the posterior structure (sacral canal). The free hand screw insertion is technically demanding particularly when it is not supported by navigation systems. The simple intraoperative 2D X-ray control is often troublesome and misleading.

Fracture or bone graft resorption was observed in a small number of cases (less than 10%) [21]. As fracture prevention, a double plate for each column or a long plate across sacroiliac joint, innominated line and pubis may be used but it can be dangerous to the sciatic nerve and iliac vessels.

The allograft may also be reinforced:

1. Pressurizing liquid cement in the space between the two cortex through a hole in the acetabulum and using a flanged cage for support;
2. Implanting an 'ice cream' shaped (i.e. Mc Minn cup) prostheses fully immersed in the allograft or with the distal conus extremity press fitted in the host bone as a primary implant. More appropriately we name these implants composite allo-prostheses.

The use of a cemented cup within the allograft to restore hip joint reduces the risk of implant loosening and dislocation compared to bipolar cup [3].

To prevent instability, artificial ligaments or mesh wrapped around the prosthetic neck are recommended [24]. Also dual mobility, snap fit or retentive cup are commonly used to increase stability.

Beyond the good outcomes, grafts are affected by some limitations: they are hard to find, to process and to preserve. However, the graft era contributed with no doubt in better understanding the reconstruction pitfalls bringing unique anatomical and mechanical knowledge in terms of resection lines and stabilization.

An alternative to biological reconstructions is represented by **pelvic endoprosthesis**. These devices were born during the boom of arthroplasty and their design provided only the geometry recovery of bone resected omitting load forces distribution and implant stability; for this feature some authors called it as 'geometric pelvic endoprostheses' [29]. The first was implanted in 1970 by Scales and Rodney and, despite the implant was removed for infection a few years later, they open the way for the development of new implant designs and manufactures. Gradinger, some years later, applied the custom-made concept on pelvic endoprosthesis after tumour removal, but the patients' outcomes were unsatisfactory due both to the low accuracy of planning and to the long surgeon learning curve especially for the periacetabular reconstruction [21, 30, 31]. After that, at the end of the last century, there was a phase of transition in which the implantation of saddle prostheses became popular in pelvic resection with iliac residual bone [32, 33]. Their spread led to biomechanical refinements and to the definition of 'modularity' concept, inherited from second and third generation saddle prostheses (Mark II and PAR). The evolution of technique led then to the birth of the so-called *Structural pelvic endoprostheses* distinguished from the previous ones since based on pelvic distributions of loads. In this category, we find the iliac stem endoprostheses, from the first Pedestal cup developed by Zimmer to the more recent LUMiC® (Implantcast, 2003). This modular device, requiring iliac neck integrity, presents an 'ice cream' shape and it is composed by an acetabular cup and a cemented or not iliac stem. Low dislocation rates and good functional outcomes still make these prostheses a valid alternative in II or II + III type pelvic reconstruction [34, 35].

The others type of '*Structural pelvic endoprostheses*' are the modular pelvic endoprostheses. Their small size allowed soft tissues coverage and this could reduce infective complications. However clinically outcomes were unsatisfactory especially for their structural stiffness [36].

In this scenario **3D printing technology** and bioengineering led the way to a new option for reconstruction after bone massive resection: the **custom-made prostheses 3D printed**. Nowadays custom-made implants represent an emerging alternative to biological reconstruction [37–39].

Preoperative high definition CT scan images are processed using CAD software in order to design a titanium implant that assumes the exact shape and geometry of the patient's bone, creating a perfect copy of the anatomical part that will be sacrificed. In oncological setting, MRI and PET can be performed in order to improve understanding of neoplasm extension in the soft tissues and metabolic activity. The preoperative planning includes bioengineers' biomechanical studies, that are crucial in order to obtain a resistant and stable implant. Peg, flag and support plates are insert in 3D design (primary stability). Type of fixation in pelvic reconstruction is based on the osteotomy level: if it is proximal to iliac neck—at the pole of a sciatic notch—implant stability is achieved with surface contact plus two antirotational stems. In case the osteotomy is at the iliac neck, which is a thick structure, a simple ice cream shape modular prosthesis may be sufficient, as reported by *De Paolis* [35]. If the osteotomy crosses the sacroiliac joint, plates and plug must be used.

In order to choose the anchorage areas, bone thickness and closeness to susceptible structures should be considered. In pelvis the thicker bone areas for better implant anchorage are the sacroiliac area (Fig. 2.2), the innominate line and above all the iliac neck. It seems not crucial a contact and/or fixation with the ileum and/or ischio-pubic ramus, if the proximal contact and stability are optimal. All above are lessons learned from previous allograft replacement experience.

Still unresolved is the matter of the anchorage after hemipelvis resection. In this setting the limited bone interface contact area and the important sliding forces determining vertical shift affect implant instability. Moreover, the sacral bone is spongy and porotic and there are close dangerous areas for screw fixation. Alternatively, an 'L shaped mounting bracket' stabilized to sacrum by screws in orthogonal planes and a rotational joint centre proximally and medially shifted (to decrease lever arm and bending forces) (Fig. 2.2). In these cases, anchoring extension to the lumbar spine may be considered.

Trial components can be printed previously to evaluate how the definitive titanium implant would fit. Only after surgeon approval, the 3D model can become definitive. Since these implants cannot be modified after print, it's necessary to obtain a bone defect with shape and size completely respectful to the preoperative planning, in order to achieve an optimal match. The precision of resection is crucial also to obtain free-disease margins and 3D-printed cutting guides should be used to increase accuracy. Surgeon training on trial models can be obtained

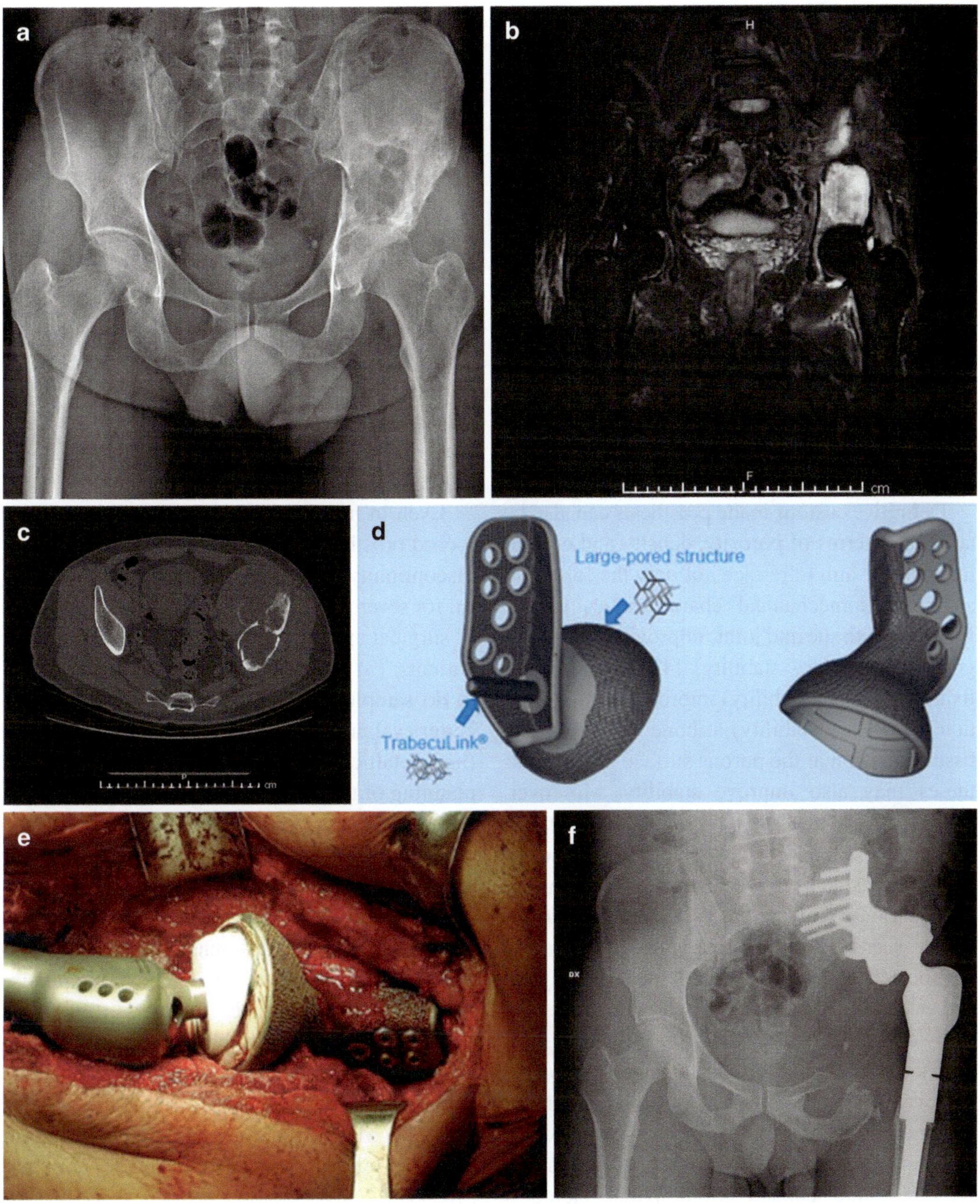

Fig. 2.2 (**a**, **b**, **c**) Preoperative X-rays, MR and CT in patient affected by pelvis chondrosarcoma involving left periacetabular region and iliac bone. (**d**) 3D–CAD model of implant prosthesis. (**e**) Intraoperative view (**f**) 1 year X-ray follow-up full weight bearing

before surgery to memorize guide plate positioning and orientation in their correct placement reducing intraoperative doubts and surgical time.

Intraoperative computed navigation is another tool that could aid precision, especially if the guides positioning requires extended soft tissue release and is close to sciatic notch or sacroiliac area [40, 41].

The perfect fit between custom-made implants and recipient site guarantees restoration of bone continuity in conformity with patient's anatomy. The absolute respect of the original shape of the bone would translate in better postoperative functional results compared to patients treated with standard prosthesis or biological bone grafts.

If all these requirements are achieved, the surgical time of reconstruction is minimal with high impact in infection control.

However, no errors are admitted in custom-made prostheses: wrong cutting planes or mismatching in contact surface are impossible to correct intraoperatively. Things are slightly different for allografts: their overall adaptability is better since they can be moulded intraoperatively in order to change their size and shape, if necessary.

Definitive custom-made prosthesis can also be tailored in terms of porosity, density and elasticity, with the aim to retrace not only the form, but also the biomechanical characteristics of the native bone tissue and joint, improving osteointegration (secondary stability) [42–44]. A stable fixation (primary stability) improve osteointegration (secondary stability) at bone interface. Soft tissue adhesion at the porous surface of the prostheses may also improve stability. Moreover, porous architecture reduces weight implant and allows inside loading of antibiotic or antiseptic solutions, reducing the infection risk. The prosthesis surface features smooth areas in order to reduce scar or neurovascular issue: these areas are located at ileopubis ramus, sacroiliac joint and at sciatic notch, where vessels and nerve typically cross.

The production of such complex implants however, in not easy. Preoperative planning, engineering studies, trials print and implant components production require long times that should be taken into consideration. When facing a chemo- or radiotherapy sensitive primary tumour, the temporal window necessary for the custom-made implant creation becomes a favourable time to perform neoadjuvant treatments. However, other malignant tumours can be locally aggressive and sometimes chemo or radiotherapy nonresponsive, so an early surgical treatment is mandatory. In these cases, the surgeon can procrastinate the implant of a custom-made prostheses, performing immediately the resection with positioning of an antibiotic loaded spacer, to keep in place until the 3D components are ready. Splitting the surgical treatment in two different operations can bring some benefits, beyond the immediate removal of the mass. The patient undergoes two procedures with shorter times compared to a unique procedure, meaning less blood loss and eventually a reduced infection risk [45]; moreover, a second surgical step gives the surgeon the opportunity to make a new staging and have a second look on margins if necessary during the reconstruction procedure. However, the choice between one or two steps procedure must be taken after specific considerations for every single case.

Even in major revision surgery of intrapelvic loosed prosthesis, with pseudotumour and pelvic discontinuity, a two steps procedures may be useful for several reasons: (1) check no skin necrosis of surgical approach, (2) reduced impact in older patients, (3) reduced blood loss, (4) opportunity to do sample culture and exclude infection, (5) better evaluation of bone loss in CT examination (no metallic artefacts) and (6) more accurate planning of the implant and cutting jigs.

Up to now reconstruction with grafts and custom-made implants seems to have comparable rates of infections and mechanical complications such as loosening and dislocation. What makes a significant difference between the two techniques is the functional outcome: the precise fit of the custom-made implants reproduces native anatomy with all the features above mentioned and this clearly influences ROM and patients' satisfaction. The clinical evaluation with the MSTS score reports higher rates for patients treated with custom-made implants [46–49].

2.2 Intercalary 3D Prosthesis

Custom-made prosthesis's popularity is also arising in another challenging field of orthopaedic oncology: intercalary reconstruction of long bone. Several techniques are described in literature, from vascularized allografts, devitalized allografts and autografts to standard or modular prosthesis. Even though good functional results have been described after the use of both biological and prosthetic reconstructions, either one of them expose patients to a certain risk of complications. Biological approaches are associated with good long term results but are also burdened with a relatively high risk of short term complications [50]. On the contrary, non-biological implants can provide good short and mid-term results and satisfying functional outcomes, but their long-term complication rate is relatively high [51]. In reason of this, the popularity of this solution is gradually declining. 3D-printed custom-made intercalary implants have the potential to represent a compromise between the two, promising to converge the early functional results of the standard prosthetic implants with the advantages of the osteointegration with the left native bone. As previously described, osteotomy should be performed using 3D-printed osteotomy guide plates in order to ensure the respect of the preoperative plan and the adequate fit of the custom-made implant within the bone loss. Nevertheless, the safety of margins and the anatomy of compartments should be always kept in mind, and the respect of preoperative planning must not take over on the dictates of orthopaedic oncological surgery. Once the osteotomies are performed, respectful of margins and preoperative planning, the implant is then inserted on site and fixed with screws to the remnant native bone [52].

There is still paucity of studies regarding this topic, but the first results described in literature are encouraging in terms of good functional scores and low complication rates at least in the short time period [53, 54].

2.3 3D Scaffolds

In addition to implants, 3D printer technology can be used to produce the so-called scaffolds, biocompatible structures of natural or synthetic origin, which can mimic the extracellular matrix to improve cells attachment and proliferation. In order to provide their function, scaffolds must be porous, to allow cell spreading and effective transport of nutrients, oxygen, waste, as well as growth factors, favouring continuous ingrowth of bone tissue. Scaffolds can be seeded with staminal cells or loaded with bioactive substances able to mimic the natural ECM and conduct the local cells to differentiate and colonize the structure.

In this logic, 3D printing technology, alongside with the latest advances in tissue engineering, can provide an alternative approach to prosthetic or graft reconstructions, with the aim not only to replace, but also to regenerate the damaged tissue.

2.4 Conclusion

1. 3D printing and bioengineering are showing an outstanding potential and custom-made prosthesis can be considered as some of the most promising reconstructive devices introduced on the market during the last years. Respect to custom-made casted conventional mega-prosthesis, 3D-printed ones show the following major advantages:
   (a) Trial components.
   (b) Perfect morphological replica of the resected bone.
   (c) Availability of cutting jigs for accurate surface fitting.
   (d) Intraoperative guides for controlled screws insertion.
   (e) Location of size, length and direction of screws, pins, plate (primary stability).
   (f) Three-dimensional porous surface allowing bone ingrowth at the osteosynthesis and soft tissue attachment (secondary stability and muscle fixation).

   This is more than a 'simple' 3D prosthesis, in fact we have to rely on a 3D philosophy reconstruction technique.
2. One of the most important limitations to the spread of this technology is represented by the cost of every single prosthesis. Nowadays the price of custom-made implants can be very high if compared to off-the-shelf prosthesis, but not respect to grafts. Paradoxically, this trouble could be circumvented with a higher

production volume: the more custom-made prosthesis are made, the lowest their price could get, allowing the producing companies to recoup the costs of printers, materials and research. Also, a slightly higher selling price, especially if compared to standard prosthesis, could be justified by the lower risk of complications and reintervention rate with better functional outcomes. In this perspective, the price difference could be seen as an investment, with the promise of saving money from future treatments [39, 55].

References

1. Ji T, Guo W, Yang RL, Tang XD, Wang YF. Modular hemipelvic endoprosthesis reconstruction–experience in 100 patients with mid-term follow-up results. Eur J Surg Oncol (EJSO). 2013;39(1):53–60.
2. Enneking WF, Dunham WK. Resection and reconstruction for primary neoplasms involving the innominate bone. J Bone Joint Surg Am. 1978 Sep;60(6):731–46.
3. Campanacci M, Capanna R, Briccoli A, Donati D, Del Ben M. Pelvic resection: the Rizzoli institute experience. In: Modern trends in pelvis and hip surgery, First International Conference; 1991. p. 71–3.
4. Grimer RJ, Aydin BK, Wafa H, Carter SR, Jeys L, Abudu A, Parry M. Very long-term outcomes after endoprosthetic replacement for malignant tumours of bone. Bone Jt J. 2016;98(6):857–64.
5. Auricchio F, Marconi S. 3D printing: clinical applications in orthopaedics and traumatology. EFORT Open Rev. 2016;1(5):121–7.
6. Brunello G, Sivolella S, Meneghello R, Ferroni L, Gardin C, Piattelli A, Zavan B, Bressan E. Powder-based 3D printing for bone tissue engineering. Biotechnol Adv. 2016;34(5):740–53.
7. Sing SL, An J, Yeong WY, Wiria FE. Laser and electron-beam powder-bed additive manufacturing of metallic implants: a review on processes, materials and designs. J Orthop Res. 2016;34(3):369–85.
8. D'Urso PS, Redmond MJ. A method for the resection of cranial tumours and skull reconstruction. Br J Neurosurg. 2000;14(6):555–9.
9. Esses SJ, Berman P, Bloom AI, Sosna J. Clinical applications of physical 3D models derived from MDCT data and created by rapid prototyping. Am J Roentgenol. 2011;196(6):W683–8.
10. Mao K, Wang Y, Xiao S, Liu Z, Zhang Y, Zhang X, Wang Z, Lu N, Shourong Z, Xifeng Z, Geng C. Clinical application of computer-designed polystyrene models in complex severe spinal deformities: a pilot study. Eur Spine J. 2010;19(5):797–802.
11. Tack P, Victor J, Gemmel P, Annemans L. 3D-printing techniques in a medical setting: a systematic literature review. Biomed Eng Online. 2016;15(1):115.
12. Wang F, Zhu J, Peng X, Su J. The application of 3D printed surgical guides in resection and reconstruction of malignant bone tumor. Oncol Lett. 2017;14(4):4581–4.
13. Ma L, Zhou Y, Zhu Y, Lin Z, Wang Y, Zhang Y, Xia H, Mao C. 3D-printed guiding templates for improved osteosarcoma resection. Sci Rep. 2016;6:23335.
14. Hugate R, Sim FH. Pelvic reconstruction techniques. Orthop Clin North Am. 2006;37(1):85–97.
15. Hillmann A, Hoffmann C, Gosheger G, et al. Tumors of the pelvis: complications after reconstruction. Arch Orthop Trauma Surg. 2003;123(7):340–4.
16. Haley RW, Culver DH, Morgan WM, et al. Identifying patients at high risk of surgical wound infection. A simple multivariate index of patient susceptibility and wound contamination. Am J Epidemiol. 1985;121:206–15.
17. Delloye C. Bone banking in orthopaedic surgery. Surgical techniques in orthopaedics and traumatology. Paris: Elsevier; 2000. p. 55–61.
18. Jaiswal PK, Aston WJS, Grimer RJ, Abudu A, Carter S, Blunn G, et al. Peri-acetabular resection and endoprosthetic reconstruction for tumours of the acetabulum. J Bone Joint Surg. 2008;90(9):1222–7.
19. Delloye C, Banse X, Brichard B, Docquier PL, Cornu O. Pelvic reconstruction with a structural pelvic allograft after resection of a malignant bone tumor. J Bone Jt Surg. 2007;89(3):579–87.
20. Capanna R, van Horn JR, Guernelli N, Briccoli A, Ruggieri P, Biagini R, Bettelli G, Campanacci M. Complications of pelvic resections. Arch Orthop Trauma Surg. 1987;106:71–7. Erratum in: Arch Orthop Trauma Surg., 106:262.
21. Ozaki T, Hoffmann C, Hillmann A, Gosheger G, Lindner N, Winkelmann W. Implantation of hemipelvic prosthesis after resection of sarcoma. Clin Orthop Relat Res. 2002;396:197–205.
22. Campanacci D, Chacon S, Mondanelli N, Beltrami G, Scoccianti G, Caff G, Frenos F, Capanna R. Pelvic massive allograft reconstruction after bone tumour resection. Int Orthop. 2012;36(12):2529–36.
23. Bell RS, Davis AM, Wunder JS, Buconjic T, McGoveran BR, Gross AE. Allograft reconstruction of the acetabulum after resection of stage-IIB sarcoma. Intermediate-term results. J Bone Jt Surg. 1997;79(11):1663–74.
24. Langlais F, Lambotte JC, Thomazeau H. Long-term results of hemipelvis reconstruction with allografts. Clin Orthop Relat Res. 2001;388:178–86.
25. Schwameis E, Dominkus M, Krepler P, Dorotka R, Lang S, Windhager R, Kotz R. Reconstruction of the pelvis after tumor resection in children and adolescents. Clin Orthop Relat Res. 2002;402:220–35.
26. Beadel GP, McLaughlin CE, Wunder JS, Griffin AM, Ferguson PC, Bell RS. Outcome in two groups of patients with allograft-prosthetic reconstruc-

tion of pelvic tumor defects. Clin Orthop Relat Res. 2005;438:30–5.
27. Sys G, Uyttendaele D, Poffyn B, Verdonk R, Verstraete K. Extracorporeally irradiated autografts in pelvic reconstruction after malignant tumour resection. Int Orthop. 2002;26(3):174–8.
28. Roberts TT, Rosenbaum AJ. Bone grafts, bone substitutes and orthobiologics: the bridge between basic science and clinical advancements in fracture healing. Organogenesis. 2012;8:114–24.
29. Ji T, Guo W. The evolution of pelvic endoprosthetic reconstruction after tumor resection. Ann Joint. 2019;4:29.
30. Gradinger R, Rechl H, Ascherl R, Plötz W, Hipp E. Partial endoprosthetic reconstruction of the pelvis in malignant tumors. Der Orthopade. 1993;22(3):167–73.
31. Windhager R, Karner J, Kutschera HP, Polterauer P, Salzer-Kuntschik M, Kotz R. Limb salvage in periacetabular sarcomas: review of 21 consecutive cases. Clin Orthop Relat Res. 1996;331:265–76.
32. Menendez LR, Ahlmann ER, Falkinstein Y, Allison DC. Periacetabular reconstruction with a new endoprosthesis. Clin Orthop Relat Res. 2009;467(11):2831.
33. Nieder E, Keller A. The saddle prosthesis mark II, Endo-Modell®. In: New developments for limb salvage in musculoskeletal tumors. Tokyo: Springer; 1989. p. 481–90.
34. Fisher NE, Patton JT, Grimer RJ, Porter D, Jeys L, Tillman RM, Abudu A, Carter SR. Ice-cream cone reconstruction of the pelvis: a new type of pelvic replacement: early results. J Bone Joint Surg. 2011;93(5):684–8.
35. De Paolis M, Biazzo A, Romagnoli C, Alì N, Giannini S, Donati DM. The use of iliac stem prosthesis for acetabular defects following resections for periacetabular tumors. Sci World J. 2013;2013:717031.
36. Guo W, Li D, Tang X, Yang Y, Ji T. Reconstruction with modular hemipelvic prostheses for periacetabular tumor. Clin Orthop Relat Res. 2007;461:180–8.
37. Rengier F, Mehndiratta A, von Tengg-Kobligk H, et al. 3D printing based on imaging data: review of medical applications. Int J Comput Assist Radiol Surg. 2010;5:335–41.
38. Semba J, Mieloch A, Rybka J. Introduction to the state-of-the-art 3D bioprinting methods, design, and applications in orthopedics. Bioprinting. 2020;18:e00070.
39. Wong KC. 3D-printed patient-specific applications in orthopedics. Orthop Res Rev. 2016;8:57–66.
40. Wong KC, Kumta S, Chiu K, Antonio G, Unwin P, Leung KSK. Precision tumour resection and reconstruction using image-guided computer navigation. J Bone Joint Surg. 2007;89:943–7.
41. Chen X, Xu L, Wang Y, Hao Y, Wang L. Image-guided installation of 3D-printed patient-specific implant and its application in pelvic tumor resection and reconstruction surgery. Comput Methods Programs Biomed. 2016;125:66–78.
42. Cunniffe G, O'Brien F. Collagen scaffolds for orthopedic regenerative medicine. J Miner Metals Mater Soc. 2011;63:66–73.
43. Ryan G, Pandit A, Apatsidis DP. Fabrication methods of porous metals for use in orthopaedic applications. Biomaterials. 2006;27:2651–70.
44. Lopez-Heredia MA, Goyenvalle E, Aguado E, et al. Bone growth in rapid prototyped porous titanium implants. J Biomed Mater Res A. 2008;85(3):664–73.
45. Temple H, O'Keefe RJ, Scully SP, Mankin HJ. Limb salvage and allograft reconstruction for pelvic tumors. In: Proceedings of the 8th international symposium on limb salvage, vol. 79; 1995.
46. Angelini A, Trovarelli G, Berizzi A, et al. Three-dimension-printed custom-made prosthetic reconstructions: from revision surgery to oncologic reconstructions. Int Orthopaed (SICOT). 2019;43:123–32.
47. Dai KR, Yan MN, Zhu ZA, Sun YH. Computer-aided custom-made hemipelvic prosthesis used in extensive pelvic lesions. J Arthroplasty. 2007;22:981–6.
48. Wang B, Hao Y, Pu F, Jiang W, Shao Z. Computer-aided designed, three dimensional-printed hemipelvic prosthesis for peri-acetabular malignant bone tumour. Int Orthop. 2018;42(3):687–94.
49. Liang H, Ji T, Zhang Y, Wang Y, Guo W. Reconstruction with 3D-printed pelvic endoprostheses after resection of a pelvic tumour. Bone Joint J. 2017;99-B:267–75.
50. Aponte-Tinao L, Ayerza MA, Muscolo DL, Farfalli GL. Survival, recurrence, and function after epiphyseal preservation and allograft reconstruction in osteosarcoma of the knee. Clin Orthop Relat Res. 2015;473:1789–96.
51. Dotan A, Dadia S, Bickels J, et al. Expandable endoprosthesis for limb-sparing surgery in children: long-term results. J Children Orthopaed. 2010;4:391–400.
52. Liu W, Shao Z, Rai S, Hu B, et al. Three-dimensional-printed intercalary prosthesis for the reconstruction of large bone defect after joint-preserving tumor resection. J Surg Oncol. 2020;121:570–7.
53. Guder WK, Hardes J, Gosheger G, Nottrott M, Streitbürger A. Ultra-short stem anchorage in the proximal tibial epiphysis after intercalary tumor resections: analysis of reconstruction survival in four patients at a mean follow-up of 56 months. Arch Orthop Trauma Surg. 2017;137:481–8.
54. Wong KC, Kumta SM. Joint-preserving tumor resection and reconstruction using image-guided computer navigation. Clin Orthop Relat Res. 2013;471:762–73.
55. Unwin PS, Eshraghi A. Custom implants. In: Ritacco LE, Milano FE, Chao E, editors. Computer-assisted musculoskeletal surgery: thinking and executing in 3D. Cham: Springer; 2016. p. 181–98.

3 The 3D Printing Production Procedure

Maurizio Scorianz, Lorenzo Guariento, and Domenico Andrea Campanacci

3.1 Introduction

Additive manufacturing technology (AM), or 3D printing, was developed in the 1980s of the last century [1]. Before then, only the subtractive manufacturing was available.

Subtractive manufacturing involves the removal of material from a solid block. This process was at first performed manually and subsequently it was automated by machines. In the beginning, those machines were controlled by mechanical methods, like cams; then, numerical controlled machines used punched cards containing the manufacturing data.

In the late 1950s, Computer Numerical Control machines (CNC) were introduced, making data management more flexible since punched cards were no longer necessary [2]. But it wasn't until the 1960s, when computers became more affordable, that this technique increased popularity.

In 1981, Hideo Kodama developed the first 3D printer, which was used to build a model house and a relief map (Fig. 3.1) [1]. Later, in 1986, Chuck Hull independently developed a 3D printer and patented the process, coining the term Stereolithography [3].

At first, AM was used to produce prototypes, then, in the last decades, it became more and more popular as the number of different technologies and materials became available. The low cost of some 3D printers and materials allowed their sale by retail stores and their diffusion to non-professional users.

AM is a viable process to manufacture single parts or small series and this is ideal for prototyping. Moreover, there are no limitations concerning the geometry and it allows to manufacture complex internal structures. This technology allows for a high design flexibility and customizability: the same 3D printer can produce very different parts, changing the design geometry and choosing different building materials (Fig. 3.2).

Limitations and advantages of subtractive manufacturing and additive manufacturing are summarized in (Table 3.1).

3.2 From Diagnostic Imaging to the Anatomical Model

It is not possible to obtain a good quality 3D-printed object from poor quality medical imaging. Therefore, the first step is to obtain good quality radiological images with high spatial resolution and contrast, which are the key factors directly impacting 3D model accuracy.

M. Scorianz (✉) · D. A. Campanacci
Orthopaedic Oncology and Reconstructive Surgery Unit, Azienda Ospedaliero Universitaria Careggi, Department of Health Sciences, University of Florence, Florence, Italy
e-mail: scorianzm@aou-careggi.toscana.it; domenicoandrea.campanacci@unifi.it

L. Guariento
Department of Industrial Engineering, University of Florence, Florence, Italy
e-mail: lorenzo.guariento@unifi.it

C. Zoccali et al. (eds.), *3D Printing in Bone Surgery*, https://doi.org/10.1007/978-3-030-91900-9_3

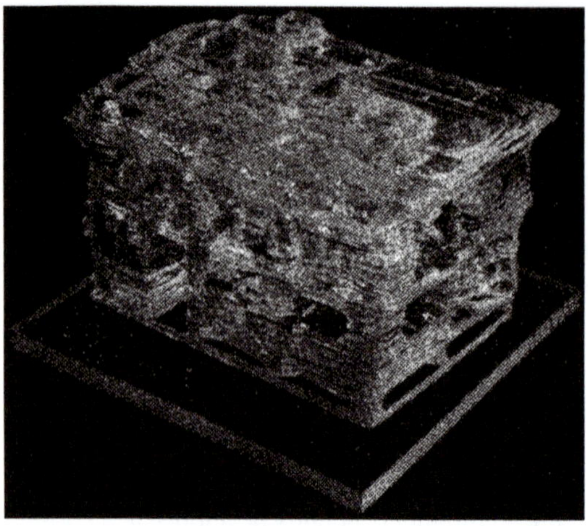

Fig. 3.1 3D-printed house model fabricated by Hideo Kodama (Reproduced from Automatic method for fabricating a three-dimensional plastic model with photo-hardening polymer, Review of Scientific Instruments, Vol. 52, No. 11, pp. 1770–73, November 1981, with the permission of AIP Publishing)

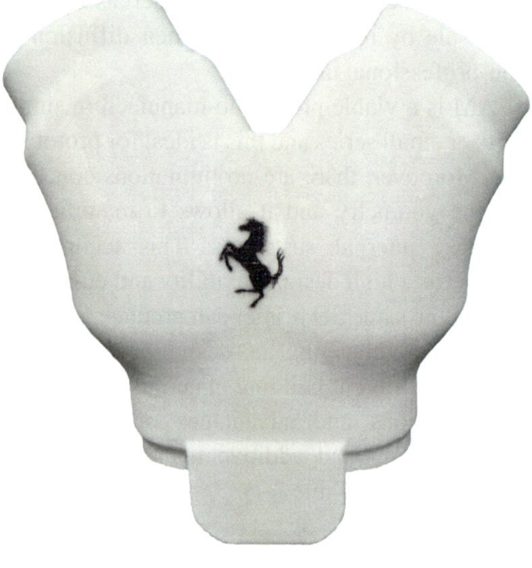

Fig. 3.2 A 3D-printed adapter designed by Solid Energy and manufactured by Ferrari. During the COVID-19 pandemic, Ferrari used the 3D printers at its Maranello plant to produce respirator valves and fittings for protective masks (Courtesy of Solid Energy S.r.l. and Ferrari S.p.A)

Spatial resolution depends on the minimum distance between two details of an image that can be resolved, and thus affects the minimum size of the object that can be detected (Fig. 3.3). Image contrast, for a grayscale image, is the difference of luminosity between pixels, which affects the

Table 3.1 Main advantages and limitations of subtractive and additive manufacturing

	Subtractive manufacturing	Additive manufacturing
PROS	High accuracy	No need for specific tooling
	High surface finishing	Relatively low machine cost
	Low cost for a big volume production	No manufacturing constraints
	High productivity levels	Low changeover cost and minimal setup
CONS	High machine and tooling cost	Relative low accuracy and surface finishing
	Low production flexibility	High cost for large production volume
	Production of waste material	Manual finishing is often necessary
	Limitations regarding manufacturable geometries	

ability to discern different densities of two adjacent regions.

CT scans are usually sufficient for some procedures, like designing customized osteotomy guides to correct axial deformities [4], while others need both the data from CT and MRI, for example to highlight a bone tumor [5]: in such cases, the bone tissue is acquired by CT, while soft tissues are usually more efficiently visualized on MRI. The acquisition of the appropriate MRI sequences and, in some cases, the use of a contrast medium is necessary to perform the subsequent steps of the 3D printing process.

Image registration is a critical step to correctly overlay the sequences with one another. Image registration is typically performed with manual or semiautomatic algorithms that involve the manual selection of corresponding landmarks respectively on CT and MRI scans. This process requires at least three couples of non-aligned points; a higher number of points increase the accuracy (Fig. 3.4).

Image fusion allows to enhance the information provided by each imaging technique.

Image fusion is carried out by specialized software which combines multiple diagnostic images within a single data set to improve the information content and clinical applicability [6].

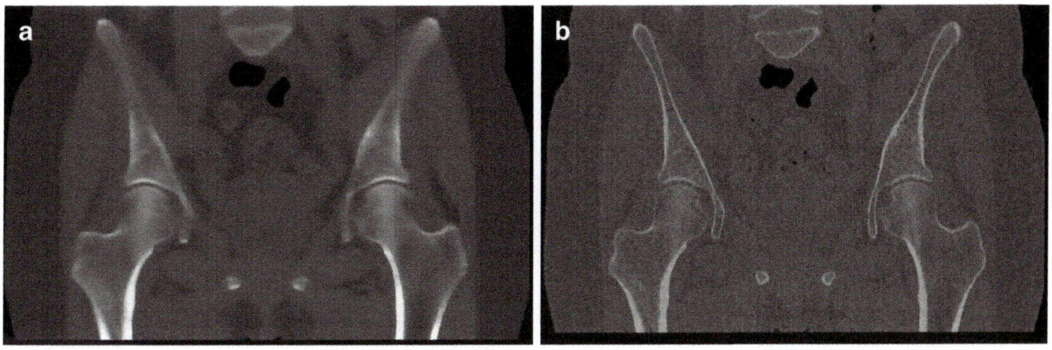

Fig. 3.3 An example of a low resolution (**a**) and a high-resolution CT image of the pelvis (**b**)

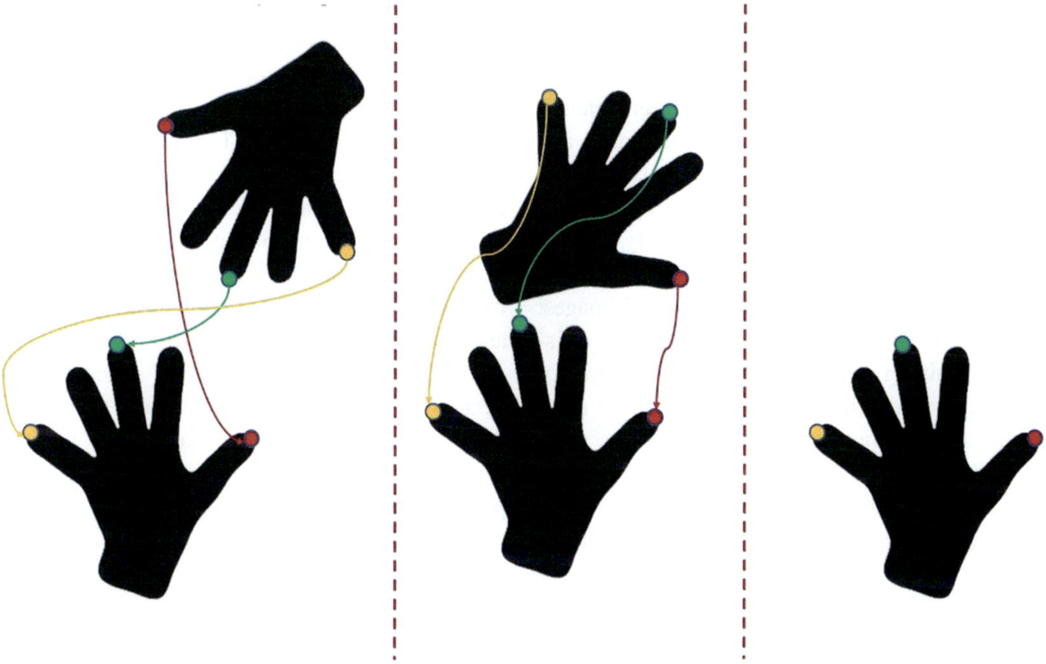

Fig. 3.4 An example of alignment in 2D. At least three corresponding points are necessary to perform the alignment without ambiguities. The same principle is valid in 3D

The next step involves the segmentation of the images. Diagnostic images segmentation is an essential process that allows to outline the geometric features of the structures of interest and it is the first step for the production of a 3D anatomical model. Image segmentation separates a 2D or 3D image into unconnected regions (segments) which are homogenous for specific signal characteristics, typically geometric and intensity-based features of pixels [7]. More specifically, 3D image segmentation splits the volume into sub-volumes composed by voxels with uniform characteristics; then each region is labeled to classify every anatomical area into bone, vessels, or pathological areas like tumors or other lesions.

A 3D anatomical model should provide clinicians with useful and readily usable information; therefore, it is a good practice to perform the segmentation only on the anatomical regions of interest to reduce the computational cost and preparation time. While designing models for 3D printing, the operator should find the best compromise between the model's complexity and its effectiveness in supporting surgeons' decisions. In most cases, a 3D anatomical reconstruction with a small number of elements might be more useful than a very complex model, which guarantees an accurate anatomical reproduction but, on the other hand, it might result less useful in assessing the anatomical relationship between the structures of interest.

To date, there is no standard segmentation method capable of producing satisfactory results for all imaging applications.

Manual image segmentation is a challenging time-consuming task, requiring a long learning curve and presenting interdiscipline and interobserver variations [8]. Several automatic segmentation tools were developed to reduce the human input. The quality of the automatic segmentation depends on the quality of the original image and the algorithm selected by the user; the parameters of the algorithm could be fine-tuned by the user and the results can be further manually refined. Threshold is one of the most commonly used automatic segmentation tool of orthopedics CT images; this method analyzes the different density of tissues, obtaining the automatic segmentation of bone segments. Other traditional methods of automatic segmentation struggle to work on more complex tissues, like tumors, where most of the segmentation must be done by the operator. In the last decade, deep learning automatic segmentation techniques obtained promising results in those complex tasks [9]. Deep learning uses artificial neural networks consisting of parallel computing systems inspired by biological neural networks. Those networks learn by analyzing example images that have been manually segmented by humans, then using the data acquired to perform automatic segmentation of new images.

After the segmentation, the following phase is the meshing process. A 3D polygonal mesh is created, which encloses the volume corresponding to the segmented anatomical region. A polygonal mesh is defined by an ordered collection of vertices, edges, and faces. The most popular format to represent a mesh is the STL format.

The STL file is a proprietary format that was developed by 3D System in 1988 [10] to be used with stereolithography. STL, being openly documented, was later adopted by almost all other 3D printing technologies. There is no agreement on the original meaning of the file extension STL; the most commonly accepted are STereo Lithography, Standard Tessellation Language, and Standard Triangle Language.

An STL file is composed of a series of connected ordered triangles and each triangle is defined by the facet normal and three vertices (Fig. 3.5). The process of covering a surface with polygons (triangles in the STL format) is called tessellation.

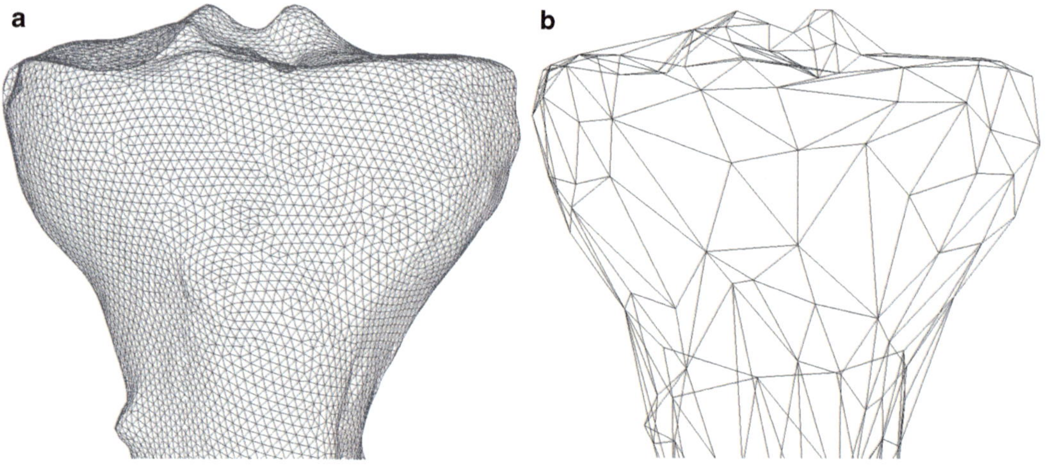

Fig. 3.5 A 3D triangular mesh of a tibia (**a**). The surface is represented with connected triangles. By decreasing the triangle size, the approximation error decreases (**b**)

The approximation of a smooth surface with a triangular mesh inevitably introduces the facetting error, which is depicted in (Fig. 3.6). Such error is defined as the average distance between the original surface and the result of the facetting operation; it can be reduced by increasing the facets number, especially in curved regions, though the file size is increased too, as well as the computational cost. According to the specific case, the facets number should represent the best compromise between facetting error and computational cost. The STL file is compatible with most CAD software and 3D printers, though some corrections are often required before 3D printing. The most common operations performed on an STL file are hole fixing, facet normal correction and intersecting faces correction, procedures intended to create a "watertight" mesh free of errors.

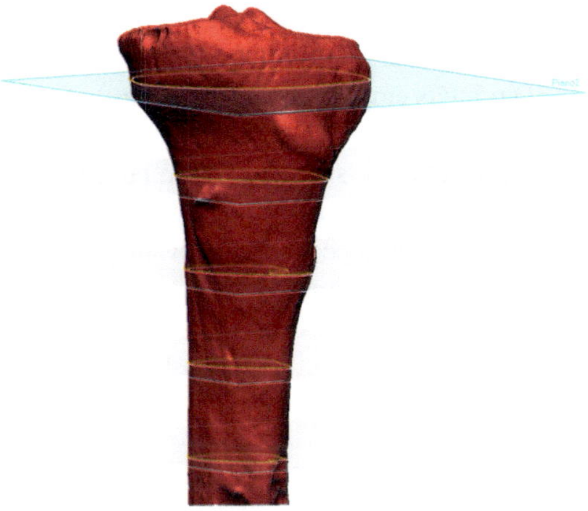

Fig. 3.7 Illustration of the slicing process. The 3D mesh is intersected with a series of parallel planes, and the sections are extracted. The path of each section is passed to the 3D printer which reproduces the model layer by layer

AMF (Additive Manufacturing File Format) is the official open standard for AM [11]. Despite this file contains information about texture and material, it is only compatible with professional high-end 3D printers and consequently it is unsupported by most manufacturers and CAD software.

3MF (3D Manufacturing Format) and VRLM (Virtual Reality Modeling Language) are popular AM formats, both able to integrate details about texture and material properties in a very compact file.

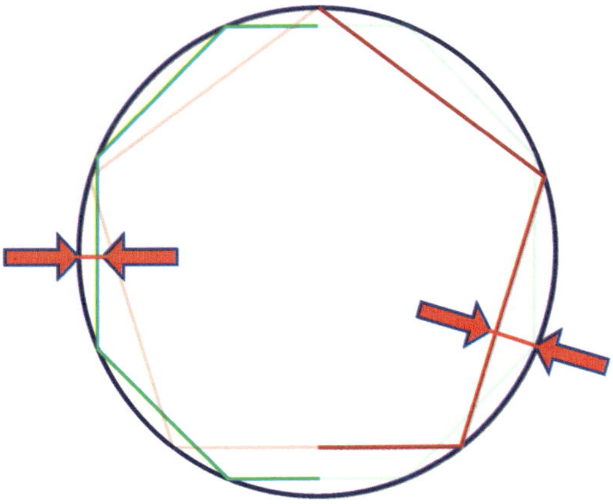

Fig. 3.6 Facetting error in 2D. When a continuous curve, like the circle in blue, is approximated with a polygon, a representation error is made, which is called facetting error. By increasing the number of sides of the polygon, the error decreases. The same concept is valid in 3D, where a smooth surface is represented by a collection of polygons (triangles for the .STL format)

A 3D model should be designed with its purpose and the manufacturing technology in mind. If the model contains details smaller than the 3D printer resolution, it might be convenient to smooth the 3D mesh. At the same time, when multiple objects need to be printed during the same process, specific supports are used to maintain the parts in the correct relative position. Once prepared, the mesh is processed by the 3D printer software for manufacturing. Most 3D printer software performs an operation called slicing (Fig. 3.7), in which the software intersects the mesh with a series of parallel planes; each intersection represents the path for the 3D printer head on each layer.

Using the 3D anatomical model as a reference and Computer-aided design (CAD) software, it is possible to design an orthopedic implant or a surgical cutting guide.

3.3 3D Printing Technology Used in Orthopedics

The ISO/ASTM 52900 international standard [12] developed in 2015 clears definitions for terms and nomenclature associated with additive manufacturing technology, making possible to classify the different types of 3D printers.

3D printers employed in orthopedics have different advantages and limitations determining their application in surgery, patient education or surgical simulation. The most commonly used 3D printers in orthopedics take advantages of the following technologies: Stereolithography (SLA), Selective Laser Sintering (SLS), Electron Beam Melting (EBM), Selective Laser Melting (SLM), Fused Deposition Modeling (FDM).

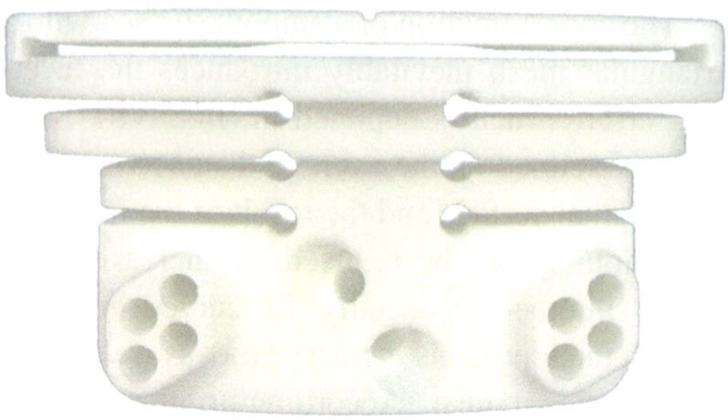

Fig. 3.8 SLS printed cutting guide (Courtesy and © Adler Ortho S.p.A)

3.3.1 Stereolithography

SLA (Stereolithography Apparatus) models are built from a photosensitive resin which is selectively cured by a UV light beam. The process is repeated for each layer, and once the part is finished, it is placed into an UV oven until complete polymerization of the resin. SLA printers can cover a wide range of applications due to the broad spectrum of available resins with different mechanical properties. In the medical field, SLA is mainly used in orthodontics and for dental surgical guides, but it is also widely employed to manufacture high-precision anatomical models. SLA printers build parts with very high dimensional accuracy (small slice thickness) and excellent surface finish. The main drawback of this technology is the high cost of the resin, and thus of the printed part.

3.3.2 Selective Laser Sintering

SLS (Selective Laser Sintering) is one of the most popular AM technologies because it provides parts with fine details and excellent surface finish at a relatively low cost (Fig. 3.8). The component is built from a thin layer of polymeric powder, which is selectively fused by a high-power laser. The building chamber is sealed and maintained at a temperature close to the melting point of the powder, in order to minimize the laser power necessary to fuse the material. Once the laser has sintered the first section of the model, the elevator moves in the build direction and the printer deposits a new layer of powder. The process continues until completion of the piece (Fig. 3.9). One of the main advantages provided by SLS, compared to other technologies, is that the unsintered powder acts as a support material for the part, which makes the post-processing very straightforward and reduces the waste material. SLS machines are quite large and expansive, but the large printing volume allows to efficiently build many different parts in the same process, which decreases the cost for a single component.

3.3.3 Electron Beam Melting

Electron Beam Melting (EBM) is one of the most commonly employed powder bed printing techniques to manufacture custom implants and surgical cutting guides (Fig. 3.10).

The working principle of Electron Beam Melting (EBM) is similar to SLS, with the difference that the building material is a metal powder, usually titanium and cobalt-chromium alloys powder. An electron beam selectively fuses the powder, then a new layer of powder is deposed and the process continues layer by layer. The temperature inside the build chamber is close to the melting point of the powder to reduce the laser energy necessary to melt the material. EBM, thanks to the support provided by the non-fused powder, can manufacture complex internal structures with tunable porosity to promote bone ingrowth and reduce the global stiffness, to match the bone mechanical properties and reduce stress shielding effect. In

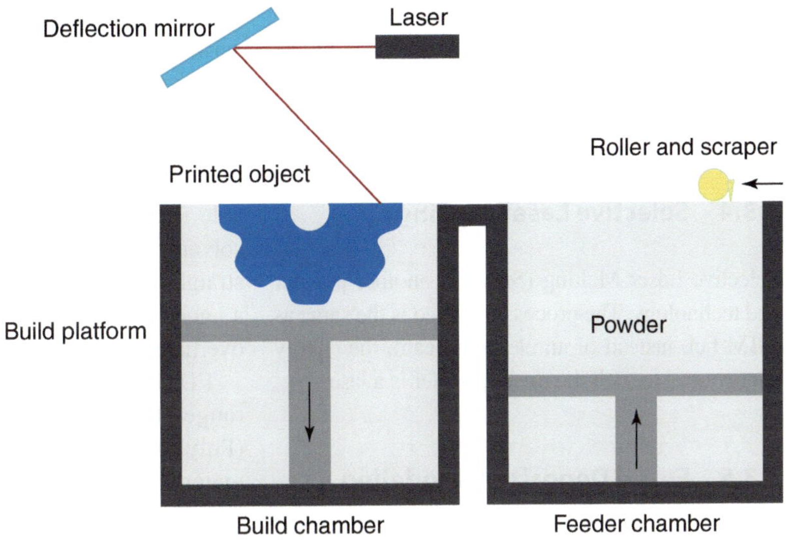

Fig. 3.9 Scheme of a SLS printer. A thin layer of powder is deposited on the build platform and sintered thanks to the high-power laser, which melts the particles. The build platform is lowered and a new layer of fresh powder is provided by the feeder chamber and leveled by a scraper, then the process continues until completion

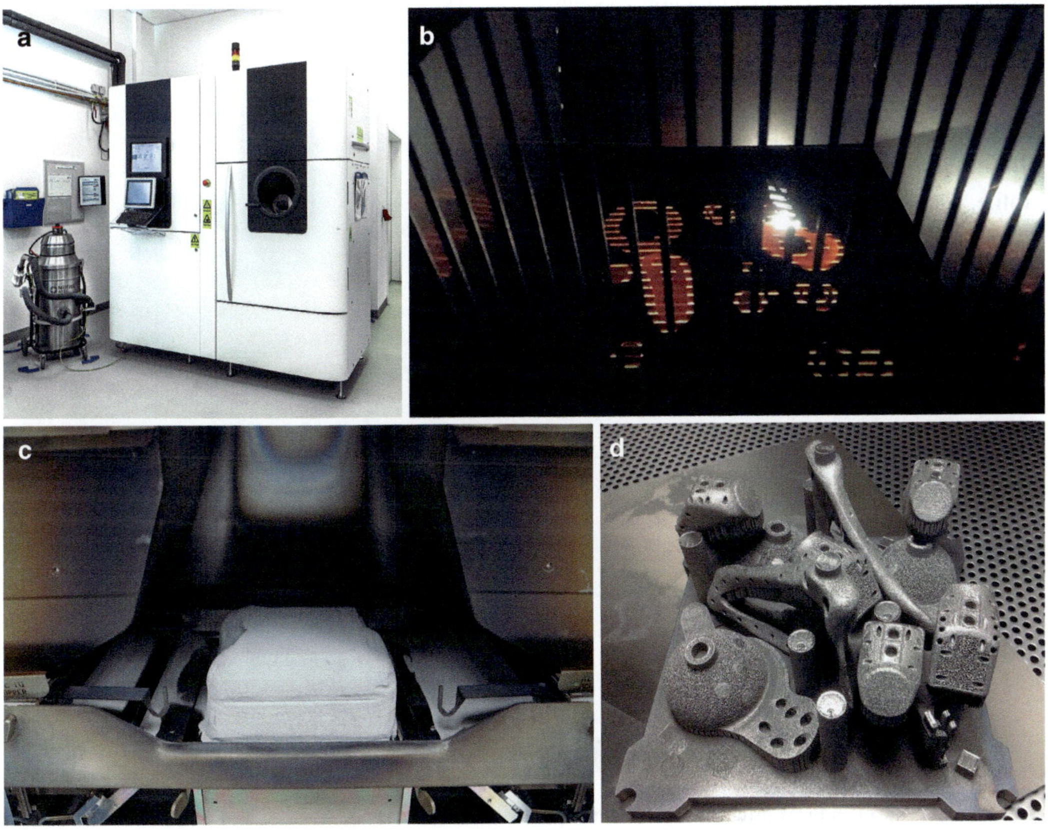

Fig. 3.10 (**a**) EBM Printer (Courtesy and © of Dr. Prang and Waldemar Link GmbH & Co.). (**b**) EBM printing process (Courtesy and © Implantcast GmbH). (**c**) Building block before the residual powder removal (Courtesy and © Implantcast GmbH). (**d**) The 3D printed component after the residual powder removal. Several pieces are manufactured from a single build tank, thus reducing time and material (Courtesy and © Implantcast GmbH)

some cases, EBM models require the creation of specific supports to avoid shrinkage and thermal deformation during cooldown, especially for small and thin parts.

3.3.4 Selective Laser Melting

Selective Laser Melting (SLM) is another powder bed technology. The process involved is the same as EBM but, instead of an electron beam, the energy source used to melt the metal powder is a laser.

3.3.5 Fused Deposition Modeling

Fused Deposition Modeling (FDM) is one of the most popular and low-cost AM technology. The affordable price of both equipment and materials made FDM very popular also to a non-specialist audience.

The building material is provided in spools and the filament is forced through a heated nozzle, placed in the printing head, which selectively deposits the fused filament creating the section profile. Then, the process continues layer by layer (Fig. 3.11). While low-end FDM machines are provided with just one extruder and have low surface finish (Fig. 3.12), professional 3D printers have one or more extruders for the building material, and one for the support material: this allows to use different materials for the part and the supports. High-end FDM printers use solvable support material, typically in hot water or solvent, which makes the cleaning operation very straightforward and allows to manufacture, with a good surface finish, complex parts with overhangs.

FDM technology is compatible with a wide range of materials: the most common are PLA (PolyLactic Acid), a low-cost biodegradable material made of renewable resources, and ABS (Acrylonitrile Butadiene Styrene), a hard and durable polymer. For medical applications, the main materials compatible with FDM are ULTEM, ABS-M30i, PEEK and PC-ISO.

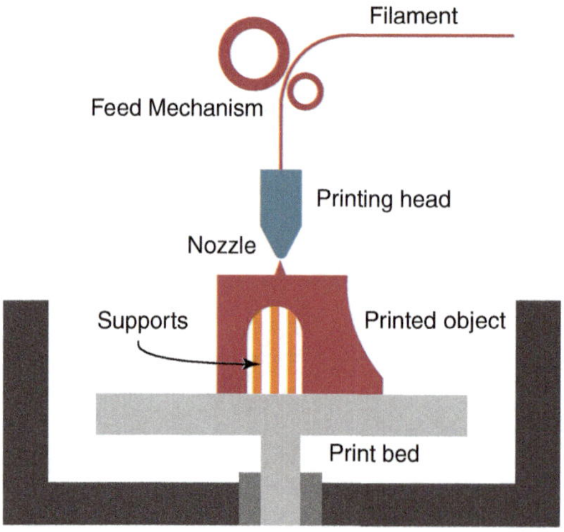

Fig. 3.11 Scheme of an FDM printer. The filament is fed to the printing head and forced through the heated nozzle. Layer by layer the print bed is lowered and the fused filament is selectively deposed, creating the model

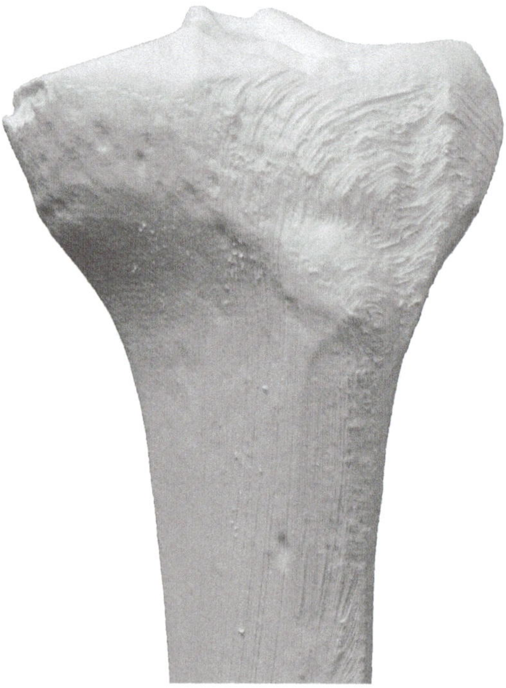

Fig. 3.12 Proximal tibia built in PLA with a low-end FDM printer. Note the poor surface finish quality of this low-cost model

3.4 Materials Used to Print Surgical Devices and Implants

The variety of available materials for AM is continuously growing, ranging from polymers to resins and metals. Additive manufacturing materials for Medical Devices must satisfy specific requirements as biocompatibility and sterilizability. As stated by Williams, [13] "biocompatibility is intended as the ability of a material to perform with an appropriate host response in a specific application."

In Table 3.2 are presented the most popular AM biocompatible materials and the relative AM technology.

Polymeric AM materials are employed for a variety of medical applications. The most common are anatomical models for training, custom surgical guides, customized orthosis, cartilage and bone replacement. PEEK is gaining more and more interest in orthopedics to manufacture custom implants because of its mechanical properties very close to that of the bone [14].

Polyamide (PA 2200), a polymer of nylon family, is one of the most versatile AM materials and SLS technology enables to design very complex geometries with good dimensional accuracy. It is widely employed to create patient-specific surgical guides and non-structural implants like cranial plates.

Metal alloys, namely Ti64Al and Cobalt-Chromium, due to the high cost and weight, are mainly used to manufacture load-bearing implants, custom fixations and long-lasting implantable devices. EBM and SLM allow to manufacture metal implants with very complex internal geometries with no need of supports. These technologies are providing clinicians and engineers with high-performance, customized implants (Fig. 3.13).

3.5 Finishing and Cleaning of the 3D Printed Piece

Most 3D printed parts need a manual post-processing before use. The most common operation is to remove the supports and polish the part.

Sintered models require the most demanding operations. First, the unsintered powder must be removed; typically, 3D printers that rely on sin-

Table 3.2 AM biocompatible materials and relative AM technology

AM technology	SLA	FDM	SLS	SLM	EBM
Biocompatible material	Photopolymer resin	PC-ISO, ABS-M30i, PEEK, ULTEM 1010	PA 2200	Titanium alloy, cobalt-chromium alloy	Titanium alloy, cobalt-chromium alloy

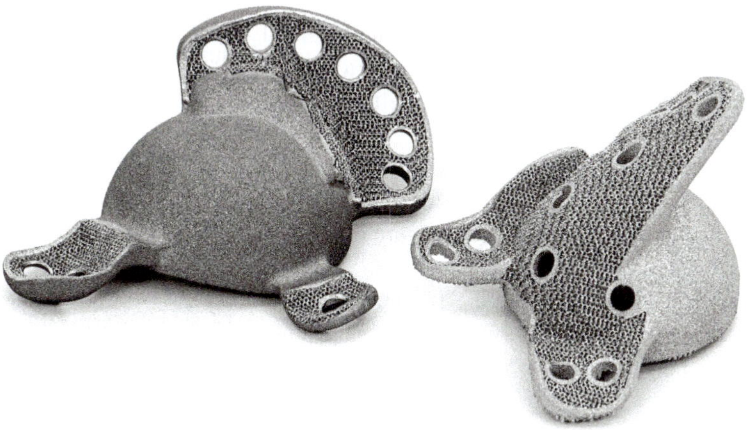

Fig. 3.13 3D printed implant. Note the different smooth and porous surfaces (Courtesy and © of Dr. Prang and Waldemar Link GmbH & Co.)

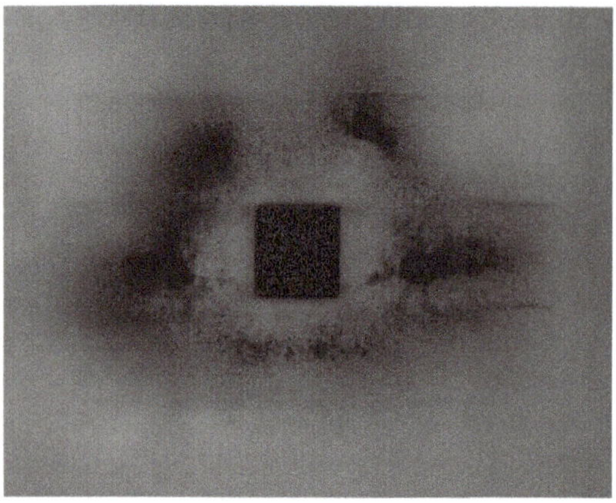

Fig. 3.14 Demonstration of production residues removal during the first cycle of cleaning process with ultrasonic waves of a porous material (Courtesy and © Implantcast GmbH)

tering or fusion of powder are provided with a dedicated module for powder removal and recycling. Such operation can be performed with a pressurized air jet or by specially designed ultrasonic cleaners. These machines use the energy of ultrasonic waves to remove the particles in the 3D printed structure (Fig. 3.14).

In case of implantable parts, special care must be taken during cleaning operations, especially for metal implantable devices. During the manufacturing process, some partially melted particles are bonded to the model [15], with deleterious effects to the mechanical properties and fatigue resistance [16]. Moreover, those particles may be released into the biological system, increasing the risk of infections. Heat treatment, followed by sandblasting, improves both the surface finish and the mechanical properties, reducing stress concentrations and removing most of the residual unmelted powder [17].

Care must be taken in the design of the porous structure of an implant to consider not only the osseointegration, but also the cleaning process to create a porous structure easy to clean.

Metal 3D printed parts are suitable for CNC machining for polishing, milling, and any other required mechanical processing.

3.6 Sterilization Methods Available for 3D Printing Materials

Sterilization is a process that involves the use of heat, radiations or chemicals to destroy all microorganisms, as viruses, bacteria, and fungi, to prevent infections and disease transmission. Sterility is typically defined with the Sterility Assurance Level (SAL), which is the probability that a single unit, that has been subjected to sterilization, nevertheless remains nonsterile. For medical devices and injections, FDA requires a SAL of at least 10^{-6}. Sterilization methods can be classified as follows [18]:

- high temperature/pressure sterilization,
- chemical sterilization,
- radiation sterilization.

The most commonly used techniques to sterilize medical devices and equipment are steam under pressure (autoclave), ethylene oxide gas, hydrogen peroxide gas plasma, gamma radiation (Table 3.3). A summary of the available sterilization methods for each of the biomaterials described in this chapter is presented in (Table 3.4).

3.6.1 Steam Autoclave

Steam autoclave is the most widely used and most dependable sterilization method for medical products [19]. The part is directly exposed to pressurized steam at a precise temperature, pressure level and for a specified period of time to ensure the sterilization effectiveness. Steam sterilization is nontoxic and cost-effective. The microbicidal action is ensured at specific temperatures, namely 121 °C and 132 °C, with a minimal exposure time respectively of 30 min, in a gravity displacement sterilizer, and 4 min, in a pre-vacuum sterilizer [20]. The main drawback of steam sterilization is its incompatibility with heat-sensitive materials.

Table 3.3 Advantages and disadvantages of the different sterilization processes

	Advantages	Disadvantages
Steam autoclaves	– Short processing time – Process simplicity – Efficacy – Nontoxicity	– High operating temperature (121 °C or 132 °C) – Possible corrosion
Ethylene oxide gas	– Low operating temperature – High microbicidal activity – Penetrates porous materials	– Long processing time (10–24 h) – Toxic, flammable and carcinogenic gas
Hydrogen peroxide gas plasma	– Low operating temperature – Medium processing time	– Very expensive – Damages to nylon based materials
Gamma radiation	– Low operating temperature – No toxic agents are involved – High penetration, also through packaging	– The use of a radioisotope requires shielding for the safety of the operators while both in use and in storage – Long processing time – Radioactive waste

Table 3.4 Sterilization methods for 3D printable biomaterials

	Steam autoclaves	Ethylene oxide gas	Hydrogen peroxide gas plasma	Gamma radiation
PA 2200	✓	✓	Not available	✓
PC-ISO	✓	✓	✓	✓
ABS-M30i	✓	✓	✓	✓
PEEK	✓	✓	✓	✓
ULTEM 1010	✓	Not available	Not available	✓
Metals	✓	✓	✓	✓

3.6.2 Ehylene Oxide Gas

Ethylene Oxide Gas (ETO) is a colorless gas with microbicidal power. It is an alkylating agent that disrupts the DNA of microorganisms, preventing them from reproducing, and is compatible with most materials. ETO effectiveness depends on the following parameters: gas concentration (450 to 1200 mg/L), temperature (37 to 60 °C), relative humidity (40 to 80%) and exposure time (1 to 6 h). ETO gas sterilization is a low-temperature method because it operates below 60 °C, making it suitable for heat- or moisture-sensitive medical equipment without deleterious effects [21]. This characteristic makes ETO widely used in the industry to sterilize heat-sensitive components, such as cutting masks and trial implants SLS printed.

Sterilized parts must be well aerated after sterilization and this process is expansive and requires dedicated equipment.

The main disadvantages associated with ETO are the high cost, long processing time, and its toxicity.

3.6.3 Hydrogen Peroxide Gas Plasma

An alternative for low-temperature sterilization is Hydrogen Peroxide Gas Plasma.

The sterilization chamber is evacuated, then a hydrogen peroxide solution is injected and ionized by an electrical field created by radio frequencies, which generates a highly reactive plasma. Microbicidal free radicals are generated in the plasma, which interacts with cell components disrupting the metabolism of microbes. The cycle duration is 55 min at a maximum temperature of 55 °C [22].

3.6.4 Gamma Radiation

Gamma radiation is a low-temperature sterilization method and the most commonly employed radioisotope is Cobalt-60.

Due to the radiation hazard, Gamma Radiation is not commonly used in hospitals, but is one of the most used sterilization methods by industries manufacturing orthopedic 3D printed custom-made implants. Gamma radiation has a high penetrating power that allows the components to be sterilized through their packaging. The gamma rays kill or inactivate microorganisms by destroying their DNA [23]. The exposure time of the specimen to the radioactive source is not predetermined but depends on the absorbed radiation.

Most sterilization facilities store the radioisotope into a water-filled source storage pool, which absorbs radiation and allows maintenance personnel to enter the radiation chamber. The applicable standard to sterilize medical devices is the ISO 11137 [24]. Gamma radiation sterilization is a relatively low-cost method, even though the radioisotopes must be safely shielded when not in use, requiring very expensive facilities.

3.7 Conclusion

3D medical printing is a complex process that contains several steps performed by specialists of different disciplines.

The different characteristics and costs of the materials used in 3D printing make it possible to use this technology in different areas, from surgery to patient education and surgery rehearsal.

It is essential that every specialist involved in the design, production, and final use of custom-made 3D printed devices knows the fundamentals of the 3D printing process explained in this chapter to make the most of this technology.

References

1. Kodama H. Automatic method for fabricating a three-dimensional plastic model with photo-hardening polymer. Rev Sci Instrum. 1981;52(11):1770–3.
2. Bright JR. Automation and management. Boston: Division of Research, Graduate School of Business Administration Harvard University; 1958.
3. Hull C. Apparatus for production of three-dimensional objects by stereolithography, US Patent 4,575,330. 1986.
4. Arnal-Burró J, Pérez-Mañanes R, Gallo-Del-Valle E, Igualada-Blazquez C, Cuervas-Mons M, Vaquero-Martín J. Three dimensional-printed patient-specific cutting guides for femoral varization osteotomy: do it yourself. Knee. 2017;24(6):1359–68.
5. Wong KC. 3D-printed patient-specific applications in orthopedics. Orthop res rev. 2016;8:57–66. Published 2016 Oct 14.
6. James AP, Dasarathy BV. Medical image fusion: a survey of the state of the art. Inf Fusion. 2014;19:4–19.
7. Bankman IN. Segmentation. In: Bankman IN, editor. Handbook of medical image processing and analysis. 2nd ed. Academic Press; 2009. p. 71–2.
8. Ng SP, Dyer BA, Kalpathy-Cramer J, et al. A prospective in silico analysis of interdisciplinary and interobserver spatial variability in post-operative target delineation of high-risk oral cavity cancers: does physician specialty matter? Clin Transl Radiat Oncol. 2018;12:40–6.
9. Hesamian MH, Jia W, He X, Kennedy P. Deep learning techniques for medical image segmentation: achievements and challenges. J Digit Imaging. 2019;32(4):582–96.
10. 3D Systems Inc. Stereolithography Interface Specification, 3D. Valenci, CA: Systems Inc.; 1988.
11. ISO/ASTMS. International Organization for Standardization/American Society for Testing and Materials 52915:2016. Geneva: ISO/ASTMS; 2016.
12. ISO/ASTMS. International Organization for Standardization/American Society for Testing and Materials 52900:2015. Geneva: ISO/ASTMS; 2015.
13. Williams DF, editor. Definitions in biomaterials. Amsterdam: Elsevier; 1987. 72 pp.
14. Ortega-Martínez J. Polyetheretherketone (PEEK) as a medical and dental material. A literature review. Med Res Arch. 2017;5:1–16.
15. Yan C, Hao L, Hussein A, Raymont D. Evaluations of cellular lattice structures manufactured using selective laser melting. Int J Mach Tools Manuf [Internet]. 2012;62:32–8.
16. Hrabe NW, Heinl P, Flinn B, Körner C, Bordia RK. Compression-compression fatigue of selective electron beam melted cellular titanium (Ti-6Al-4V). J Biomed Mater Res Part B Appl Biomater. 2011;99B(2):313–20.
17. Yan C, Hao L, Hussein A, Young P. Ti-6Al-4V triply periodic minimal surface structures for bone implants fabricated via selective laser melting. J Mech Behav Biomed Mater. 2015;51:61–73.
18. Govindaraj S, Muthuraman M. Systematic review on sterilization methods of implants and medical devices. Int J ChemTech Res. 2015;8:974–4290.

19. Adler S, Scherrer M, Daschner FD. Costs of low-temperature plasma sterilization compared with other sterilization methods. J Hosp Infect. 1998;40(2):125–34.
20. Rutala WA, Weber DJ. Guideline for disinfection disinfection and sterilization in healthcare facilities. In: Bennett Brachman's hospital infections. 6th ed; 2019.
21. Rutala WA, Weber DJ. Guideline for disinfection disinfection and sterilization in healthcare facilities. In: Ethylene oxide "Gas" sterilization Bennett Brachman's hospital infections. 6th ed; 2019.
22. Rutala WA, Weber DJ. Guideline for disinfection disinfection and sterilization in healthcare facilities. In: Hydrogen peroxide gas plasma in Bennett Brachman's hospital infections. 6th ed; 2019.
23. West C, McTaggart R, Letcher T, Raynie D, Roy R. Effects of gamma irradiation upon the mechanical and chemical properties of 3D-printed samples of polylactic acid. J Manuf Sci Eng Trans ASME. 2019;141(4):1.
24. Sandle T. Application of sterilization by gamma radiation for single-use disposable technologies in the biopharmaceutical sector. J GXP Compliance. 2012;16:1–8.

4 The Engineer's Point of View

Simone Di Bella and Rosalia Mineo

4.1 Introduction

In the last decade, industrial technological development has made great progress in the additive manufacturing production both in the fields of industrial manufacturing and in the medical-surgical device industry ones.

Initially created for making of prototypes and models for demonstration use ("Rapid Prototyping"), 3D Additive technologies have begun a rapid rise in the sectors of production of finished components, becoming rapidly a reference product for the medical sector.

In this chapter will be analyzed in detail, all phases of the production process of a customized medical device obtained with 3D technology in the application of bone surgery and will be explored the technical and engineering aspects related. The first important step is the images acquisition, nowadays it's possible to have diagnostic exams with high resolution, important feature for obtaining a device with a good fit with the host bone. The second step is the planning and design. During the planning, it's possible to anticipate the surgical challenge and to have the best understanding of the clinical case, throughout 3D virtual or printed models. During the designing, patient-specific implants and anything is needful for its implantation, such as guide templates or surgical instruments, are developed. The final step is the production of the device set.

S. Di Bella (✉) · R. Mineo
MT Ortho Srl, Aci Sant'Antonio (CT), Italy

University of Catania, DICAR, Catania (CT), Italy
e-mail: simone.dibella@mtortho.com; rosalia.mineo@mtortho.com

4.2 3D Technologies and Medical Application

Additive manufacturing technologies are increasingly used in the medical field to improve the clinical conditions of patients.

A 3D printing machine allows obtaining 3D physical parts by adding successive layers of material to recreate the virtual cross section. The 3D printing technologies used in medicine can be classified according to the technique of manufacturing and includes stereolithography apparatus (SLA), fused deposition modeling (FDM), selective laser sintering (SLS) and electron beam melting (EBM).

The technology of 3D printing has the potential to solve many design challenges. This technique has been applied successfully to a variety of surgical problems, and has shown promising results in improving outcomes, decreasing morbidity, and shortening surgical time [1].

Medical additive manufacturing is not only about devices that have direct application in the body, there are a lot of useful indirect application.

C. Zoccali et al. (eds.), *3D Printing in Bone Surgery*, https://doi.org/10.1007/978-3-030-91900-9_4

The direct applications regard implantable devices both custom-made and [2–4] off-the-shelf ones, above all in orthopedics, neurosurgery, maxillo and dental field, but also orthoses throughout the production of personalized busts, orthotics and exoskeletons. A charitable example is the use of 3D technologies in the production of transradial prosthesis, that allows children, who have lost limbs because of sociopolitical conflicts, to have an artificial limb thanks to a reduction of costs related [5].

About the indirect application, 3D printing techniques can generate models that give a better understanding of the complex anatomy and pathology of the patients and aid in education and surgical training, but also can produce patient-specific instruments and surgical cutting guides.

The latest and most innovative application concerns the bioprinting technologies (BT). In tissue engineering and regenerative medicine, BT provides an automated and advanced platform to fabricate various biomaterials through precise deposition of cells and polymers in a premeditated fashion. The common applications are the bioprinting of cell-laden constructs, bone and cartilage cells and tissues constructs, skin cells and tissues, blood vessels, and neuronal tissues [6].

This technology is widely used also for screening of drugs and cancer research [7]. It offers several advantages such as precise and controlled deposition of cells, hormones, drugs, and growth factors. Further, it provides a base for development of tissues constructs, organs and organoids, and organ-on-a-chip, mimicking natural ones [8].

4.3 Production Flow of a Custom-Made Medical Device

In traditional orthopedic procedures, surgeons have to combine all preoperative two-dimensional (2D) images and formulate a 3D surgical plan. These processes are particularly difficult when surgeons meet very complex anatomy or severe deformity as in bone tumor surgery. So, the experience of the surgeon and his ability to image the three-dimensional anatomy, play a key role in planning the surgery and in the result of the surgical intervention.

The combination of the potential offered by imaging technologies and the freedom of production of additive manufacturing, allows to overcome these limits obtaining custom-made devices that improve diagnosis, planning, surgery, and clinical outcomes.

A custom-made implant is a medical device specifically conceived, designed, and produced for a single patient, so it matches his unique anatomy and it's based on the patient's own medical images. They are used when patient's bony geometry falls outside the range of standard implants with respect to implant size or disease-specific requirements or when the custom-made solution could obtain a better clinical outcome.

The whole process of ideation and development of a custom-made device can be divided into three phases (Fig. 4.1):

1. image acquisition,
2. planning/design,
3. 3D printing.

Each of these phases, is directly controlled by a surgeon or an engineer or by the cooperation of them.

Essential to the successful process is the interprofessional cooperation and communication between the orthopedic surgeon and the engineer as they have technological and educational differences. For example, the engineer may not be familiar with anatomy, epidemiology, surgical approach, and resection/reconstruction procedures. In contrast, the orthopedic surgeon may not know the numerous steps of the fabrication process of a 3D-printed physical model.

4.3.1 Image Acquisition

Medical images are the key link between 3D printing technology and patient-specific orthopedic implant [9].

Accurate medical imaging data must be obtained to represent better the real condition of

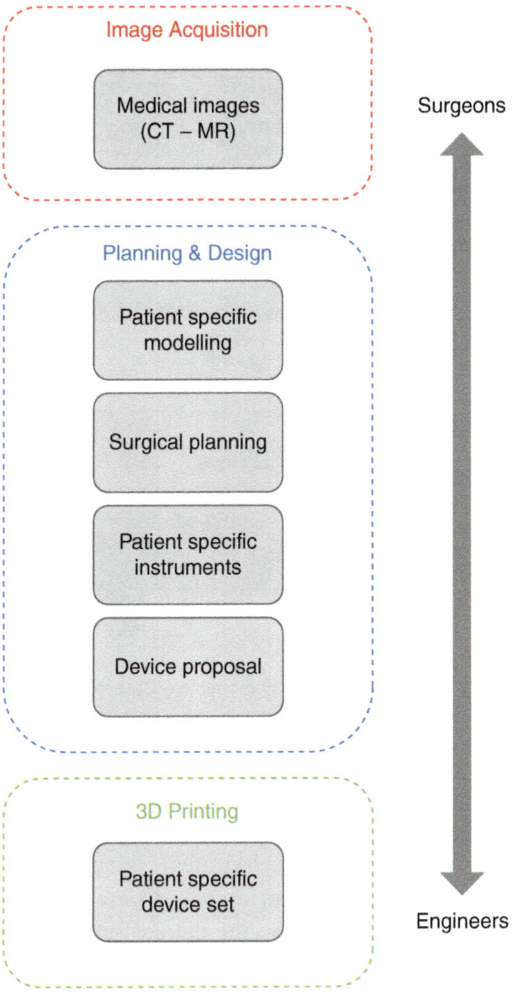

Fig. 4.1 This image summarizes the clinical workflow of patient-specific orthopedics from image acquisition to 3D-printed models and implants

the patient. The modern multirow detector computer tomography (MDCT) and magnetic resonance imaging (MRI) provide fast and accurate 3D image with high resolution.

The resolution of the 3D model obtained by the medical images depending on some parameter of the detector used for the analysis. The optimal condition is to produce thin-section axial image with slice thickness of less than 1 mm and isotropic voxel.

CT scan images are ideal when bones are the region of interest due to its high contrast, instead MRI is superior to CT in delineating soft tissue anatomy, such as that of articular cartilage in joint disease and intramedullary or extraosseous extension in orthopedic tumors.

All the acquired medical images are saved in a standard data format to store exchange and transmit images (DICOM "digital imaging and communications in medicine").

Before the image acquisition, the engineer provides to the hospital structure, often represented directly by the surgeon or the head of radiology, the parameters for obtaining images as precise as possible and suitable for the type of application to be made.

To create a 3D model using DICOM images as starting data, it needs to use special software that convert these files into a format suitable for three-dimensional design such as stereolithography (STL StereoLithography). For this purpose the Mimics software (Materialize, Belgium) is often used; it allows, thanks to specific segmetation operations (to group areas in the images whose pixels have a gray value included in a certain range that identifies that of region of interest), to obtain surfaces and contours of the desired portions (Fig. 4.2).

4.3.2 Planning & Design

In traditional preoperative planning, orthopedic surgeon utilized 2D plain X-ray and CT scan images to assess the bony anatomy and pathology of the patient and defines, basing on them the best strategy to be follow during the surgery.

In 3D printing bone surgery, the surgical planning phase is a process carried out by the surgeon and by the team of engineers of the device manufacturer. The surgeon give his indications as the type of prosthesis, the surgical access, the fixing strategy, and the engineer analyzes the problem from a technical point of view, looking for the best engineering solution, studying the loads and forces that the prosthesis will be support.

All communications between these two figures usually take place through telematic channels, with sharing of images and technical drawings.

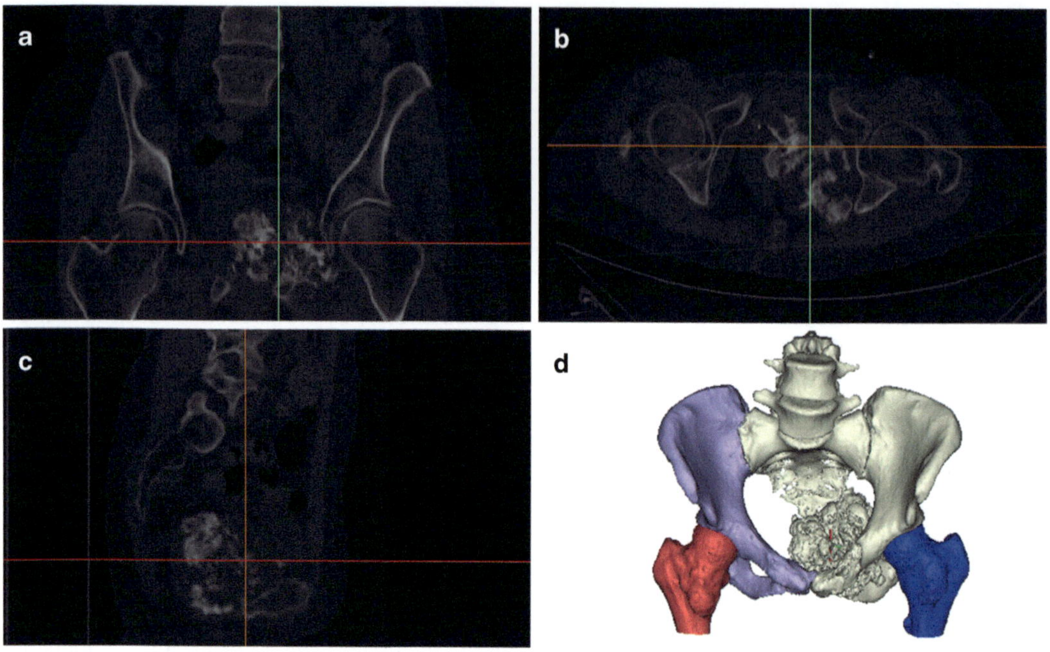

Fig. 4.2 CT scan images imported into a CAD engineering program to obtain 3D CAD model. (**a**) Coronal view, (**b**) Axial view, (**c**) Sagittal view, and (**d**) Tridimensional view

4.3.2.1 Anatomic Models for Surgical Planning

Patient-specific, physical bone models can be recreated from patients' CT image data by 3D printing.

The models not only allow surgeons to have tactile and visual understanding of the patient-specific anatomy and pathology, but also anticipate the operative challenges they will aid in the planning of orthopedic procedures. These models can also be sterilized so that the surgeon can manipulate the model on the operative field while performing the procedure [10].

These models can also be used to perform simulated operations directly on the plastic component and verify that all imagined steps are truly applicable. If the surgery requires the implantation of adaptable metal components, such as plates, these models can be used as real molds where is possible to recreate the correct matching geometry. Maxillofacial prostheses are often used in this field, where is often necessary to create plates or mesh that can be modified directly in the operating room [11].

Patient-specific 3D-printed models can be also used for education and preoperative discussions about surgical strategies and options among care providers across different disciplines. It may increase the patient satisfaction as patients and their families can easily understand their medical conditions with real physical model.

4.3.2.2 Blood Vessels Visualization

Three-dimensional printed models can provide effective preoperative planning, the geometry of nearby vessel could be obtained to determine most accurate osteotomy and most appropriate prosthesis, resulting in decreased operative time and decreased blood loss [12].

By working on the same CT images it is possible to "isolate" the gray values corresponding to the blood vessels, so obtaining their three-dimensional models. This could be useful to the surgeon to evaluate the best access strategy both through digital visualization and through 3D scale reproduction of the model (Fig. 4.3).

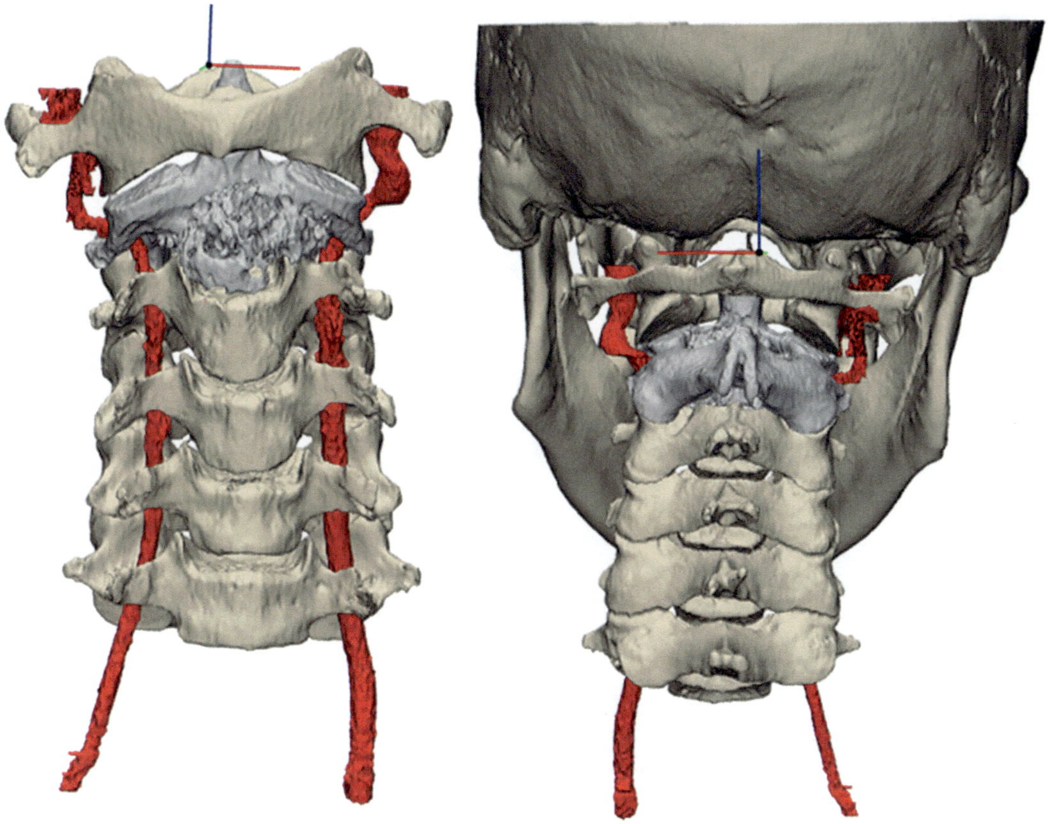

Fig. 4.3 Blood Vessels 3D Visualization

4.3.2.3 Anatomical Cutting Guides

In the oncology and sometimes in complex orthopedics revision cases the first planning phase is the definition of the surfaces that delimit the bone parts to be removed. The three-dimensional cutting planes are therefore defined to remove the pathological parts with an appropriate safety margin (Fig. 4.4).

This operation could be performed using dedicated software that allows the fusion of CT and MR images so that both bone and soft tissues can be visualized together. However, these technologies are not easily available, therefore the surgeon have to perform a manual check between the images provided by CT and MR ones to define the regions to be removed. At the end of this phase, an osteotomy simulation can be performed. To reproduce the virtual cut during the surgery, the engineer designs specific anatomical cutting guides that ensure univocal positioning on the bone [13] (Fig. 4.5).

A series of Boolean operation on the CAD model are conducted to create the contact interface between the bone and guides and no soft tissue, as muscle insertion or cartilages tissue, are evaluated during the design process. For this reason, it's important to perform an accurate skeletonization of the matching surfaces bone before performing the osteotomies.

Often, for complex cases, multiple versions can be designed to perform the same osteotomies. So, the surgeon during the surgery, have the opportunity to choose the better of these, according to the surgical access or difficulty in placing.

Anatomical cutting guides are made with AM technology using plastic materials such as ABS, PA or metal materials. Due their intended use, materials must be certified to be short-term

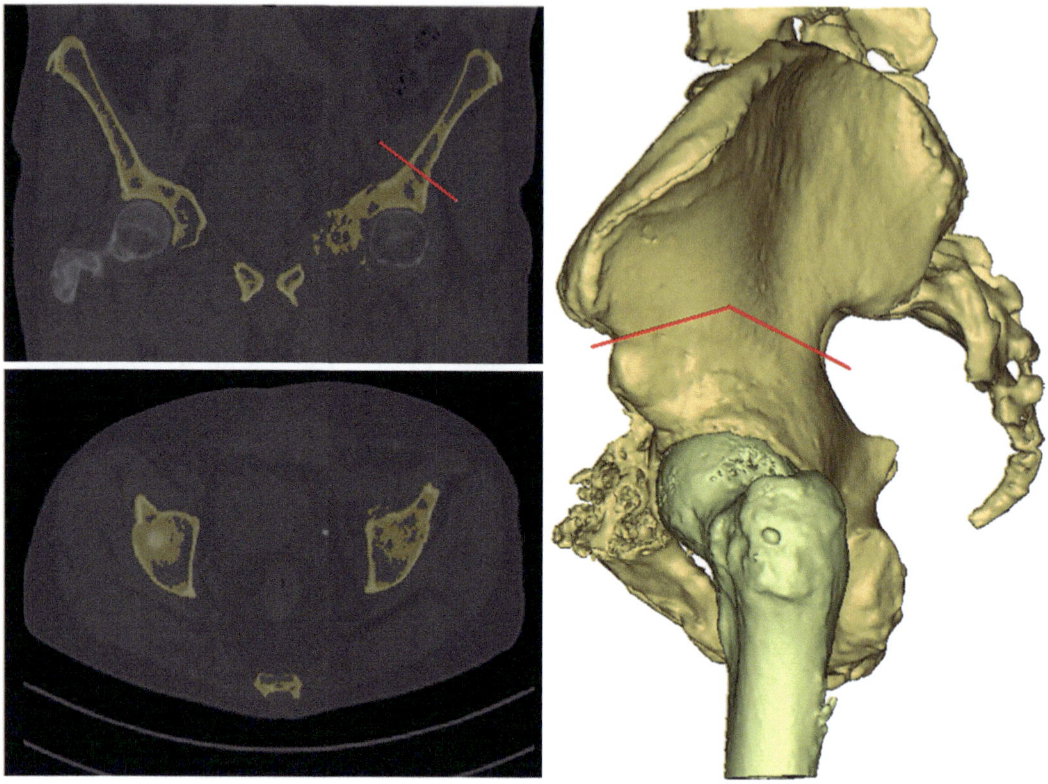

Fig. 4.4 Planning of cutting plane for osteotomy

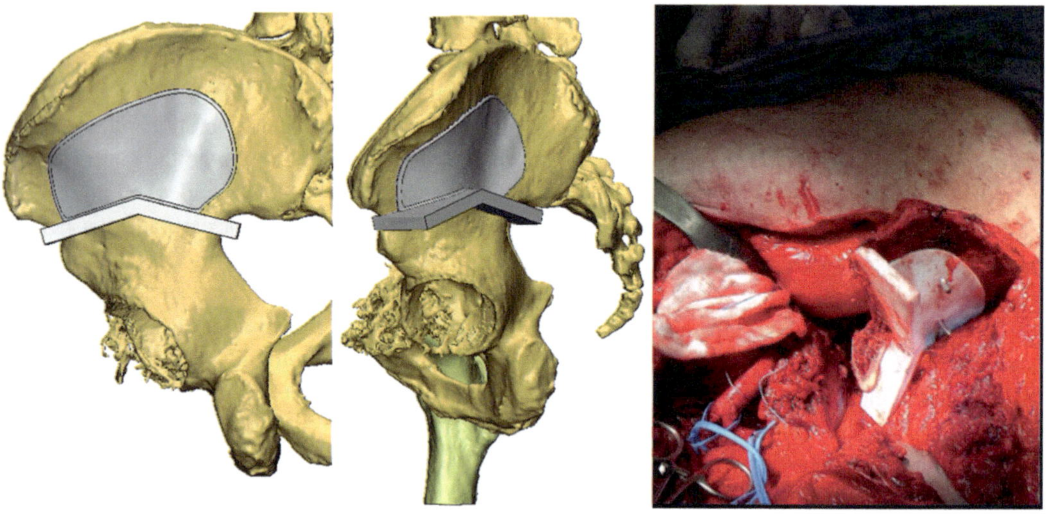

Fig. 4.5 Planning or anatomical resection guides

implantable medical devices and must be sterilizable.

4.3.2.4 Design of Patient-Specific Implant and Instruments

The goal of designing customized device is to restore the functionality and anatomy of the pathological skeletal site treated and to ensure its stability and durability.

The intended use of the device carries with it a lot of important information during the design phase. The engineer's task is to translate the doctor's indications and turn them into a feasible technical project.

The different aspects that must be considered for the correct design of a custom-made prosthesis are the following:

1. *Materials*:

   In bone surgery different kind of printed materials can be used, both metallic and polymeric ones. Among metallic materials, Titanium alloys offer the best compromise between biological properties (biocompatibility and osseointegration) and mechanical ones (elasticity close to the bones) [14]. Titanium is widely used in bone filling or replacement prostheses and in arthrodesis cases where a high osseointegrating capability is required. When articular condition has to be maintained, Cobalt–Chrome alloy is the best choose thanks to its lower friction coefficient compared to other metallic materials. Polymeric materials, on the other hand, are used in surgical support instruments such as cutting guides or implant positioning template.

2. *Geometry*:

   In the case of filling and replacement implants, this aspect results into the choose to restore or not the exact geometry of the removed bone tissue. For large osteotomies, a perfectly anatomical prosthesis could lead to a heavy, bulky, and hard to implant device. Also, anatomical geometry reconstruction could be result in an incorrect suturing of the soft tissues over the device with the risk of infection and rejection of the implant.

   The solutions adoptable are for example the elimination of nonfunctional parts, the creation of hollow structures and the realization of a geometry with an offset in minus compared to the anatomical shape (Fig. 4.6). Another aspect to consider is the interaction with an off-the-shelf prosthesis, in this case it is essential to have the related technical drawings and/or operating techniques. In this phase, specific

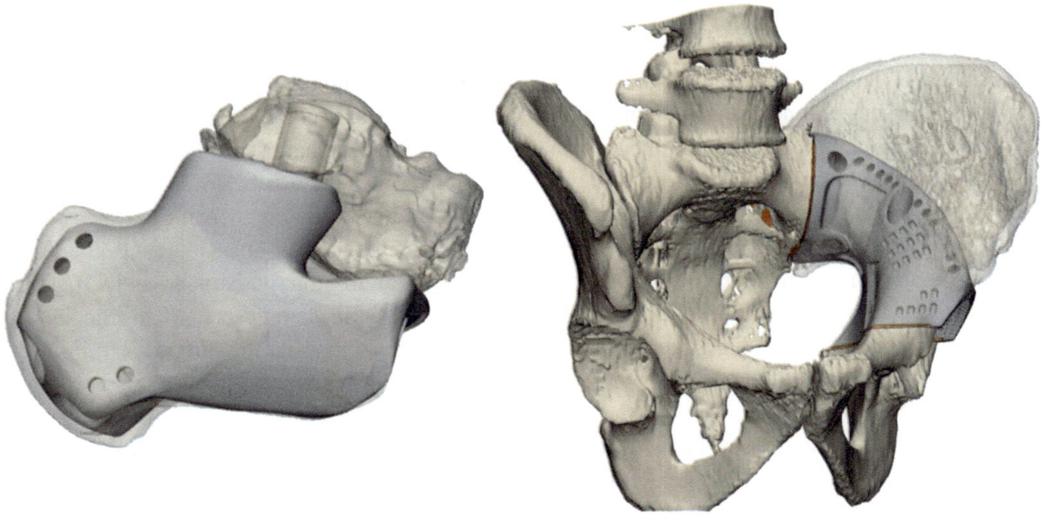

Fig. 4.6 In minus offset surfaces (left), hollowed and not anatomical part with structures for tendons and ligaments fixing (right)

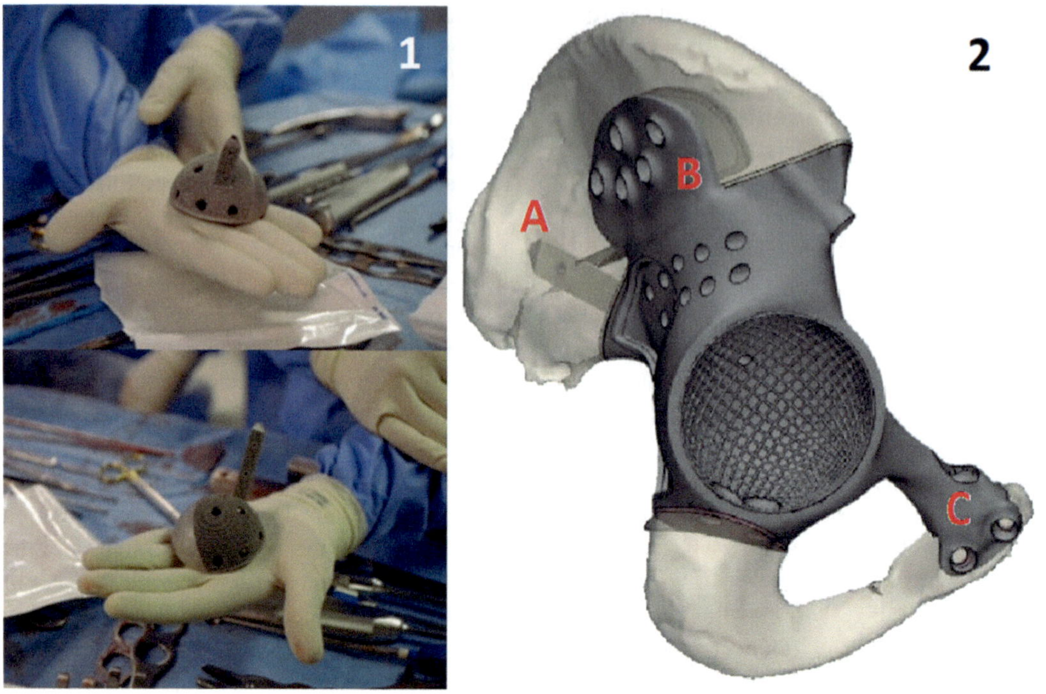

Fig. 4.7 Intramedullary triangle trabecular post (left), different kind of fixing system (right): (A) intramedullary post, (B) sandwich structures with symmetrical plates blocked with screws and nuts, (C) plates with bone screws

structures for fixing tendons, ligaments, or soft structures could also be designed.

3. *Surgical approach*:

   Knowing the surgical access is important to ensure the implantability of the device. From the design point of view, it involves important assessments in terms of positioning of plates, orientation of screws and encumbrance surfaces (to evaluate the impingement with soft tissues or other bone structures). The type of surgical access also influences the design of the anatomical cutting templates or specific surgical instruments.

4. *Fixing system*:

   In the design of an orthopedic prosthesis, it is necessary to ensure the stability of the device both in the early stages following surgery (primary stability) and over time (secondary stability).

   Primary stability can be obtained through different types of fixing system, such as screws and plates, intramedullary post, sandwich structures with symmetrical plates blocked with screws and nuts (Fig. 4.7).

   Secondary stability is ensured by osteointegrating surfaces at the bone/implant interface with structures that stimulate osseointegration of the implant, such as trabecular structures (Fig. 4.11).

5. *Loading condition*:

   The design of a device must be included evaluations in terms of resistance to the physiological loads that the device will be subjected in vivo, once implanted. First of all, it's necessary to know the biomechanics of the skeletal site to image the correct loading condition. The goal of this study is to reduce stress-shielding effect, to ensure homogeneous distribution of loads at the interface, to limit the risk of subsidence and to avoid risk of breaking due to fatigue.

   Preliminary evaluation in terms of distribution of stresses and deformations can be obtained through finite element analysis [15,

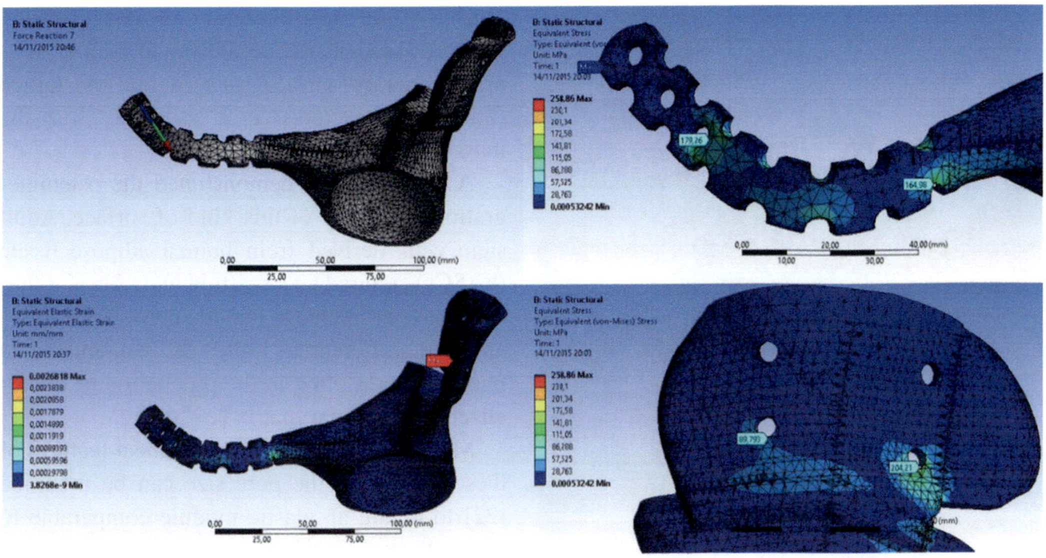

Fig. 4.8 Preliminary FEM (Finite element analysis) evaluation for a custom hip implant

16]. These analyzes allow to predict, by setting constraints and loads conditions, which will be the most stressed areas and if the tensions and deformations, reached in the worst cases, fall within the material safety coefficients (Fig. 4.8).

Collected all necessary information, the engineer proceeds to design the device using special three-dimensional software. Although the design phase is a specific task of the engineer, the process involves a continuous exchange of feedback between the engineer and the surgeon. The definitive approval of the project is the responsibility of the prescriber surgeon, and once obtained the manufacture of the device's set can start.

4.4 Intraoperative Execution

3D bone model can allow a better understanding of many complex aspect in the preoperative, intraoperative (Fig. 4.9) e post-operative phases. In the operative field the models can provide to surgeon both visual and tactile useful informations [17].

Moreover, the using of CT-based navigation allows accurate execution of the intended bone resection, above all in tumor resection due to the distorted surgical anatomy. Studies have shown an accuracy between the achieved bone resection and the planned ones less than 2 mm [18].

Image-guided computer navigation allows reproducing surgical planning with less error also in the reconstruction phase [19]. Custom-made prosthesis CAD could be seen in the navigation system (through image fusion of the virtual CT data sets with the custom prosthesis), to suggest to the surgeon the orientation and position of the implant as planned and thus obtaining a precise fitting of the custom prosthesis to the residual bone segment after resection [20] (Fig. 4.10).

4.5 Advantages of 3D-Printed Custom Implants

The additive manufacturing production of prostheses allows to obtain any complex shape without geometric limits; this is impossible using traditional subtractive manufacturing techniques.

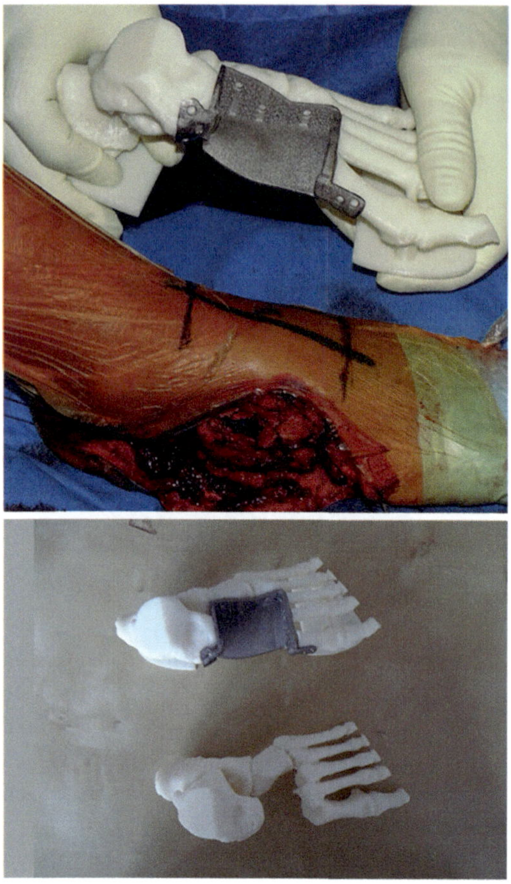

Fig. 4.9 3D plastic model help the surgeon during the positioning phase

One of the most important advantages of the AM prostheses is the possibility to realize complex free-form surface such as scaffold lattice (trabecular structures) in a continuity with the massive part (Fig. 4.11).

A lot of studies demonstrated the osteointegration capability of this kind of surface. Adult stem cells derived from human adipose tissue (hASCs) cultured on a scaffold on trabecular titanium have been able to join the network, proliferate and differentiate into an osteoblast-like phenotype, resulting in the production of mineralized extracellular matrix [21].

Moreover, focusing on mechanical features of these structures, the pore size can be modified [22] to obtain an elastic module comparable to that of the patient's bone.

Regarding the advantages of using a patient-specific prosthesis, the accuracy of the surgery is considerably improved respect to the traditional orthopedic procedures. A custom-made implant allows to have a precise implant shape matching the bone site and accurate guides and templates that ensure the optimal implantation of the device [23].

Another aspect is the important reduction of the surgical time, due to the possibility of the 3D preoperative planning (through the direct visualization of the malformation and better anticipa-

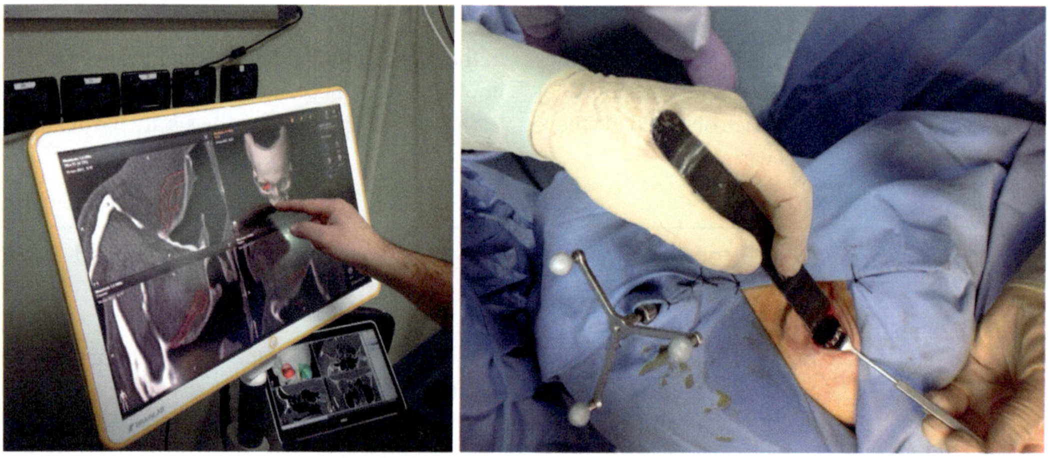

Fig. 4.10 Custom-made prosthesis CAD could be seen in the navigation system (in red on the left side), to allow the best positioning of the implant

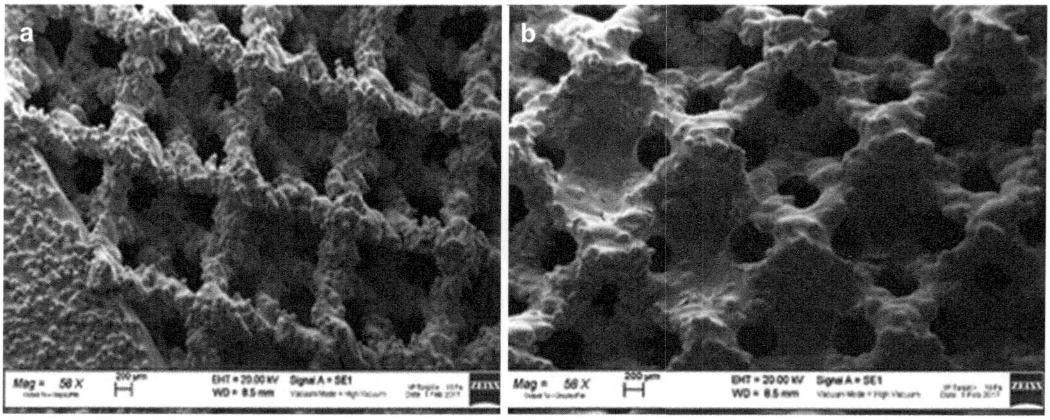

Fig. 4.11 Scansion electron microscopy of empty cage (**a**) and of cage seeded with hASCs and cultured in growth medium (**b**) and osteogenic medium

tion of anatomic difficulties) and no correction or manipulation of the implant are needed [23].

4.6 Limitations and Potential Future Development

Although the high performance and the satisfactory clinical outcomes of 3D-printed custom-made implants, there are some limitations related to their use, that are useful to evaluate in order to rational choose of this, for a specific patient.

The concerns include the costs of implants due to the high technological contents of the 3D printing processes that includes Cad software, 3D printing machine, Project engineer, etc.

Moreover, 3D software (for planning and design) requires specific skills that most surgeons don't have, despite the huge responsibility played by themselves at the critical stage of preoperative planning. It's important in this highly specialized field that the surgeons have a 3D visual tendency and accept the support of external technicians without fearing loss over their leadership.

The time required to plan and produce the 3D object could be also a limitation when there's the need to meet a surgical deadline so this aspect could be unsuitable for use in emergency cases.

Unlike to the off-the-shelf implants, that are available in differ size and shape intraoperatively, the patient-specific implants don't allow the same flexibility due to their specific intended use. In addition to that, there's a difficult of placement of the implants [24] due to the minimal surgical approach, the complex site anatomy and the presence of the soft tissues, especially in the cases of orthopedic revision where the guided osteotomy is not required and the implant have to match the existing bone tissue.

Other disadvantages are related to imaging phase. Some artifacts were found to have likely affected the acquisition parameters and resolution of the image, leading to final errors in volume. Another aspect is the difficult to building a 3D model of soft tissue than bony structures one, because of the resolution of the current imaging acquisition technology.

Above all in the oncology, a potential future development could be in the new MRI Scanner feature sequences that may allow both bone and soft tissue to be reconstructed from a single image set without any registration. This would be beneficial in reduce patient radiation exposure.

Potential future benefits could result from the choice of hybrid devices. Combining different kind of materials such as metallic parts and bone graft [25] could be obtained a device that ensures optimal mechanical stability and biological performance.

Finally, to increase the use of 3D printing technology in bone surgery, an online integrated platform could be developed to allow for easy cooperation among radiologists, orthopedic surgeons, engineers, and implant companies. All the digital designing data could be integrated to facilitate customized patient treatments. Surgeons may then choose which 3D-printed solutions are most appropriate for their patients [26].

References

1. Tack P, Victor J, Gemmel P, et al. 3D-printing techniques in a medical setting: a systematic literature review. Biomed Eng Online. 2016;15:115. https://doi.org/10.1186/s12938-016-0236-4.
2. Tartara F, Bongetta D, Pilloni G, Colombo EV, Giombelli E. Custom-made trabecular titanium implants for the treatment of lumbar degenerative discopathy via ALIF/XLIF techniques: rationale for use and preliminary results. Eur Spine J. 2019;29(2):314–20. https://doi.org/10.1007/s00586-019-06191-y.
3. Francaviglia N, Maugeri R, Contino AO, Meli F, Fiorenza V, Costantino G, Giammalva RG, Iacopino DG. Skull bone defects reconstruction with custom-made titanium graft shaped with electron beam melting technology: preliminary experience in a series of ten patients. Acta Neurochir Suppl. 2017;124:137–41. https://doi.org/10.1007/978-3-319-39546-3_21.
4. Angelini A, Trovarelli G, Berizzi A, Pala E, Breda A, Ruggieri P. Three-dimension-printed custom-made prosthetic reconstructions: from revision surgery to oncologic reconstructions. Int Orthop. 2018;43:123–32. https://doi.org/10.1007/s00264-018-4232-0.
5. Gretsch KF, Lather HD, Peddada KV, Deeken CR, Wall LB, Goldfarb CA. Development of novel 3D-printed robotic prosthetic for transradial amputees. Prosthet Orthot Int. 2016;40(3):400–3. https://doi.org/10.1177/0309364615579317.
6. Waeljumah A, Muhammad W, Xianglin Z. Bioprinting and its applications in tissue engineering and regenerative medicine. Int J Biol Macromol. 2018;107:261–75. https://doi.org/10.1016/j.ijbiomac.2017.08.171.
7. Lee J, Cho D. 3D printing technology over a drug delivery for tissue engineering. Curr Pharm Des. 2015;21(12):1606–17. https://doi.org/10.2174/1381612821666150115125324.
8. Jipeng L, Mingjiao C, Xianqun F, Huifang Z. Recent advances in bioprinting techniques: approaches, applications, and future prospects. J Transl Med. 2016;14:271. https://doi.org/10.1186/s12967-016-1028-0.
9. Rengier F, Mehndiratta A, von Tengg-Kobligk H, et al. 3D printing based on imaging data: review of medical applications. Int J Comput Assist Radiol Surg. 2010;5:335–41. https://doi.org/10.1007/s11548-010-0476.
10. Kim H, Liu X, Noh K. Use of a real-size 3D-printed model as a preoperative and intraoperative tool for minimally invasive plating of comminuted midshaft clavicle fractures. J Orthop Surg Res. 2015;10:91. https://doi.org/10.1186/s13018-015-0233-5.
11. Novelli G, Tonellini G, Mazzoleni F, Bozzetti A, Sozzi D. Virtual surgery simulation in orbital wall reconstruction: integration of surgical navigation and stereolitho graphic models. J Craniomaxillofac Surg. 2014;42:2025–34. https://doi.org/10.1016/j.jcms.2014.09.009.
12. Punyaratabandhu T, Liacouras P, Pairojboriboon S. Using 3D models in orthopedic oncology: presenting personalized advantages in surgical planning and intraoperative outcomes. 3D Print Med. 2018;4:12. https://doi.org/10.1186/s41205-018-0035-6.
13. Wong KC, Kumta S, Sze K, Wong CM. Use of a patient-specific CAD/CAM surgical jig in extremity bone tumor resection and custom prosthetic reconstruction. Comput Aided Surg. 2012;17(6):284–93. https://doi.org/10.3109/10929088.2012.725771.
14. Mirone G, Barbagallo R, Corallo D, Di Bella S. Static and dynamic response of titanium alloy produced by electron beam melting. Procedia Struct Integr. 2016;2:2355–66. https://doi.org/10.1016/j.prostr.2016.06.295.
15. La Rosa G, Clienti C, Di Bella S, Rizza F. Numerical analysis of a custom-made pelvic prosthesis. Procedia Struct Integr. 2016;2:1295–302. https://doi.org/10.1016/j.prostr.2016.06.165.
16. Epasto G, Distefano F, Mineo R, Guglielmino E. Subject-specific finite element analysis of a lumbar cage produced by electron beam melting. Med Biol Eng Comput. 2019;57:2771–81. https://doi.org/10.1007/s11517-019-02078-8.
17. Niikura T, Sugimoto M, Lee S, Sakai Y, Nishida K, Kuroda R, Kurosaka M. Tactile surgical navigation system for complex acetabular fracture surgery. Orthopedics. 2014;37(4):237–42. https://doi.org/10.3928/01477447-20140401-05.
18. Wong KC, Kumta S. Computer-assisted tumor surgery in malignant bone tumors. Clin Orthop Relat Res. 2013;471(3):750–61. https://doi.org/10.1007/s11999-012-2557-3.
19. Wong KC, Kumta S, Chiu K, Cheung K, Leung K, Unwin P, Wong M. Computer assisted pelvic tumor resection and reconstruction with a custom-made prosthesis using an innovative adaptation and its validation. Comput Aided Surg. 2007;12(4):225–32. https://doi.org/10.3109/10929080701536046.
20. Wong KC, Kumta SM, Leung KS, Ng KW, Ng EWK, Lee KS. Integration of CAD/CAM planning into computer assisted orthopaedic surgery. Comput Aided Surg. 2010;15(4–6):65–74. https://doi.org/10.3109/10929088.2010.514131.
21. Gastaldi G, Asti A, Scaffino M, Visai L, Saino E, Cometa A, Benazzo F. Human adipose-derived stem cells (hASCs) proliferate and differentiate in osteoblast-like cells on trabecular titanium scaffolds. J Biomed Mater Res A. 2010;94A(3):790–9. https://doi.org/10.1002/jbm.a.32721.
22. Epasto G, Palomba G, Di Bella S, Mineo R, Guglielmino E, Traina F. Experimental investigation of rhombic dodecahedron micro-lattice structures manufactured by electron beam melting. Mater Today

Proc. 2019;7:578–85. https://doi.org/10.1016/j.matpr.2018.12.011.

23. Martelli N, Serrano C, Van den Brink H, Pineau J, Prognon P, Borget I, El Batti S. Advantages and disadvantges of 3-dimensional printing in surgery: a systematic review. Surgery. 2016;159(6):1485–500. https://doi.org/10.1016/j.surg.2015.12.017.
24. Baauw M, Van Hellemondt G, Van Hooff M, Spruit M. The accuracy of positioning of a custom-made implant within a large acetabular defect at revision arthroplasty of the hip. Bone Joint J. 2015;97-B:780–5. https://doi.org/10.1302/0301-620X.97B6.35129.
25. Ferracini R, Bistolfi A, Garibaldi R, Furfaro V, Battista A, Perale G. Composite Xenohybrid bovine bone-derived scaffold as bone substitute for the treatment of tibial plateau fractures. Appl Sci. 2019;9:2675. https://doi.org/10.3390/app9132675.
26. Wong KC. 3D-printed patient specific applications in orthopedics. Orthop Res Rev. 2016;8:57–66. https://doi.org/10.2147/ORR.S99614.

3D Pelvis/Hip Prosthesis

5

Andrea Angelini and Pietro Ruggieri

5.1 Introduction

Surgery around the bony pelvis and in the acetabular area is challenging given the complexity of pelvic anatomy, deep exposures and to presence of critical neurovascular and visceral structures. With the increasing use of arthroplasty, the increased life expectancy and functional performance required by patients with hip osteoarthritis, the incidence of revision surgery is becoming a current problem [1, 2]. The most frequent complications requiring acetabular revision include aseptic loosening, wear and periprosthetic osteolysis, pseudo-tumors, instability, and infection. Excluding the infective setting, the collective aspect is represented by the acetabular bone loss compromising implant fixation and stability. Due to the wide range of osteolysis and bone defect, pelvic reconstruction is challenging and different strategies have been used including both non-biologic and biologic fixation. In recent years, with the improvement of 3D printing technology, new approaches have been introduced to manage complex reconstructions. Custom-made metal 3D-printed patient-specific implants and surgical tools have been studied for revision hip arthroplasties with favorable results [3–7] and then applied for pelvic oncologic resection and reconstruction [3, 8–11]. The surgical goal in limb salvage surgery is to resect bone tumors with adequate margins while sparing the host bone for functional reconstruction [12–14]. With the 3D printing technology is possible to improve precision surgery and to realize a custom implant on patient's anatomy [15–21]. Recently, there has been increasing interest in applying 3D-printing techniques for pelvic reconstruction [3–11, 22, 23] with satisfactory results in term of functional and oncologic outcomes. Principles, concepts, and applications of 3D-printed technology in pelvic reconstruction will be analyzed in the following paragraphs. Major limitations and advantages are summarized in Table 5.1.

5.2 How to Create a Medical 3D-Printed Implant for Pelvic Reconstructions

5.2.1 Step 1: Ideation

The first step in the process of a creating a 3D-printed implant is strictly correlated with the surgical indications based on patient's anatomy, amount of osteolysis or planned resection and quality of residual bone. In musculoskeletal oncology, the indications for pelvic reconstruction are mainly based on tumor site and type of pelvic resection. Surgical areas have been classi-

A. Angelini · P. Ruggieri (✉)
Department of Orthopedics and Orthopedic Oncology, University of Padova, Padova, Italy
e-mail: andrea.angelini@unipd.it; pietro.ruggieri@unipd.it

C. Zoccali et al. (eds.), *3D Printing in Bone Surgery*, https://doi.org/10.1007/978-3-030-91900-9_5

Table 5.1 Limitations and advantages of 3D printing technology in reconstruction for pelvic defect

Major limitations	Advantages
Mechanical safety of 3D-printed implant at long term is obviously not guaranteed	3D-printed models are useful to better understand the surgical procedure
Pelvic prostheses are usually large and there is a maximum printable size limited by metal 3D printer	Accurate resection and reconstruction with patient-specific instrumentation
Studies on cost-effectiveness are required	The possibility to produce anatomic implants with a wide freedom in terms of shapes and structure
Sterilization of implants with large trabecular thickness	The bony ingrowth in the porous structure of the prosthesis may reduce mechanical failures at long-term follow-up
Composite materials[a]	Potential developments in 3D-printed technology to decrease infective complications

[a]A single titanium alloy is generally used for implant fabrication, combined with conventional orthopedic surgical instruments for arthroplasty

fied by Enneking and Dunham [24] in four zones: type I involves resection of the ilium; type II involves resection of the acetabulum; and type III involves resection of the ischium and pubic rami; type IV refers to a lesion involving a portion of the sacrum. Multiple combinations of these types were used depending on the tumor location and extent of bony invasion. Angelini et al. recently reported an algorithm to guide the reconstructive strategies primarily based on the abovementioned classification of surgical resection [3]. In our experience, a 3D-printed custom-made prosthesis should be used in pelvic resections involving the entire iliac bone or part of the sacrum, and when the residual part of the ilium is not adequate to accommodate a modular stemmed acetabular cup. In surgical revision of acetabular complex bone defects, the indication is directly related with the extent of osteolysis, absence of structural bone support and discontinuity of pelvic ring. With the advent of 3D printing technology, surgeons have the possibility to create a 3D model of patient's anatomy to plan the revision surgery in complex cases where the anatomy is too complex to be understood from conventional imaging studies [19, 25, 26]. Once the decision to realize a custom 3D-printed prosthesis as better reconstructive solution has been made, it is important to move through the subsequent steps in the process [27, 28]: image acquisition, multidisciplinary work on virtual model and printing of prostheses and surgical tools (Fig. 5.1).

5.2.2 Step 2: Image Acquisition

The next step is the conversion of the imaging data (Digital Imaging and Communications in Medicine–DICOM) into a digital 3D model. The CT DICOM images are preferred for implant design because CT has good sensitivity for identifying bone stock, if performed with 1 mm cut every 1 mm step to have a voxel size of 1 mm square that define the level of accuracy of the plan [20, 29]. In revision surgery we strongly suggest a two stages procedure: first the removal of the prosthetic components, then the acquisition of the images without artifacts and finally to program the reconstruction with the customized implant. The alternative is the use of an artifact subtraction algorithm on CT scans (Fig. 5.2). In pelvic bone tumors there is a need of an accurate analysis of tumor extension and image acquisition is followed by the "segmentation" process. Segmentation is the delineation of tumor volume and anatomic structures on the CT (or combined with MRI) scan by defining their contours. The fusion of CT and MRI scans superimposes the images of one modality over the other thus combining the accuracy in depicting soft tissue and bone medullary involvement seen mainly on MRI scans with the higher resolution CT data set [20]. Segmentation can be performed automatically on a dedicated software platform, with the possibility of manual changes (slice-by-slice), in an acceptable time-frame of 20–30 min. These images are then sent to the company for the subsequent analysis on a computerized 3D virtual model.

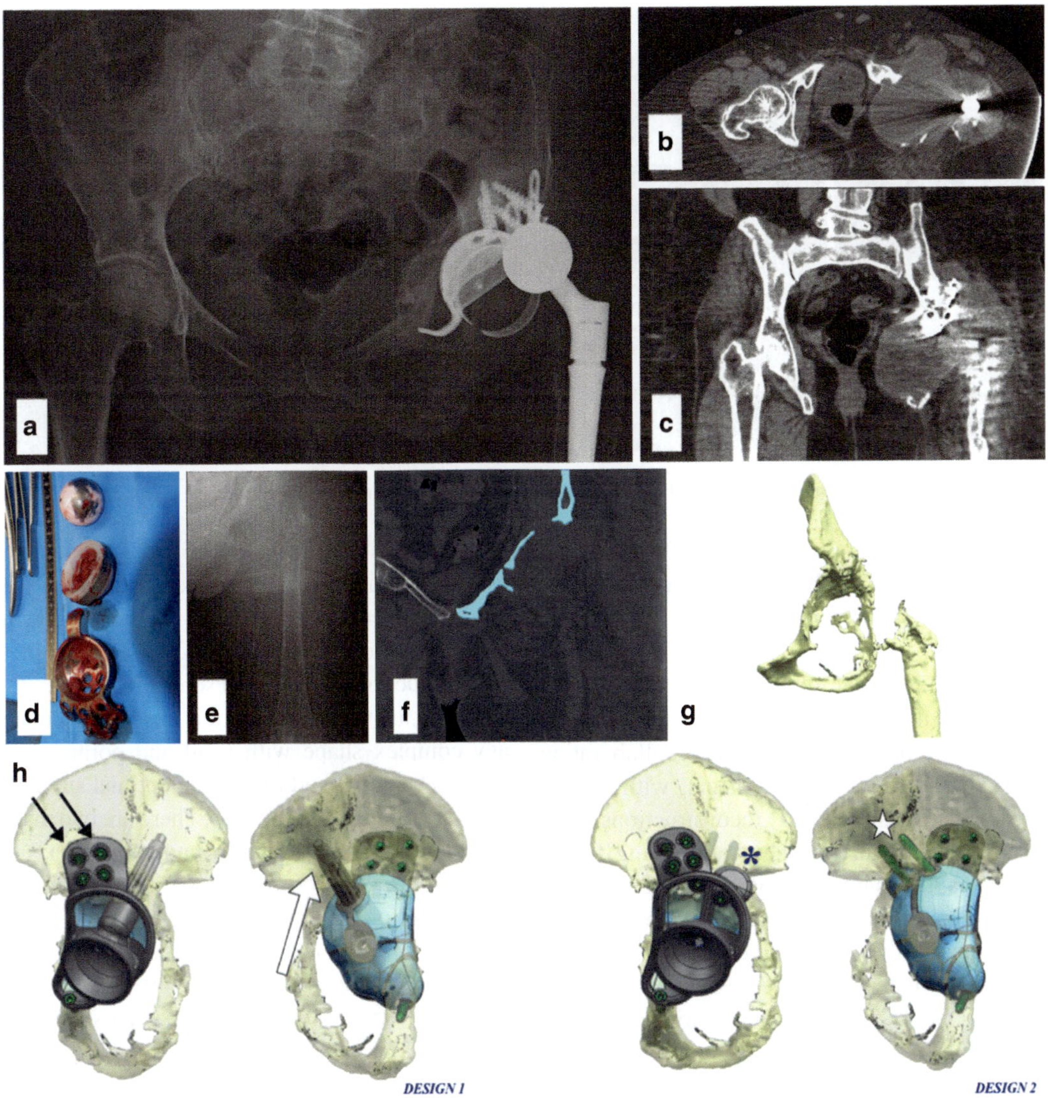

Fig. 5.1 Pseudotumor and dislocation of hip arthroplasty in 63 years old woman. (**a**) Pelvic plain radiograph demonstrating the implant loosening with large periacetabular osteolysis. (**b**) Axial and (**c**) Coronal pelvic CT scan showing involvement of the left acetabular region by the large pseudotumor. (**d**) Implant removal during the surgical excision of the pseudotumor. (**e**) Plain radiograph in the two-stage procedure. (**f**) Segmentation process with the delineation of residual bone on the CT (**g**) 3D CT scan reconstruction shows the bone defect. (**h**) Multidisciplinary work on transparent virtual 3D-model with two different strategies for primary fixation to host bone of custom prosthesis: a press-fit stem (white arrow) with short cortical screws (black arrows) in the "design 1" or two parallel screws in the load direction (asterisk) and small posterior flange to avoid rotation around longitudinal axis (white star) in the "design 2" (Implant designed with Promade, Lima Corporate Medical Systems, Villanova San Daniele del Friuli, Italy)

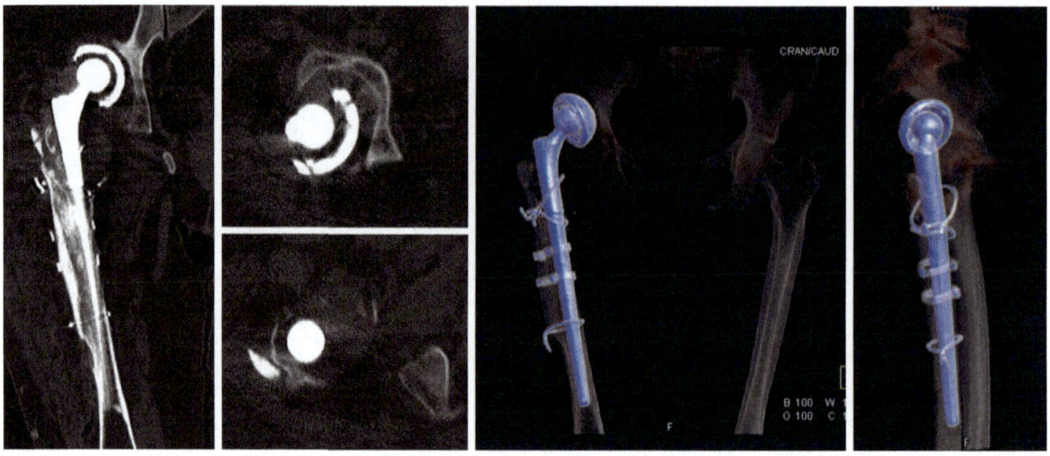

Fig. 5.2 Coronal, axial, and 3D pelvic CT with artifact subtraction algorithm in the preoperative planning of revision arthroplasty

5.2.3 Step 3: Multidisciplinary Work on 3D Virtual Model

A virtual 3D model allows to plan the surgical procedure and the type of prosthetic implant through a close multidisciplinary collaboration involving surgeons and engineers, with greater accuracy than simple CT reconstructions [30]. The surgeon contributes by transferring to the engineers the anatomical landmarks that can be reached in the surgical approach, the resection planes and, in the case of tumor lesions, the needs related to achieving the oncological outcomes of tumor removal with adequate margins [31–36]. In our experience there is a difference in approaching a reconstruction for oncologic disease compared to revision surgery. Angelini et al. reported a preliminary analysis on the use of 3D-printed technology in 13 cases including revisions of total hip arthroplasty (3 patients) and oncologic surgeries (10 patients) [3]. In a multicentric series on 41 cases including 29 pelvic reconstructions, the Authors underlined a differentiated approach between the 7 non-oncologic patients and the 24 patients mainly treated for their malignant bone tumors [10]. While the anatomy of bone loss will not change over time between image acquisition and the surgical procedure in non-oncological settings, this aspect must be considered in cancer surgery [3, 37]. In planning the resection planes for tumor removal, it is important to take into consideration the worst-case scenario, foreseeing a possible growth of the tumor during the required time of prosthesis' production and surgical schedule.

Using the virtual model, it is possible to create any complex shape with solid and porous sections to be combined to provide optimal strength and performance [15, 16, 38]. There are two main aspects to be considering in implant design: (1) porous surfaces to improve implant integration with bone for the long-term mechanical strength and (2) specific textured surfaces for a strict adherence of the soft tissues as well as smooth areas in close proximity to the vascular structures [3, 10, 22, 39]. Based on these principles of matching the geometry, required functional objectives and mechanical properties, the production process of a customized prosthesis is well established.

5.2.4 Step 4: Printing

With the use of 3D-printed technology, it is possible to print numerous different materials including plastics, polymers, glass, ceramic, metals, and biological materials [19, 40]. The virtual 3D models can be printed with sterilizable polymerics materials fulfilling biocompatibility standards in a 1:1 scale and can be used to improve the surgeon's understanding of the surgical procedure

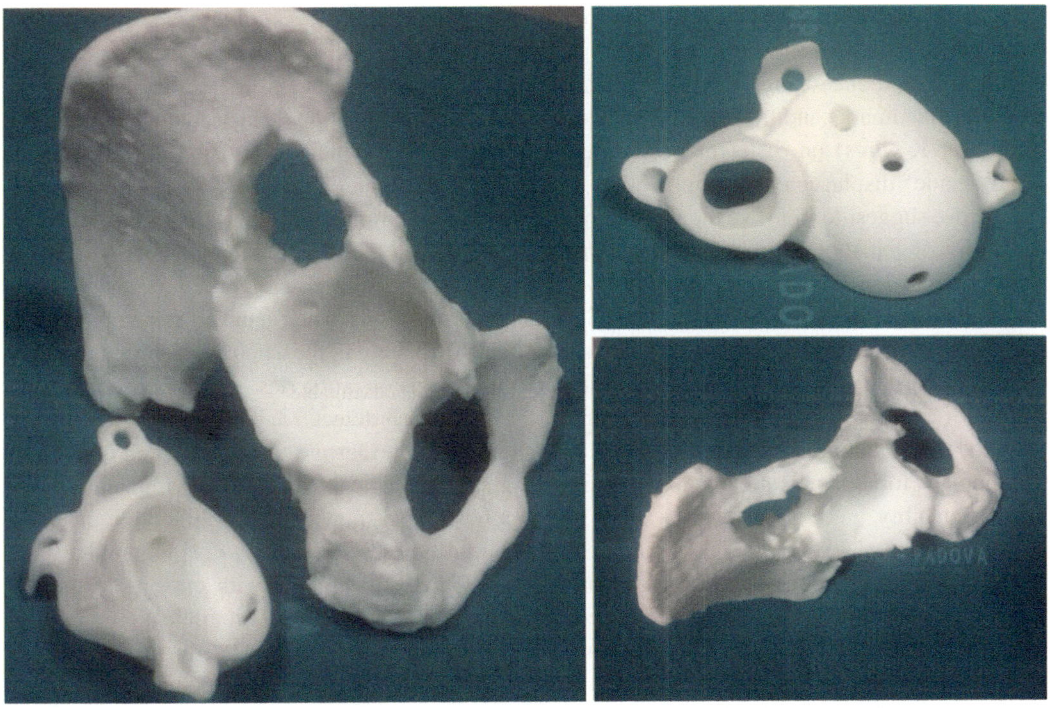

Fig. 5.3 Bone model and acetabular implant printed in a biocompatible sterilizable material (1:1 scale)

and to test the specific tools (Fig. 5.3). Bone models can be printed from transparent material in order to visualize the extent of tumor within the bone or can contain detachable parts. For implant fabrication, 3D printing can be realized in titanium metal with increasingly popularity and low reduction of cost and time. Metal implants are made with an industrial process using laser metal sintering technologies (DMLS) or a powder-based layer-by-layer electron beam melting (EBM).

5.3 Patient-Specific Tools and Guides

With the customization of reconstructive implant, it is possible to realize patient-specific instrumentation (PSI) to increase the precision of prosthetic placement. The types of 3D-printed tools used in revision surgery and orthopedic oncology include mainly cutting jigs and drilling guides, and should be considered a less-expensive and time-saving alternative to computer navigation [41–43]. These tools realized in biocompatible materials can be sterilized for surgery without being deformed or breaking. Historically, standard cutting jigs have been widely used in primary and revision arthroplasty to help the surgeon in the realization of surgical plan based on preoperative imaging. The custom-made 3D-printed prostheses need the absolute precision in performing the multi-planar osteotomies [19, 43, 44] and, on the other hand, the accuracy of surgical margin in musculoskeletal oncology represents one of the main prognostic factors on the risk of local recurrence and overall survival [31–36].

Custom planned cutting jigs are guides for oscillating saws and osteotomes for ensuring a correct osteotomy line. Obviously, the cutting jigs reduce the errors derived from the freehand use of oscillating saw-blades and un-correct directions, but there are aspects to consider in their production. First of all, they should be planned ahead for a specific oscillating saw blade, because of the potential risk of underestimating the surgical margin. In fact, due to the vibrations and tendency to bend, a 1 mm thick saw blade will make a 2 mm cut in bone. Furthermore, the jigs should be easily aligned with the host bone using specific and easily accessible landmarks and then fixed with at least 3 pins (or K-wires) on different trajectories to avoid guide displacement during bone cut. Finally, we suggest to improve the intraoperative versatility of the tool, with detachable parts to show the position of cutting PSI or the correct placing of definitive implant. Drill guides PSI are specific tools designed to guide drill holes for improving correct alignment of screws and stems planned on the virtual model. These can be mounted on the cutting jigs and/or on the definitive implant for bone fixation, maximizing the primary stability.

In the authors' experience, 3D-printed PSIs are realized after a detailed preoperative planning together with engineers and routinely used in real-life surgery. A wide surgical exposure is mandatory for the correct guide placement, soft tissue cleaning from bone landmarks and accessibility of surgical instrumentation without compromising neurovascular structures.

5.4 3D-Printed Prostheses in Pelvic Reconstructions: Revision Surgery

Total hip arthroplasty (THA) is one of the most successful orthopedic procedures performed today indicated for end-stage osteoarthritis of the hip. Its increasing use is inevitably associated to revision procedures, that in half of the cases involve the acetabular cup [45, 46]. In these cases, the amount and quality of acetabular bone stock plays an important role in the success of revision and in the surgical strategy (Fig. 5.4). The commonly used systems to evaluate the degree of acetabular bone defect are the AAOS (American Academy of Orthopaedic Surgeons) classification of bone defects and Paprosky classification [46, 47]. These classification systems are useful as a guide to choose between the different biologic and non-biologic options, even if it is not clear for complex and large types of bone defects. Non-biologic fixation refers to a construction that achieves initial stability through a mechanical implant, especially between the acetabular component and the residual host bone. Cementless fixation has become the preferred method for acetabular revision considering the low complication rate reported compared to cemented implants [1, 48, 49]. In this scenario, customized 3D-printed implants are indicated and have been successfully used for revision total hip arthroplasty when standard implant size does not adequately fit the extensive bone loss, in multiple revision surgeries with poor bone stock (Paprosky 3 defects) and pelvic discontinuity [4, 10, 19, 50]. Despite the difficulty in comparing results in patients with custom implants, recent reports have shown a low likelihood of mechanical failures [17, 50]. Liang [22] reported a series of 35 patients treated with custom 3D-printed prosthesis with low complication rate at 6–30 months follow-up. Angelini et al. reported a higher incidence of complications in non-oncologic settings compared with patients primarily treated for oncologic disease, even if the need of implant removal was rarely required [3, 10]. This can be justified by the fact that adapting a custom implant to an iliac osteotomy line is easier and has greater primary stability than seeking contact with an inhomogeneous acetabular residual bone.

5.5 3D-Printed Prostheses in Pelvic Reconstructions: Tumors

The goal of surgery in the treatment of pelvic bone tumors is the complete removal of tumor mass with a surrounding margin of healthy tissue. In the past decades various methods have been used to restore large bone defects in limb salvage surgery, including megaprostheses or structural allografts [12, 51–56]. In recent years, with the advent of 3D printing technology, it is possible to reconstruct bone defects using custom implants [3, 10, 22, 39, 57]. A 3D-printed titanium implant is preferred due to the possibility to create a biocompatible porous structure of the exact size to fill the bone defect [3, 58–60]. One

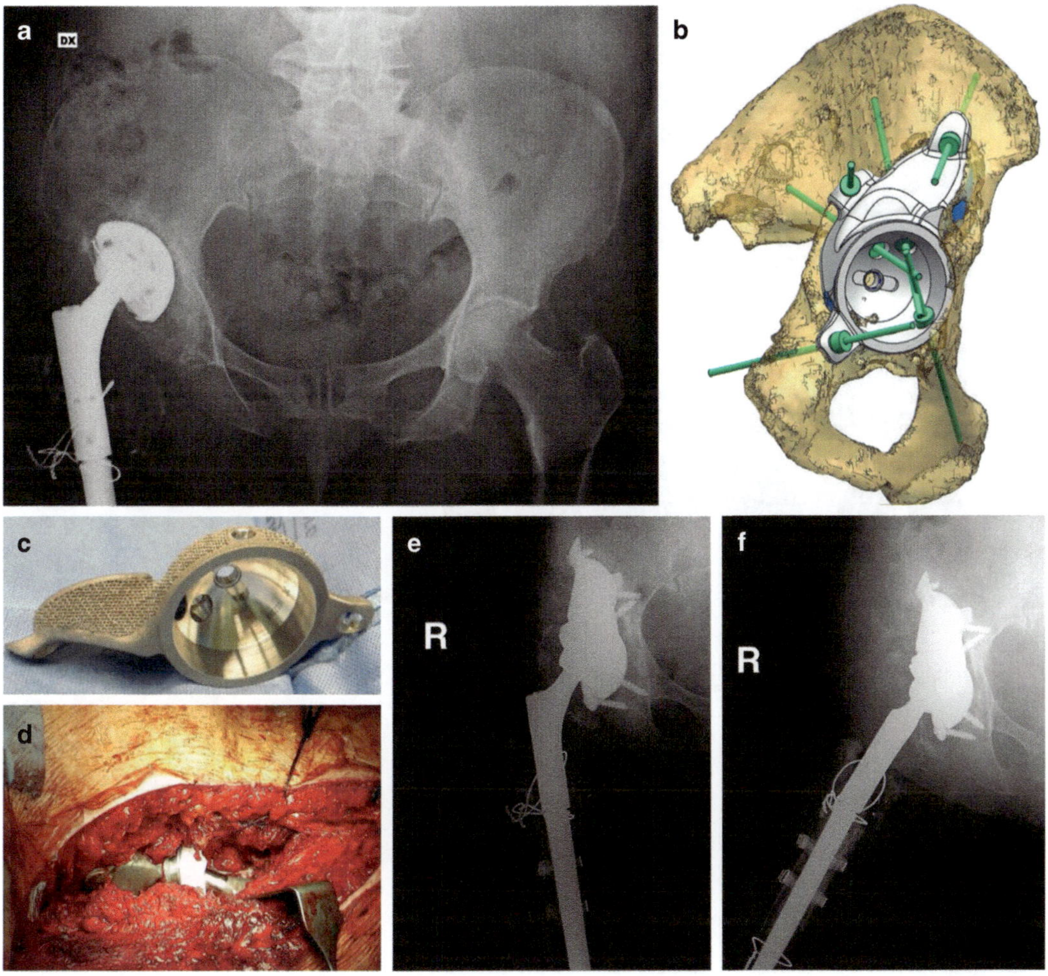

Fig. 5.4 Aseptic loosening after multiple revision surgeries for loosening and periprosthetic fracture in a 66-year-old woman. (**a**) Pelvic plain radiograph shows the iliac migration of the acetabular cup and the extensive bone loss. (**b**) Creation of a digital 3D-model after segmentation process with planning of the custom implant. (**c**) Custom-made 3D-printed prosthesis. (**d**) Intraoperative photograph showing the definitive implant. (**e**) Anteroposterior and (**f**) Axial plain radiographs show the good implant stability at 2 years follow-up

of the main differences with the non-oncologic settings is the accuracy in the reconstruction of the defect after resection of the bone tumor [3, 61], as well as the correct definition of cutting plans [10]. Tumors which arise and grow in bone cannot always be fully viewed and palpated in surgery, making complete resection challenging. Furthermore, the surgeon must consider a possible tumor growth between the surgical planning and the moment in which it will be possible to perform the surgery, which will be correlated with the time of the availability of the implant. The planned bone cuts should always account for a worst-case scenario, outside are where cancer cells may still be viable despite chemotherapy (Fig. 5.5). In our recently reported experience, 29 out of 41 patients were treated with pelvic reconstruction with custom-designed 3D-printed prostheses in different oncologic and non-oncologic settings [10]. It took approximately 3–4 weeks for the design and manufacture of each personalized 3D-printed prosthesis. In all patients with bone tumors (mainly chondrosarcomas, osteosarcomas, and Ewing's sarcomas) the

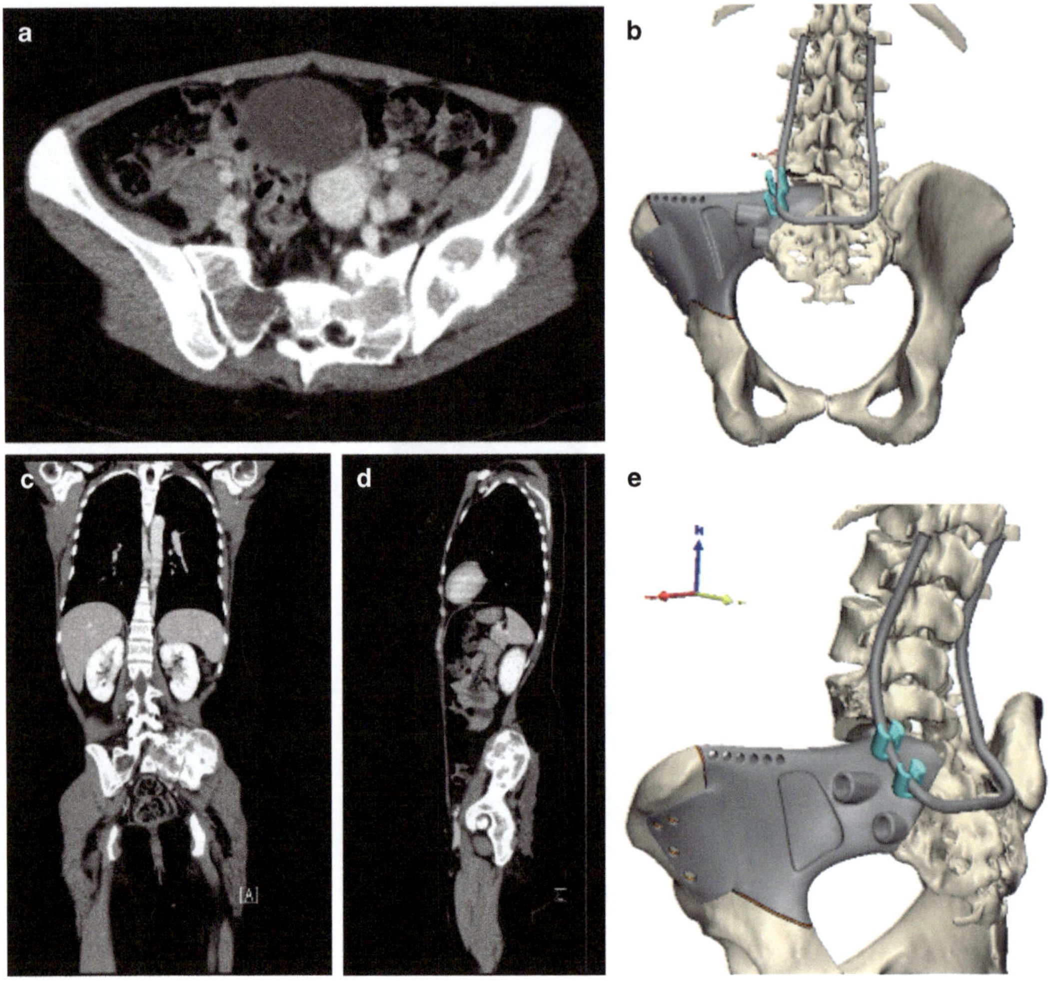

Fig. 5.5 Osteosarcoma of the iliac wing in a 26-years-old woman. (**a**) Axial, (**b**) Coronal, and (**c**) Sagittal CT scans show a tumor the left hemipelvis from the supracetabular area to the sacrum. Note the extensive extraosseous mass. (**d**) Anteroposterior and (**e**) Oblique views of the digital 3D-model show the definitive planning of a 3D-printed custom prosthesis with spinopelvic fixation

planned margins have been successfully obtained with the use of cutting jigs, with no significant difference in terms of tumor growth [10].

Other relevant aspects are the need of a stable fixation with host bone and optimal soft tissue reattachment to reduce the complication rate. In fact, the length of hospitalization, wound related complications and repeated surgery are adverse prognostic factors in oncologic patients, especially in chemo-sensitive histotypes [62–64]. Different strategies for primary fixation to host bone have been reported, including long cancellous screws, cortical screws, press-fit porous stems and small hooks for stabilization, often used in combination [3, 10, 11, 15]. We strongly suggest the use of porous surfaces in implant/bone interface for long-term bony ingrowth, combined tools for primary fixation and counter screws as safety locking to avoid screws mobilization. When resection involves the proximal part of the ilium, sacroiliac joint or the sacrum, we improve stability with a posterior pedicle screw-rod fixation connected to tulip-head screws directly designed on the custom prosthesis

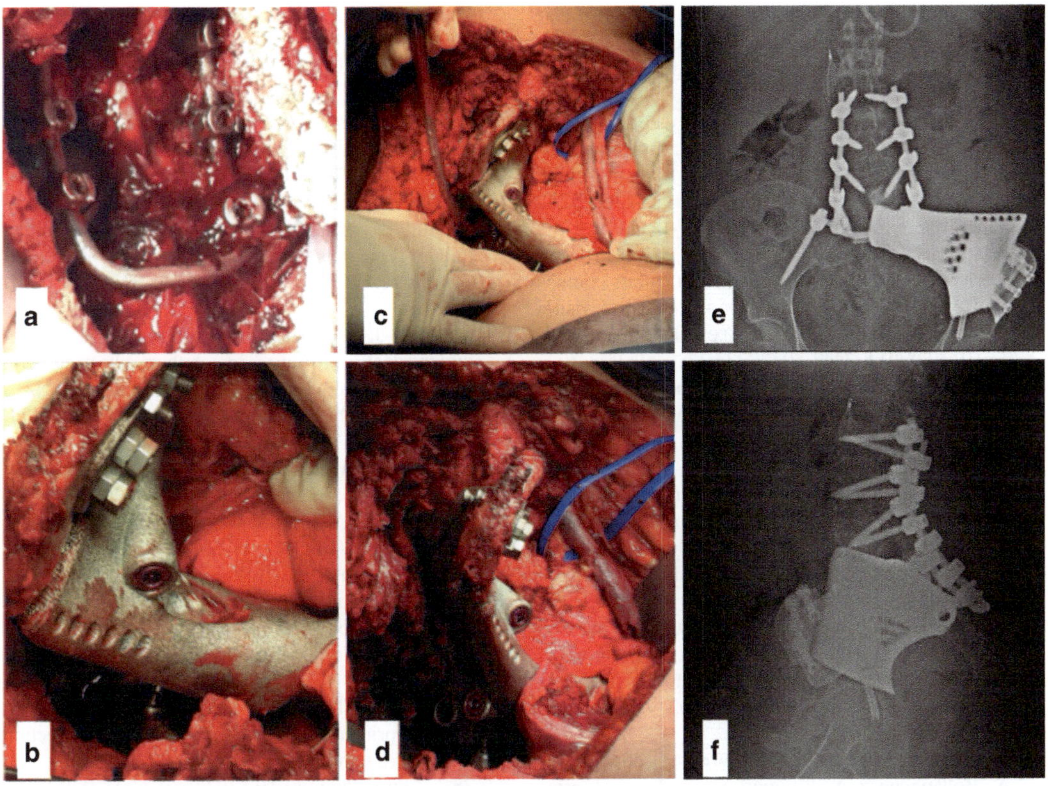

Fig. 5.6 Osteosarcoma of the iliac wing in a 26 years old woman (same patient). Intraoperative photographs showing (**a**) the spinal instrumentation with custom 3D-printed rod; (**b**) the implant fixation to the residual iliac bone; (**c**) the relations with anatomical structures; (**d**) the posterior extension to the sacrum, with fixed tulip cups. (**e**) Anteroposterior and (**f**) lateral radiographs show the definitive implant

(Fig. 5.6). About implant designs, in the preliminary reports it is possible to observe a wide spectrum of prostheses, that reflect the concepts and experiences of individual surgeons [3, 10, 11, 22, 57, 65, 66]. With the increase in numbers, follow-up knowledge and collaboration with engineers, the prosthetic design (especially in specific site such as the periacetabular area) of the prosthesis is becoming a "conventional" custom: in other words the shape and fixation tools are mainly based on the resection plans [3, 10, 11].

5.6 Conclusions

3D-printed prostheses represent at today a viable reconstructive method for complex and large pelvic bone defects in both revision hip arthroplasty and oncologic settings. These implants have the potential aims to improve pelvic stability with acceptable complication rate and satisfactory functional results. Mid-term results indicate that 3D-printing is a very advantageous technology and will become increasingly accessible in the next decades.

References

1. Sporer SM, Paprosky WG, O'Rourke MR. Managing bone loss in acetabular revision. Instr Course Lect. 2006;55:287–97.
2. Sheth NP, Nelson CL, Springer BD, Fehring TK, Paprosky WG. Acetabular bone loss in revision total hip arthroplasty: evaluation and management. J Am Acad Orthop Surg. 2013;21(3):128–39. https://doi.org/10.5435/JAAOS-21-03-128.
3. Angelini A, Trovarelli G, Berizzi A, Pala E, Breda A, Ruggieri P. Three-dimension-printed custom-made prosthetic reconstructions: from revision surgery to oncologic reconstructions. Int Orthop. 2019;43(1):123–32. https://doi.org/10.1007/s00264-018-4232-0.

4. Li H, Qu X, Mao Y, Dai K, Zhu Z. Custom acetabular cages offer stable fixation and improved hip scores for revision THA with severe bone defects. Clin Orthop Relat Res. 2016;474(3):731–40.
5. Berasi CC 4th, Berend KR, Adams JB, Ruh EL, Lombardi AV Jr. Are custom triflange acetabular components effective for reconstruction of catastrophic bone loss? Clin Orthop Relat Res. 2015;473(2):528–35. https://doi.org/10.1007/s11999-014-3969-z.
6. Wind MA Jr, Swank ML, Sorger JI. Short-term results of a custom triflange acetabular component for massive acetabular bone loss in revision THA. Orthopedics. 2013;36(3):e260–5. https://doi.org/10.3928/01477447-20130222-11.
7. Wyatt MC. Custom 3D-printed acetabular implants in hip surgery—innovative breakthrough or expensive bespoke upgrade? Hip Int. 2015;25(4):375–9. https://doi.org/10.5301/hipint.5000294.
8. Wong KC, Kumta SM, Geel NV, Demol J. One-step reconstruction with a 3D-printed, biomechanically evaluated custom implant after complex pelvic tumor resection. Comput Aided Surg. 2015;20(1):14–23. https://doi.org/10.3109/10929088.2015.1076039.
9. Wei R, Guo W, Ji T, Zhang Y, Liang H. One-step reconstruction with a 3D-printed, custom-made prosthesis after total en bloc sacrectomy: a technical note. Eur Spine J. 2017;26(7):1902–9. https://doi.org/10.1007/s00586-016-4871-z.
10. Angelini A, Kotrych D, Trovarelli G, Szafrański A, Bohatyrewicz A, Ruggieri P. Analysis of principles inspiring design of three-dimensional-printed custom-made prostheses in two referral centres. Int Orthop. 2020;44(5):829–37. https://doi.org/10.1007/s00264-020-04523-y.
11. Wang B, Hao Y, Pu F, Jiang W, Shao Z. Computer-aided designed, three dimensional-printed hemipelvic prosthesis for peri-acetabular malignant bone tumour. Int Orthop. 2018;42(3):687–94. https://doi.org/10.1007/s00264-017-3645-5.
12. Angelini A, Calabrò T, Pala E, Trovarelli G, Maraldi M, Ruggieri P. Resection and reconstruction of pelvic bone tumors. Orthopedics. 2015;38(2):87–93. https://doi.org/10.3928/01477447-20150204-51.
13. Ayvaz M, Bekmez S, Mermerkaya MU, Caglar O, Acaroglu E, Tokgozoglu AM. Long-term results of reconstruction with pelvic allografts after wide resection of pelvic sarcomas. Sci World J. 2014;27(2014):605019. https://doi.org/10.1155/2014/605019.
14. Campanacci M, Capanna R. Pelvic resections: the Rizzoli institute experience. Orthop Clin North Am. 1991;22(1):65–86.
15. Shah FA, Snis A, Matic A, Thomsen P, Palmquist A. 3D printed Ti6Al4V implant surface promotes bone maturation and retains a higher density of less aged osteocytes at the bone-implant interface. Acta Biomater. 2016;30:357–67. https://doi.org/10.1016/j.actbio.2015.11.013.
16. Sing SL, An J, Yeong WY, Wiria FE. Laser and electron-beam powder-bed additive manufacturing of metallic implants: a review on processes, materials and designs. J Orthop Res. 2016;34(3):369–85. https://doi.org/10.1002/jor.23075.
17. Sun W, Li J, Li Q, Li G, Cai Z. Clinical effectiveness of hemipelvic reconstruction using computer-aided custom-made prostheses after resection of malignant pelvic tumors. J Arthroplasty. 2011;26(8):1508–13. https://doi.org/10.1016/j.arth.2011.02.018.
18. Mumith A, Thomas M, Shah Z, Coathup M, Blunn G. Additive manufacturing: current concepts, future trends. Bone Joint J. 2018;100-B(4):455–60. https://doi.org/10.1302/0301-620X.100B4.BJJ-2017-0662.R2.
19. Mulford JS, Babazadeh S, Mackay N. Three-dimensional printing in orthopaedic surgery: review of current and future applications. ANZ J Surg. 2016;86(9):648–53. https://doi.org/10.1111/ans.13533.
20. Ritacco LE, Milano FE, Farfalli GL, Ayerza MA, Muscolo DL, Aponte-Tinao LA. Accuracy of 3-D planning and navigation in bone tumor resection. Orthopedics. 2013;36(7):e942–50.
21. Wong TM, Jin J, Lau TW, Fang C, Yan CH, Yeung K, To M, Leung F. The use of three-dimensional printing technology in orthopaedic surgery. J Orthop Surg (Hong Kong). 2017;25(1):2309499016684077. https://doi.org/10.1177/2309499016684077.
22. Liang H, Ji T, Zhang Y, Wang Y, Guo W. Reconstruction with 3D-printed pelvic endoprostheses after resection of a pelvic tumour. Bone Joint J. 2017;99-B(2):267–75. https://doi.org/10.1302/0301-620X.99B2.BJJ-2016-0654.R1.
23. Imanishi J, Choong PF. Three-dimensional printed calcaneal prosthesis following total calcanectomy. Int J Surg Case Rep. 2015;10:83–7. https://doi.org/10.1016/j.ijscr.2015.02.037.
24. Enneking WF, Dunham WK. Resection and reconstruction for primary neoplasms involving the innominate bone. J Bone Joint Surg Am. 1978;60:731–46.
25. Mobbs RJ, Coughlan M, Thompson R, Sutterlin CE, Phan K. The utility of 3D printing for surgical planning and patient-specific implant design for complex spinal pathologies: case report. J Neurosurg Spine. 2017;26(4):513–8. https://doi.org/10.3171/2016.9.SPINE16371.
26. AlAli AB, Griffin MF, Butler PE. Three-dimensional printing surgical applications. Eplasty. 2015;14(15):e37. PMID: 26301002.
27. Song B, Zhao X, Li S, Han CJ, Wei QS, Wen SF, Liu J, Shi Y. Differences in microstructure and properties between selective laser melting and traditional manufacturing for fabrication of metal parts: a review. Front Mech Eng. 2015;10(2):111–25.
28. Palmquist A, Shah FA, Emanuelsson L, Omar O, Suska F. A technique for evaluating bone ingrowth into 3D printed, porous Ti6Al4V implants accurately using X-ray micro-computed tomography and histomorphometry. Micron. 2017;94:1–8.
29. Caracciolo JT, Letson GD. Radiologic approach to bone and soft tissue sarcomas. Surg Clin N Am. 2016;96(5):963–76.

30. Fadero PE, Shah M. Three dimensional (3D) modelling and surgical planning in trauma and orthopaedics. Surgeon. 2014;12(6):328–33. https://doi.org/10.1016/j.surge.2014.03.008.
31. Angelini A, Guerra G, Mavrogenis AF, Pala E, Picci P, Ruggieri P. Clinical outcome of central conventional chondrosarcoma. J Surg Oncol. 2012;106(8):929–37. https://doi.org/10.1002/jso.23173.
32. Loh AH, Wu H, Bahrami A, Navid F, McCarville MB, Wang C, Wu J, Bishop MW, Daw NC, Neel MD, Rao BN. Influence of bony resection margins and surgicopathological factors on outcomes in limb-sparing surgery for extremity osteosarcoma. Pediatr Blood Cancer. 2015;62(2):246–51. https://doi.org/10.1002/pbc.25307.
33. He F, Zhang W, Shen Y, Yu P, Bao Q, Wen J, Hu C, Qiu S. Effects of resection margins on local recurrence of osteosarcoma in extremity and pelvis: systematic review and meta-analysis. Int J Surg. 2016;36(Pt A):283–92. https://doi.org/10.1016/j.ijsu.2016.11.016.
34. Albergo JI, Farfalli GL, Ayerza MA, Ritacco LE, Aponte-Tinao LA. Computer-assisted surgery (CAS) in orthopedic oncology. Which were the indications, problems and results in our first consecutive 203 patients? Eur J Surg Oncol. 2021;47:424–8. https://doi.org/10.1016/j.ejso.2020.06.008.
35. Abraham JA, Kenneally B, Amer K, Geller DS. Can navigation-assisted surgery help achieve negative margins in resection of pelvic and sacral tumors? Clin Orthop Relat Res. 2018;476(3):499–508. https://doi.org/10.1007/s11999.0000000000000064.
36. Ahmad S, Stevenson J, Mangham C, Cribb G, Cool P. Accuracy of magnetic resonance imaging in planning the osseous resection margins of bony tumours in the proximal femur: based on coronal T1-weighted versus STIR images. Skeletal Radiol. 2014;43(12):1679–86. https://doi.org/10.1007/s00256-014-1979-2.
37. Sternheim A, et al. Navigated pelvic osteotomy and tumor resection: a study assessing the accuracy and reproducibility of resection planes in sawbones and cadavers. J Bone Joint Surg Am. 2015;97(1):40–6.
38. Xiu P, Jia Z, Lv J, Yin C, Cheng Y, Zhang K, Song C, Leng H, Zheng Y, Cai H, Liu Z. Tailored surface treatment of 3D printed porous Ti6Al4V by microarc oxidation for enhanced Osseointegration via optimized bone in-growth patterns and interlocked bone/implant interface. ACS Appl Mater Interfaces. 2016;8(28):17964–75. https://doi.org/10.1021/acsami.6b05893.
39. Wang J, Min L, Lu M, Zhang Y, Wang Y, Luo Y, Zhou Y, Duan H, Tu C. Three-dimensional-printed custom-made hemipelvic endoprosthesis for primary malignancies involving acetabulum: the design solution and surgical techniques. J Orthop Surg Res. 2019;14(1):389. https://doi.org/10.1186/s13018-019-1455-8.
40. Rengier F, Mehndiratta A, von Tengg-Kobligk H, Zechmann CM, Unterhinninghofen R, Kauczor HU, Giesel FL. 3D printing based on imaging data: review of medical applications. Int J Comput Assist Radiol Surg. 2010;5(4):335–41. https://doi.org/10.1007/s11548-010-0476-x.
41. Fang C, Cai H, Kuong E, Chui E, Siu YC, Ji T, Drstvenšek I. Surgical applications of three-dimensional printing in the pelvis and acetabulum: from models and tools to implants. Unfallchirurg. 2019;122(4):278–85. https://doi.org/10.1007/s00113-019-0626-8.
42. Wong KC, Niu X, Xu H, Li Y, Kumta S. Computer navigation in orthopaedic tumour surgery. Adv Exp Med Biol. 2018;1093:315–26. https://doi.org/10.1007/978-981-13-1396-7_24.
43. Gouin F, Paul L, Odri GA, Cartiaux O. Computer-assisted planning and patient-specific instruments for bone tumor resection within the pelvis: a series of 11 patients. Sarcoma. 2014;2014:842709. https://doi.org/10.1155/2014/842709.
44. Cernat E, Docquier PL, Paul L, Banse X, Codorean IB. Patient specific instruments for complex tumor resection-reconstruction surgery within the pelvis: a series of 4 cases. Chirurgia (Bucur). 2016;111(5):439–44. https://doi.org/10.21614/chirurgia.111.5.439.
45. Bozic KJ, Kurtz SM, Lau E, Ong K, Vail TP, Berry DJ. The epidemiology of revision total hip arthroplasty in the United States. J Bone Joint Surg Am. 2009;91(1):128–33.
46. D'Antonio JA. Periprosthetic bone loss of the acetabulum. Classification and management. Orthop Clin North Am. 1992;23(2):279–90.
47. Paprosky WG, Bradford MS, Younger TI. Classification of bone defects in failed prostheses. Chir Organi Mov. 1994;79(4):285–91.
48. Templeton JE, Callaghan JJ, Goetz DD, Sullivan PM, Johnston RC. Revision of a cemented acetabular component to a cementless acetabular component. A ten to fourteen-year follow-up study. J Bone Joint Surg Am. 2001;83:1706–11.
49. Gaffey JL, Callaghan JJ, Pedersen DR, Goetz DD, Sullivan PM, Johnston RC. Cementless acetabular fix- ation at fifteen years. A comparison with the same surgeon's results following acetabular fixation with cement. J Bone Joint Surg Am. 2004;86:257–61.
50. Taunton MJ, Fehring TK, Edwards P, Bernasek T, Holt GE, Christie MJ. Pelvic discontinuity treated with custom triflange component: a reliable option. Clin Orthop Relat Res. 2012;470(2):428–34. https://doi.org/10.1007/s11999-011-2126-1.
51. Abudu A, Grimer RJ, Cannon SR, Carter SR, Sneath RS. Reconstruction of the hemipelvis after the excision of malignant tumours. Complications and functional outcome of prostheses. J Bone Joint Surg Br. 1997;79(5):773–9. https://doi.org/10.1302/0301-620x.79b5.6749.
52. Bus MP, Szafranski A, Sellevold S, Goryn T, Jutte PC, Bramer JA, Fiocco M, Streitbürger A, Kotrych D, van de Sande MA, Dijkstra PD. LUMiC® Endoprosthetic reconstruction after periacetabular tumor resection: short-term results. Clin Orthop Relat

Res. 2017;475(3):686–95. https://doi.org/10.1007/s11999-016-4805-4.
53. Angelini A, Drago G, Trovarelli G, Calabrò T, Ruggieri P. Infection after surgical resection for pelvic bone tumors: an analysis of 270 patients from one institution. Clin Orthop Relat Res. 2014;472(1):349–59. https://doi.org/10.1007/s11999-013-3250-x.
54. Mankin HJ, Gebhardt MC, Jennings LC, Springfield DS, Tomford WW. Long-term results of allograft replacement in the management of bone tumors. Clin Orthop Relat Res. 1996;324:86–97. https://doi.org/10.1097/00003086-199603000-00011.
55. Traub F, Andreou D, Niethard M, Tiedke C, Werner M, Tunn PU. Biological reconstruction following the resection of malignant bone tumors of the pelvis. Sarcoma. 2013;2013:745360. https://doi.org/10.1155/2013/745360.
56. Wilke BK, Houdek MT, Rose PS, Sim FH. Proximal femoral allograft-prosthetic composites: do they really restore bone? A retrospective review of revision allograft-prosthetic composites. J Arthroplasty. 2019;34(2):346–51.
57. Wang J, Min L, Lu M, Zhang Y, Wang Y, Luo Y, Zhou Y, Duan H, Tu C. What are the complications of three-dimensionally printed, custom-made, integrative Hemipelvic Endoprostheses in patients with primary malignancies involving the acetabulum, and what is the function of these patients? Clin Orthop Relat Res. 2020;478(11):2487–501. https://doi.org/10.1097/CORR.0000000000001297.
58. Wu SH, Li Y, Zhang YQ, Li XK, Yuan CF, Hao YL, Zhang ZY, Guo Z. Porous titanium-6 aluminum-4 vanadium cage has better osseointegration and less micromotion than a poly-ether-ether-ketone cage in sheep vertebral fusion. Artif Organs. 2013;37(12):E191–201.
59. Lee YH, Chung CJ, Wang CW, Peng YT, Chang CH, Chen CH, Chen YN, Li CT. Computational comparison of three posterior lumbar interbody fusion techniques by using porous titanium interbody cages with 50% porosity. Comput Biol Med. 2016;71:35–45.
60. Li S, Li X, Hou W, Nune KC, Misra RDK, Correa-Rodriguez VL, Guo Z, Hao Y, Yang R, Murr LE. Fabrication of open-cellular (porous) titanium alloy implants: osseointegration, vascularization and preliminary human trials. Sci China Mater. 2018;61(4):525–36.
61. Kunz P, Bernd L. Methods of biological reconstruction for bone sarcoma: indications and limits. Recent results. Cancer. 2009;179:113–40.
62. Angelini A, Mavrogenis AF, Trovarelli G, Ferrari S, Picci P, Ruggieri P. Telangiectatic osteosarcoma: a review of 87 cases. J Cancer Res Clin Oncol. 2016;142(10):2197–207. https://doi.org/10.1007/s00432-016-2210-8.
63. Parry MC, Laitinen M, Albergo J, Jeys L, Carter S, Gaston CL, Sumathi V, Grimer RJ. Osteosarcoma of the pelvis. Bone Joint J. 2016;98-B(4):555–63. https://doi.org/10.1302/0301-620X.98B4.36583.
64. Grimer RJ, Carter SR, Tillman RM, Spooner D, Mangham DC, Kabukcuoglu Y. Osteosarcoma of the pelvis. J Bone Joint Surg Br. 1999;81(5):796–802. https://doi.org/10.1302/0301-620x.81b5.9241.
65. Dai KR, Yan MN, Zhu ZA, Sun YH. Computer-aided custom-made hemipelvic prosthesis used in extensive pelvic lesions. J Arthroplasty. 2007;22(7):981–6. https://doi.org/10.1016/j.arth.2007.05.002.
66. Jentzsch T, Vlachopoulos L, Fürnstahl P, Müller DA, Fuchs B. Tumor resection at the pelvis using three-dimensional planning and patient-specific instruments: a case series. World J Surg Oncol. 2016;14(1):249. https://doi.org/10.1186/s12957-016-1006-2.

Custom Reconstruction Around the Knee

6

Davide Maria Donati, Tommaso Frisoni, and Benedetta Spazzoli

6.1 Introduction

Post-traumatic osteochondral defects in the knee are common in young patients (Osteochondritis Dissecans, OD); they have good chance to repair due to the reactivity of the subchondral bone and synovial membrane cells. If the healing process is not adequate, fresh osteochondral allografts are a suitable option for reconstruction in wide defects [1].

In young patients, articular damage or defects can also be related to chemo-induced osteonecrosis (Figs. 6.1–6.3) or bone tumours treatment as well as giant cell tumour of bone or chondroblastoma that usually involves epiphyseal region of long bones around the knee mainly between age of 20 and 40 years [2, 26].

Extensive intralesional curettage and application of polymethylmethacrylate (PMMA) is the gold standard procedure, whilst for stage III lesions, a resection and reconstruction with unicondylar massive allograft can be performed [3]. The first technique has the advantages of thermal effects on remaining tumour cells, early detection of local recurrences and immediate full weight bearing after surgery. Concernings about the application of PMMA close to articular surface are related to an increased risk of damage of the subchondral bone [4, 5], due to thermal effect and the different mechanical properties (Figs. 6.4 and 6.5). Previous study have demonstrated that subchondral bone is crucial in order to avoid postoperative mechanical failure, including deformity, fracture and degeneration of the articular surface [6], which may lead to a chronic pain, functional limitation up to early osteoarthritis requiring joint arthroplasty either with standard or modular prostheses according to bone defect, but they are associated with high rates of complication such as infection and loosening.

Osteoarthritis progression depends from the thickness and quality of the hyaline cartilage as well as from the mineral content of the cartilage deep layer (transition from columnar and calcified layer). There are MRI evidences in animal and human, showing how modifications in the subchondral bone are present in a very early stage of osteoarthritis. Recent reports underline the importance of a normal subchondral bone width and permeability in maintaining the optimal cartilage nutrition [7]. Moreover, histological studies on cartilage repair specimens showed strict correlation between the quality of regenerated

D. M. Donati (✉) · T. Frisoni
Orthopedic Oncology Department, IRCCS Istituto Ortopedico Rizzoli, Bologna, Italy

Biomedical and Neuromotor Sciences Department—DIBINEM, University of Bologna, Bologna, Italy
e-mail: davidemaria.donati@ior.it; tommaso.frisoni@ior.it

B. Spazzoli
Orthopedic Oncology Department, IRCCS Istituto Ortopedico Rizzoli, Bologna, Italy
e-mail: benedetta.spazzoli@ior.it

C. Zoccali et al. (eds.), *3D Printing in Bone Surgery*, https://doi.org/10.1007/978-3-030-91900-9_6

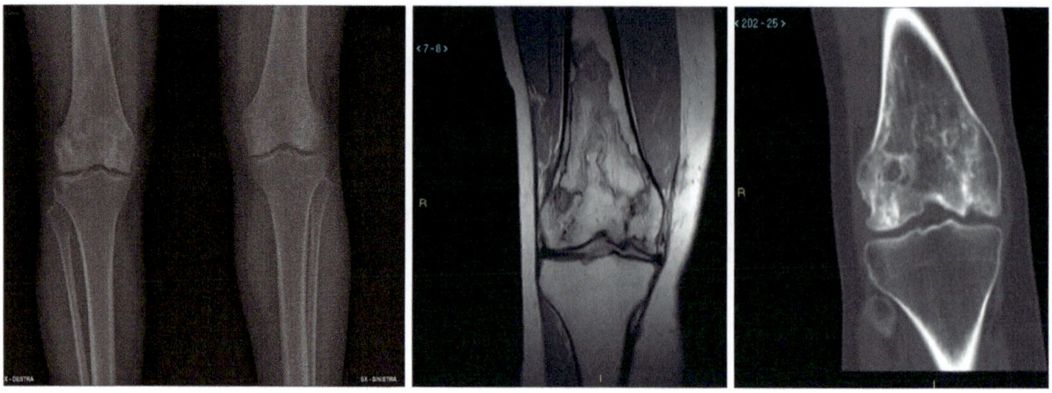

Figs. 6.1–6.3 Plan X-ray, MRI T1 sequence and coronal CT scan of a chemo-induced osteonecrosis of femoral condyle in a 15-years-old female

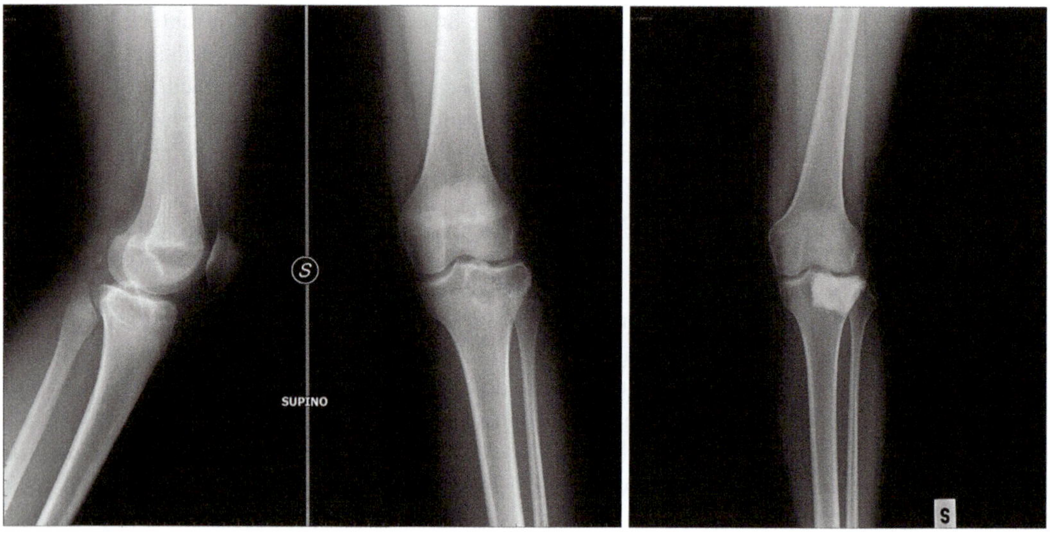

Figs. 6.4 and 6.5 Plan X-ray of a proximal tibia chondroblastoma before and after curettage and cementation

cartilage and subchondral bone. Hence, the optimal joint status will depend on good quality of the cartilage as well as the subchondral bone.

With rapid prototyping technique, an individual-based solution can be performed on the patient anatomy and his clinical needs. Different products can be obtained starting from custom-made prostheses and specific instruments.

3D printing allows to design an architecture with similar mechanical characteristic of bone [8], able to induce osteointegration and decrease the stress-shielding phenomenon due to the porosity and the elasticity of trabecular titanium [9]. Moreover, rapid prototyping can be used to develop specific instruments for each single step, minimizing the approach and bone loss, reducing the time of surgery and improving the reconstruction.

The aim of our research is to develop a new customized implant for knee repair to treat wide defects that alternatively may require commercial implants such as UKA, TKA, modular prostheses or massive allograft transplantation.

The idea is an hybrid prosthesis composed by a metallic frame with poly-caprolactone (PCL), a biodegradable material on the joint surface that be considered as a scaffold with similar mechanical characteristic of the implant itself in the short term, but potentially able to be substituted from the regenerative activity of the patient during time configuring a sort of biological prosthesis.

This procedure allows to preserve the most bone stock possible, respecting the stability given by soft tissue (ligaments) and maintaining the articular surface on the opposite.

6.1.1 Image Processing

A 3D virtual model of the bone is created based on CT scan (1 mm slice thickness ore below) of the whole segment (Figs. 6.6–6.8) using a segmentation software that allows to export data into a computer-aided design (CAD) software (Invesalius 3.1.1).

Defect identification has to be performed; more often fusion with MRI scan is required to better understand the bone quality and osteotomy level.

6.1.2 PSIs (Guides)

PSIs are then designed on the 3D virtual model based on CT according to surgical approach, desired resection margins and reconstruction requirements (fixation, soft tissue sparing or detachment/reinsertion).

PSI must have specific contact surfaces to fit into unique position on the host bone and contain holes for 2 mm Kirschner wires (K-wires) to pin the instrument onto the bone.

The instrument is shaped either with a surface to obtain the osteotomies using an oscillating saw blade and a template to prepare a footprint where a more accurate fit can be found for the guide itself and the implant can be fixed (Fig. 6.9).

6.1.3 Tools

As well as guides, additional customized tools can be developed. Commercial products are often not adequate to be used with custom products, so these instruments must be designed according to the PSIs and implant as well. Furthermore they can be provided not only to be specific for the guide but also to achieve a surgical need as progressive and controlled drilling or bone impaction (Figs. 6.10 and 6.11) in order to improve surgical accuracy and prepare a biological background.

6.1.4 Implants

Implants are designed to replace a bone/cartilage defect; the anatomy is retrieved from contralateral knee then mirrored in the affected side in order to restore the native geometry and achieve a correct mechanical axis (Fig. 6.12).

Metal back have a porous titanium architecture and are provided of fixation elements as

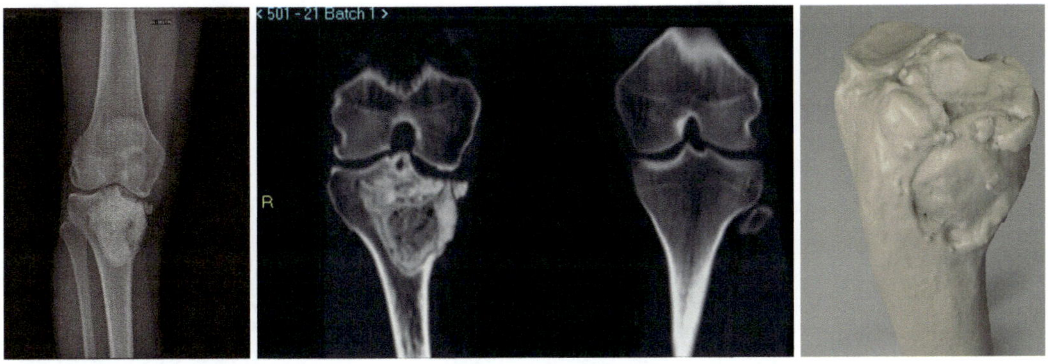

Figs. 6.6–6.8 Plan X-ray, coronal CT scan and 3D model of a large defect of medial tibial condyle after treatment for GCT in a 30-years-old male

spikes (Fig. 6.13), pre-calibrated screw insertion holes and/or external small plates to increase stability to the host bone avoiding rotation.

For wide defects in which cortical bone must be replaced, trabecular titanium was polished and increased in width.

At the edge corresponding to articular surface, a poly-caprolactone (PCL) layer is moulded. It is a synthetic biodegradable polymeric material, soluble and easy to treat.

The use of PCL requires a gamma ray sterilization in order to prevent deformation; standard sterilization process with steam or ethylene oxide is used for PSIs and the other tools which are in titanium or stainless steel alloy. A non-sterile 3D anatomical model is also provided for preoperative simulation and educational purpose; then, once sterilized, is used intraoperatively to assist the surgeon.

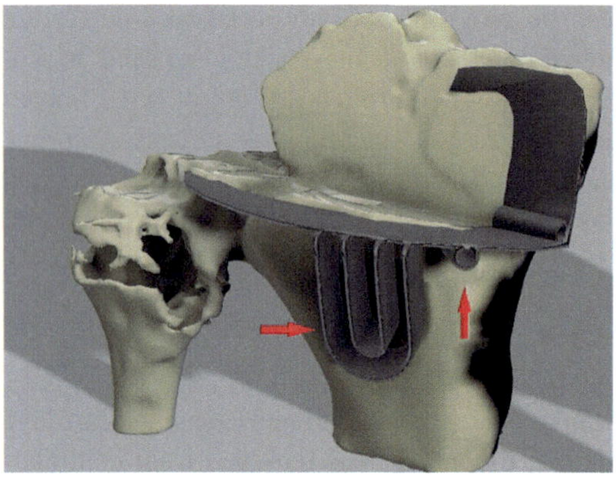

Fig. 6.9 3D model of a PSI. Red arrows indicate K-wires hole and the fixation tool guide

6.1.5 Surgery

The patient is placed on supine position. Surgical approach follows the preoperative plan already established, according to previous incisions if present or standard approach for UKA (parapatellar approach).

Once the bone and the articular surface are exposed, guides are placed as previously planned. Special attention was addressed to maintain as far as possible insertion of ligament and capsule in order to preserve the stability; when ligament detachment was necessary, a suture of these structure was planned on the prosthesis.

A brief instruction protocol is provided by the company in which all steps are explained (Fig. 6.14).

6.2 Material and Methods

From June 2015 to April 2020 6 patients underwent reconstruction around the knee with PSI guides and custom-made prosthesis at Rizzoli Orthopaedic Institute (Bologna, Italy). An

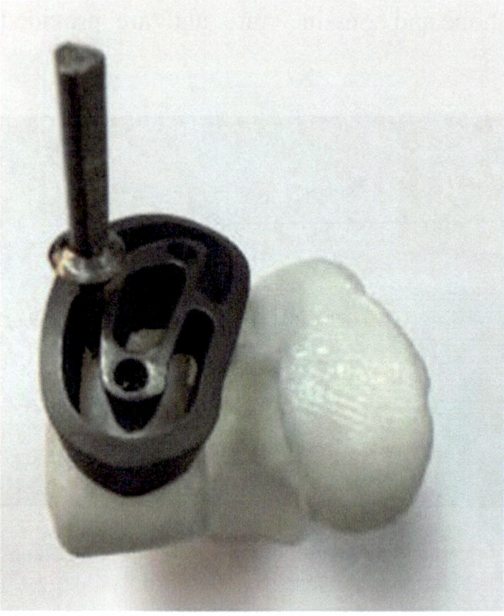

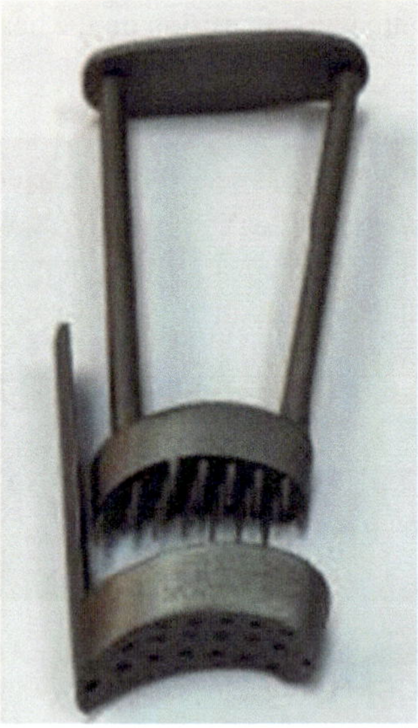

Figs. 6.10 and 6.11 Custom drill and impactor developed according to PSI

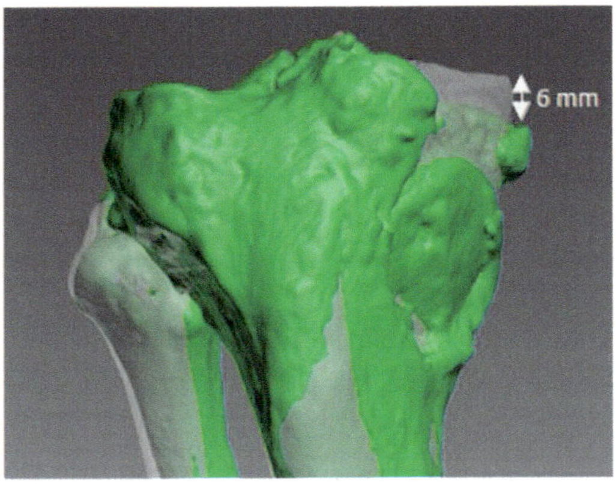

Fig. 6.12 Mechanical axis study. Fusion of affected knee 3D model (green) and contralateral mirrored knee (grey)

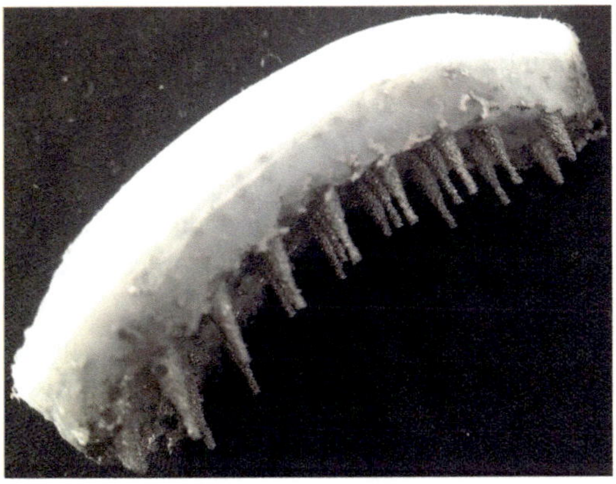

Fig. 6.13 Trabecular titanium spikes are showed

informed patient-specific consent was preliminary obtained.

Five patients had a follow-up longer than 1 year and were included in the present study. Mean follow-up was 23,6.4 months (range, 12–42). Mean age was 32 years (range, 24–46). There were 3 females and 2 males. Two of them were previously treated for oncologic condition (one for a GCT of proximal tibial, one for a chondroblastoma of proximal tibia, and one for steroid induced osteonecrosis of the femoral condyle do to previous lymphoma treatment). The other two patients were affected by early osteoarthritis after a tibial plateau fracture and juvenile osteochondritis of lateral femoral condyle respectively.

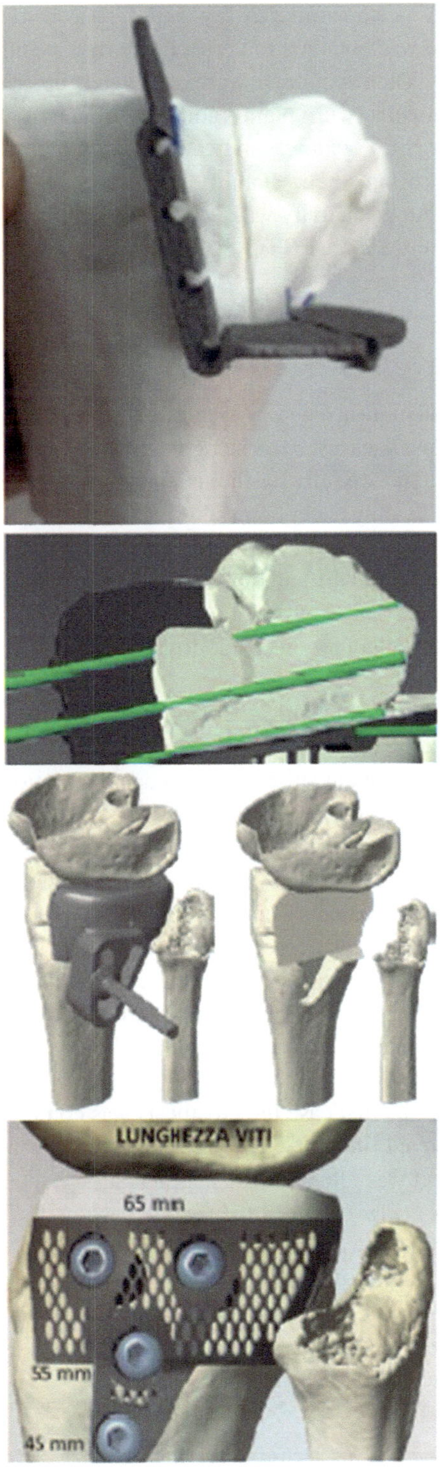

Fig. 6.14 Extraction of a "step-by-step procedure instruction"

A postoperative X-ray and CT scan of the knee was obtained to verify the correct positioning. Then patients were followed up every 3 months with plain radiographs and a dual energy CT scan was indicated every 6 months to control prosthetic stability and osteointegration. Functional activity was evaluated using the Knee Society Score (KSS).

6.3 Results

Mean surgical time was 73 min (range, 51–100 min).

In all cases but one, guides and prostheses were successfully positioned on the planned area.

The only exception was a patient in which the defect was in the posterior part of the femoral condyle and difficult to be reached. Thus the final implant had 2° of rotation but without any impact on articular motion or stability. We didn't observe any reaction to PCL.

All patients were allowed to full weight bearing at 30 days from surgery.

One patient suffered for an acute infection by Propionebacterium Acnes and a surgical wash out associated with IV antibiotic administration was needed to achieve a complete resolution.

Two patients underwent revision of the implant; in one case for synovitis due to uncontrolled rheumatoid arthritis (after 28 months), in one for prosthetic loosening after 42 months more likely due to poor bone quality in a patient with a severe steroid induced osteonecrosis.

In the first case the prosthesis was completely removed and a CCK was implanted; the bone defect was filled with an augmentation (tantalum cone) (Fig. 6.15). In the second case part of the prosthesis was left behind as wedge for a posterior stabilized TKA.

In 3 of the 5 patients considered with the reconstruction in site at final follow up, KSS score was higher than 90.

6.4 Discussion

Wide osteochondral defects around the knee are often related to traumatic event or treatment for bone tumour. Several reconstruction options are available according to the defect extension/size. Three dimensional scaffold, bone allograft and prosthetic replacement are the treatment of choice.

Three dimensional scaffolds are promising but data are controversial with low level of evidence related to long term outcomes and lack of randomize trials [10].

Although advantages in prosthetic reconstruction and massive allograft (such as surgical technique, commercial products availability, early weight bearing and biological reconstruction with restoration of bone stock respectively) are clear, many complications may occur as well as infection, loosening, periprosthetic, and allograft fracture [3, 11, 12].

3D printing technology seems to have potential benefits. Additive manufacturing (rapid prototyping of Ti-6Al-4V trough an EBM process) allows to develop customized products to restore anatomically a specific defect with architecture and mechanical characteristic similar to the bone [13–17], thus more "bone friendly" (osteointegration) and potentially helpful to decrease the above mentioned complications [18, 19].

Furthermore patient-specific instruments (PSIs) can be developed in the same production flow. These tools such as guides, impactor or drill are crucial to minimize the approach with bone stock preservation, reducing time of surgery and improving the reconstruction with better functional outcome [20–22].

The use of poly-caprolactone (PCL), which is a synthetic biodegradable polymeric material, works as a scaffold in the articular environment. In literature in vitro and preclinical studies have already demonstrated how PCL is a suitable material added to titanium implants in bone defect treatment [23–25].

This kind of reconstruction preserves the opposite articular surface and restores as far as possible the anatomy and biomechanic of the knee. We reported no evidence of reaction to this polymer in the articular space.

Our goal is a hybrid prosthesis ("bioprosthesis") composed by a metallic frame with biodegradable material on the joint surface that be considered as a scaffold potentially able to be substituted from the regenerative activity of the patient during time.

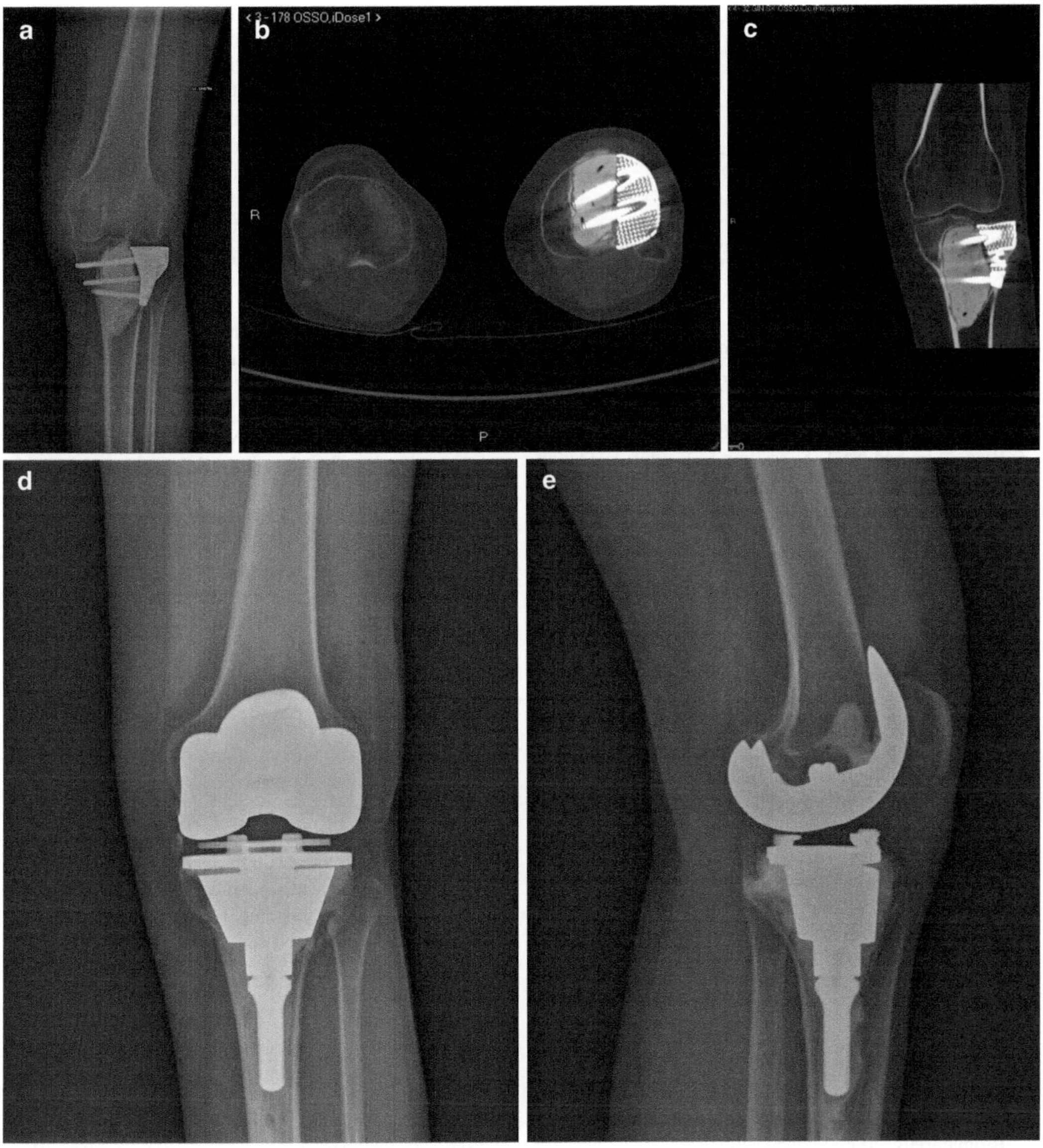

Fig. 6.15 (**a**, **b**, **c**) Postoperative X-ray and CT scan (axial and coronal view). (**d**, **e**) X-ray after knee revision surgery

Failures we reported are more likely related to patient selection; we addressed patients to this reconstruction with the aim to avoid more invasive surgery such us a TKA, modular or composite prosthesis in young patients. However in those who suffered a failure, our implant was not a contraindication to a rescue surgery with a standard reconstruction.

Patient selection bias, small number of patients and a short follow up time are the actual limitations of our study. A more comprehensive study with a longer follow up time and a wider cohort of patients is needed to understand the real potential of this reconstruction.

6.5 Conclusions

3D printing has a potential role in wide osteochondral defect treatment around the knee. It allows to restore anatomically a bone/cartilage loss with similar biomechanical features. Our prosthesis is an innovative project that may represent an alternative to standard reconstruction in selected patients.

References

1. Giorgini A, Donati D, Cevolani L, Frisoni T, Zambianchi F, Catani F. Fresh osteochondral allograft is a suitable alternative for wide cartilage defect in the knee. Injury. 2013;44(Suppl 1):S16–20. https://doi.org/10.1016/S0020-1383(13)70005-6.
2. Raskin KA, Schwab JH, Mankin HJ, Springfield DS, Hornicek FJ. Giant cell tumor of bone. J Am Acad Orthop Surg. 2013;21(2):118–26.
3. Bianchi G, Sambri A, Sebastiani E, Caldari E, Donati D. Is unicondylar osteoarticular allograft still a viable option for reconstructions around the knee? Knee. 2016;23:692–7.
4. Boyko R, Kase J, Askew M, Weiner S. Potential for thermal damage to articular cartilage by PMMA reconstruction of a bone cavity following tumor excision: a finite element study. J Biomech. 2009;42(8):1120–6 . Epub 2009 Apr. https://doi.org/10.1016/j.jbiomech.2009.02.005.
5. Farfalli G, Slulittel P, Muscolo L, Ayerza M, Aponte-Tinao L. What happens to the articular surface after curettage for epiphyseal chondroblastoma? A report on functional results, arthritis, and arthroplasty. Clin Orthop Relat Res. 2017;475(3):760–6. https://doi.org/10.1007/s11999-016-4715-5.
6. Abdelrahman M, Bassiony AA, Shalaby H, Assal MK. Cryosurgery and impaction subchondral bone graft for the treatment of giant cell tumor around the knee. HSS J. 2009;5(2):123–8.
7. Gomoll A. The subchondral bone in articular cartilage repair: current problems in the surgical management. Knee Surg Sports Traumatol Arthrosc. 2010;18:434–47.
8. Ryan G, Pandit A, Apatsidis DP. Fabrication methods of porous metals for use in orthopaedic applications. Biomaterials. 2006;27:2651–70.
9. Lopez-Heredia MA, Goyenvalle E, Aguado E, et al. Bone growth in rapid prototyped porous titanium implants. J Biomed Mater Res A. 2008;85(3):664–73.
10. D'Ambrosi R, Valli F, De Luca P, Ursino N, Usuelli G. MaioRegen osteochondral substitute for the treatment of knee defects: a systematic review of the literature. J Clin Med. 2019;8(6):783. https://doi.org/10.3390/jcm8060783.
11. Ippolito J, Campbell M, Siracuse B, Benevenia J. Reconstruction with custom unicondylar hemiarthroplasty following tumor resection: a case series and review of the literature. J Knee Surg. 2020;33(8):818–24. Epub 2019 May 8. https://doi.org/10.1055/s-0039-1688556.
12. Shehadeh A, Isleem U, Abdelal S, Salameh H, Abdelhalim M. Surgical technique and outcome of custom joint-sparing endoprosthesis as a reconstructive modality in juxta-articular bone sarcoma. J Oncol. 2019;2019:9417284. https://doi.org/10.1155/2019/9417284.eCollection.2019.
13. El-Hajje A, Kolos EC, Wang JK, et al. Physical and mechanical characterisation of 3D-printed porous titanium for biomedical applications. J Mater Sci Mater Med. 2014;25(11):2471–80.
14. Facchini L, Magalini E, Robotti P, et al. Microstructure and mechanical properties of Ti-6Al-4V produced by electron beam melting of pre-alloyed powders. Rapid Prototyp J. 2009;15(3):171–8.
15. Lewandowski JJ, Seifi M. Metal additive manufacturing: a review of mechanical properties. Annu Rev Mat Res. 2016;46:14.1–14.36.
16. Liu P, Yang Y, Liu R, et al. A study on the mechanical characteristics of the EBM-printed Ti-6Al-4V LCP plates in vitro. J Orthop Surg Res. 2014;9:106.
17. Roland L, Grau M, Matena J, Teske M, Gieseke M, Kampmann A, Beyerbach M, Murua Escobar H, Haferkamp H, Gellrich NC, Nolte I. Poly-ε-caprolactone coated and functionalized porous titanium and magnesium implants for enhancing angiogenesis in critically sized bone defects. Int J Mol Sci. 2015;17(1):1.
18. Hou G, Bingchuan Liu B, Yun Tian Y, Liu Z, Zhou F, Ji H, Zhang Z, Guo Y, Lv Y, Yang Z, Wen P, Zheng Y, Cheng Y. An innovative strategy to treat large metaphyseal segmental femoral bone defect using customized design and 3D printed microporous prosthesis: a prospective clinical study. J Mater Sci Mater Med. 2020;31:66.
19. Lu M, Wang J, Tang F, Min L, Zhou Y, Zhang W, Tu C. A three-dimensional printed porous implant combined with bone grafting following curettage of a subchondral giant cell tumour of the proximal tibia: a case report. BMC Surg. 2019;19(1):29. https://doi.org/10.1186/s12893-019-0491-y.
20. Jud L, Müller D, Fürnstahl P, Fucentese S, Vlachopoulos LF. Joint-preserving tumour resection around the knee with allograft reconstruction using three-dimensional preoperative planning and patient-specific instruments. Knee. 2019;26(3):787–93 . Epub 2019 Mar 16. https://doi.org/10.1016/j.knee.2019.02.015.
21. Vlachopoulos L, Schweizer A, Meyer DC, Gerber C, Fürnstahl P. Three-dimensional corrective osteotomies of complex malunited humeral fractures using patient specific guides. J Shoulder Elbow Surg. 2016;25:2040–7.
22. Wang J. Individualized reconstruction for severe periprosthetic fractures around the tumor prosthesis of knee under assistance of 3D printing technology. A case report. Medicine (Baltimore). 2018;97(42):e12726.
23. Grau M, Matena J, Teske M, Petersen S, Aliuos P, Roland L, Grabow N, Murua Escobar H, Gellrich NC, Haferkamp H, Nolte I. In vitro evaluation of PCL and P(3HB) as coating materials for selective laser melted porous titanium implants. Materials

(Basel). 2017;10(12):1344. https://doi.org/10.3390/ma10121344.
24. Matena J, Petersen S, Gieske M, Teske M, Beyerbach M, Kampmann A, Murua Escobar H, Gellrich N, Haferkamp H, Nolte I. Comparison of selective laser melted titanium and magnesium implants coated with PCL. Int J Mol Sci. 2015;16(6):13287–301. https://doi.org/10.3390/ijms160613287.
25. Matsumoto G, Hoshino J, Kinoshita Y, Sugita Y, Kubo K, Maeda H, Arimura H, Matsuda S, Ikada Y, Kinoshita Y. Evaluation of guided bone regeneration with poly(lactic acid-co-glycolic acid-co-ε-caprolactone) porous membrane in lateral bone defects of the canine mandible. Int J Oral Maxillofac Implants. 2012;27(3):587–94.
26. Suneja R, Grimer RJ, Belthur M, Jeys L, Carter SR, Tillman RM, Davies AM. Chondroblastoma of bone: long-term results and functional outcome after intralesional curettage. J Bone Joint Surg Br. 2005;87:974–8.

When the Bone Is Not Enough: The Role of Custom-Made Implants in Cup Revision Surgery

7

Loris Perticarini, Stefano Marco Paolo Rossi, Ron Ben Elyahu, and Francesco Benazzo

7.1 Acetabular Bone Defects Classifications and Possible Solution

Failure of total hip arthroplasty is often associated with significant acetabular bone stock loss. Norwegian Arthroplasty Register reported that the failure rate of revision hip arthroplasty is 25.6% vs. 11.4% for prinnnmary THA at 10 years follow-up, especially for acetabular component revision [1]. Ong et al. showed that patients with revision arthroplasty were five to six times more likely to undergo re-revision compared with patients with primary arthroplasty studying the 5% Medicare claims data set (1997–2006) [2]. Yu et al. presented a report on 288 revision THA where outcomes in patients who undergo multiple revisions are significantly inferior to the primary surgery, as evidenced by our 1 year 54% re-revision survival [3]. Moreover, they found that aseptic loosening was the first cause of implant failure, and that the indications for both primary and re-revision surgery was acetabular loosening in 20% and 24% of cases respectively [3].

In case of multiple revisions or severe acetabular bone defect, pelvic discontinuity or bone loss extended beyond the acetabulum, custom-made implants can be used to reduce the risk of further re-revision.

7.1.1 Severe Acetabular Bone Defect

Several classification systems have been developed to define bone defects of the acetabulum. Classification systems were proposed to permit the surgeon to plan reconstruction in the preoperative phase of revision surgery. There is no consensus as to which system of classification to use, and the utilization is geographically dependent. The American Academy of Orthopaedic Surgeons (AAOS) recommends the classification of D'Antonio [4], based on the presence of segmental, cavitary, or combined defects, whereas European surgeons tend to adopt the system developed by Paprosky [5], that is comprehensive and provides treatment recommendations based on the location and degree of bone loss. The Paprosky classification is based on four variables: location or migration of the hip center of rotation

L. Perticarini (✉) · S. M. P. Rossi
Sezione di Chirurgia Protesica ad Indirizzo Robotico—Unità di Traumatologia dello Sport, U.O. Ortopedia e Traumatologia, Fondazione Poliambulanza, Brescia, Italy

R. B. Elyahu · F. Benazzo
Sezione di Chirurgia Protesica ad Indirizzo Robotico—Unità di Traumatologia dello Sport, U.O. Ortopedia e Traumatologia, Fondazione Poliambulanza, Brescia, Italy

Università degli Studi di Pavia, Pavia, Italy
e-mail: fbenazzo@unipv.it

C. Zoccali et al. (eds.), *3D Printing in Bone Surgery*, https://doi.org/10.1007/978-3-030-91900-9_7

Type	Femoral head Center migration	Ischial osteolysis	Kohler line	Teardrop
I	None	None	Intact	Intact
IIA	Mild (<3cm)	None	Intact	Intact
IIB	Moderate (<3cm)	Mild	Intact	Intact
IIC	Mild (<3cm)	Mild	Disrupted	Moderate lysis
IIIA	Severe (>3cm)	Moderate	Intact	Moderate lysis
IIIB	Severe (>3cm)	Severe	Disrupted	Severe lysis

Fig. 7.1 Paprosky classification of acetabular bone defects

about the superior obturator line, degree of teardrop destruction, amount of ischial osteolysis, and integrity of the Kohler line (Fig. 7.1).

In our Country, AIR (Associazione Italiana Riprotesizzazione), has adopted its own classification of the acetabular defects: I in case of acetabulum enlarge, no cavitary or segmental defects; II represented by acetabulum enlarge, one wall segmental defects, III in presence of acetabulum enlarge, two or more walls segmental defects, and IV in case of massive circumferential defect.

Restoring normal anatomy and achieving stable fixation of the acetabular component, which is the goal of this challenging revision surgery, can be particularly challenging when the surgeon must deal with severe acetabular defects and/or pelvic discontinuity, as defined by preoperative classification of the case. Stable fixation may be achieved by using cementless acetabular components with screws if the contact of the component with the host bone is more than 50% [6].

Cups made of highly porous metals, whose features are high elasticity modulus with improved biomechanical properties, and proactivity toward bone with high chance of bone ingrowth and osteointegration that offer improved bone ingrowth and biomechanical properties, have also shown encouraging results for acetabular revision. However, it may be difficult or impossible to achieve stability, even with these highly technologically produced materials, if the acetabular defect is large, bone quality is poor, there is limited host bone contact, or there is pelvic discontinuity. Moreover, the variability of shape of the pelvis and the variety, size, and shape of acetabular defects make treatment with conventional off-the-shelf implants difficult. These complex situations have traditionally been treated with ilioischial cages (cup-cage). Although ilioischial cages provide excellent initial stability, their middle- to long-term failure rates are high as a result of a lack of biologic fixation [7]. Therefore, when the standard revision implants are not enough, a custom-made acetabular component has been proposed to achieve these goals.

Additive manufacturing such as electron beam melting (EBM), and laser sintering (SLM or SLS) of powered of metal such as titanium, have opened nowadays new possibilities of customized engineering of constructs aimed to help the surgeons in anatomical reconstruction of bone defects in whatever portion of the body, including pelvis.

7.1.2 Pelvic Discontinuity

Pelvic discontinuity (AAOS Type IV, Paprosky IIIB, AIR IV) is defined as a defect across the anterior and posterior columns, at different levels, but with a total separation of the superior from the inferior acetabulum. Current options for management of osteolytic pelvic discontinuity include bulk acetabular allograft with plating, standard cage reconstruction with ischial and iliac screw fixation, a cup-cage construct with a porous metal acetabular component covered by a cage fixed proximally and distally, and different techniques using porous metal augmentations and a porous metal acetabular component [8]. While the methods differ, healing of the discontinuity and a stable acetabular construct remains the challenging targets and the treatment goals. A triflange cup is a custom-designed, titanium, porous-, and/or hydroxyapatite-coated acetabular component with ilial, ischial, and pubic flanges. These flanges allow for intimate, stable contact between the implant and the host bone, for initial stability while maintaining or returning the hip center of rotation to its anatomic location. In contrast to off-the-shelf malleable reconstructive cages, which have the potential for fatigue failure particularly when used in these cases of discontinuity, the triflange components offer rigid fixation to promote healing of the discontinuity and biologic fixation of the implant itself [8].

7.1.3 Bone Defect Extended Beyond the Acetabulum

In many cases, the bone defect extends from the acetabular area far proximally and distally, reaching the ileum and the ischium, and configuring an aggressive, neoplastic like scenario. In these cases, the use of custom-made implants is strongly recommended. For this reason, we support the necessity of adopting a bone defect classification with extension over the periacetabular region.

Enneking et al. in 1978 [9] divided the pelvis into 4 zones (zone 1, represented of iliac bone, zone 2 represented by the periacetabular region, zone 3 composed by pubis or ischium and zone 4 which corresponds to hemisacrum) to help the oncology surgeons.

In our opinion, these zones are important also in acetabular revision surgery and we propose a new periprosthetic pelvic classification to help the surgeons to identify and quantify the remaining bone, and not the missing bone, and to plan the reconstruction. The pelvis can be divided into three periprosthetic zones: α (alpha) zone (acetabulum, medial wall, ilium bone valid) that we could divide in α1, (1 wall persisting, with insufficiency of 2 walls), and in α2 (where we have the pelvic discontinuity); β (beta) zone (anterior column extension), that we had divided in β1 if the iliac bone is persisting for more than 50% or β2 if less than 50%; γ (gamma) zone (posterior column extension) divided in γ1 (only the ischial spine is remaining) u and γ2 (the ischial tuberosity is unsupportive) (Fig. 7.2a, b).

The basic principle of this newly proposed classification is to consider the residual, remaining bone able to support the new engineered cup or any off-the-shelf design, in order to plan the reconstruction, and not the missing bone.

However, at the moment we cannot properly assess the quality of the remaining, supportive bone, which is the other fundamental element in the reconstructive planning. Assessment of bone quality can be merely based so far upon the experience of judgment of the surgeons of the imaging materials including radiography, CT scan, MRI, or DEXA.

7.2 PreOperative Evaluation

All patients must be assessed clinically and with radiographic images before surgery. This typically included standard hip, AP pelvis, as well as CT scans which are mandatory to create bone custom models.

The CT scan protocol consisted of images that start from the top of iliac crest up to mid-femur, or at least 3 cm below the existing femoral implant. The optimal data involves images with a thickness of 1.0 mm and spacing of 0.8 mm (maximum acceptable are 2.0 mm of thickness and 2.0 mm of spacing), with metal subtraction software with the uncompressed data recorded to send to the implant manufacturer. The CT scan slide data are used to create a computerized, three-dimensional (3D) reconstruction of the patient's hemipelvis.

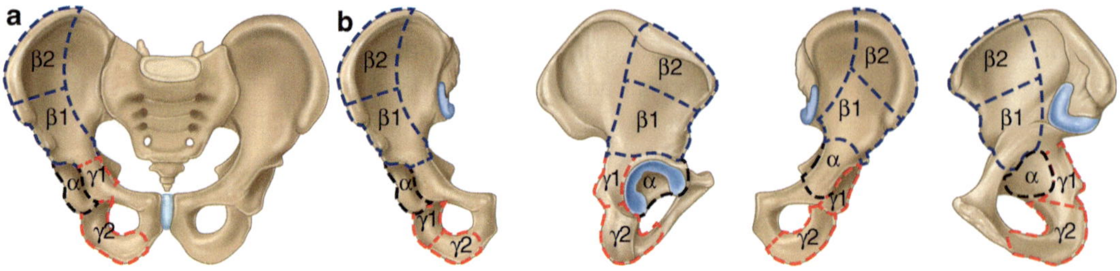

Fig. 7.2 New classification of pelvic bone defects; pelvis coronal view (**a**) and representation of hemipelvis in four different views (**b**)

7.3 Design and Construction of the Model

Unlike what happens in tumors, where the area to be resected must be considered and extramarginal osteotomies can be properly planned accordingly to accommodate the implant, in case of revision due to cup loosening, it is necessary to preserve all the bone available. The remaining pelvic landmarks, as defined by our classification, (obturator foramen, iliac wing, pubic ramus when they are available) are used to determine the hip center, the geometry of the new cup, and his orientation. The less possible amount of bone (particularly if the quality is not considered good) must be removed from the 3D model, as well cement, screws, and/or other useless components from the previous surgery, to accommodate the custom cup design.

The engineers collaborate with the surgeon to define the reference design of the cup (iliac spindle, cup-cage, triflange, a mixing of them), the head center, and cup orientation. The cup orientation is established by setting the abduction and anteversion angles of the cup, and it is based on patient-specific considerations, including leg length discrepancy, planned retention or revision of the femoral component, length of contralateral leg, and cup size. The abduction angle generally is targeted at 40° to 45° and is established using the plane of the obturator foramen as a reference. The anteversion angle is recognized using the plane of the iliac wing and the obturator foramen as references.

Subsequently, the engineers design the screw holes and paths targeting the structural, supporting bone remained. The highest number of screws, normally three to seven 6.5-mm acetabular screws, is planned; sometimes larger screws, specifically designed, can also be used.

Dedicated visual 3D tools and instrumentations to improve implants' congruency are used.

The implants are developed by subtractive or by additive manufacturing technology based on a precise analysis of patients' preoperative CT scans. Primary stability is enhanced and tailored on the patient's anatomy employing cup designs fitting the remaining anatomy, exploiting the high friction performances of the porous material matrix, in some cases with a porous-plasma spray or a hydroxyapatite coating to facilitate bone ingrowth.

7.4 Surgery

The posterior hip approach is useful for correct exposure and visualization of the pelvis. Other approaches can be used upon surgeon's preference and skill, keeping in mind that the posterior portion of the pelvis must be clearly exposed. It is possible to identify and trace the sciatic nerve from the greater sciatic notch to the ischium.

After dislocation of the hip, the femoral stem could be removed or from the top of the femur or using the transfemoral approach. In cases where the femoral component is retained, the gluteus minimum and gluteus medius are elevated from the iliac bone and space created between the muscle and the ilium, and the taper of the stem could be placed into this space. The previous cup must be removed, without sacrificing further bone.

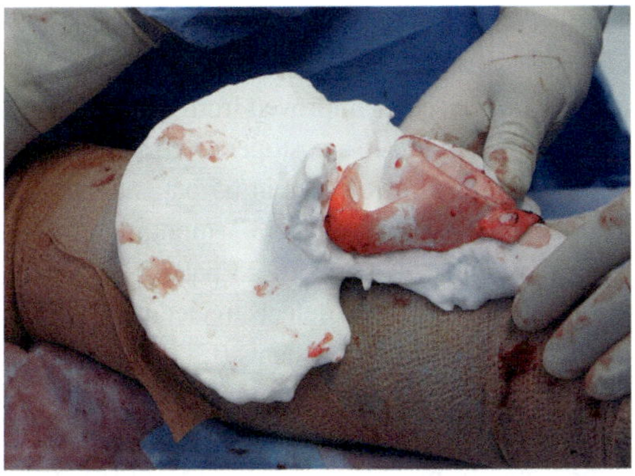

Fig. 7.3 A sterilized 3D pelvic model used like reference intraoperatively

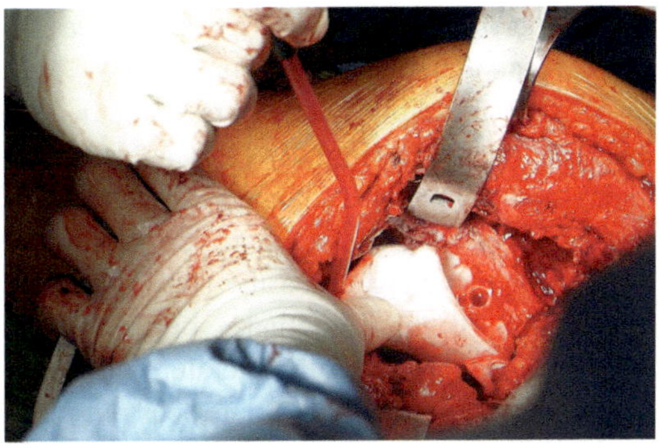

Fig. 7.4 A cup 3D trial models used to check the correct bone–implant contact and the position of the screw

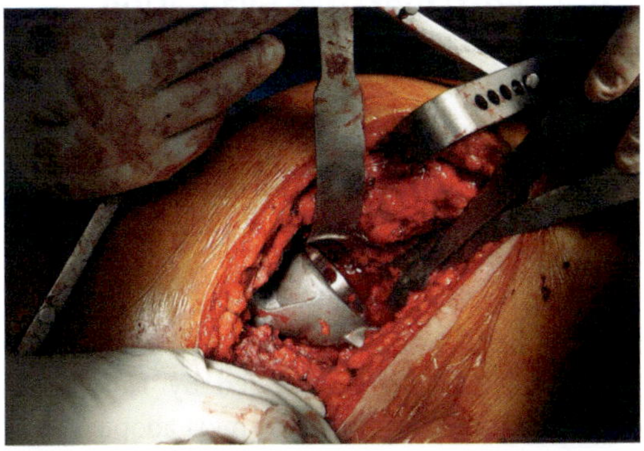

Fig. 7.5 Definitive custom cup implant: good fit and primary stability was obtained

If it is necessary for the visualization of the ilium, the gluteus medius, and minimus must be elevated off the wing of the ilium, to protect the superior gluteal artery and nerve. Ischium can be correctly exposed all the way down to the lateral insertions of hamstring tendons with partial release, taking care to protect the sciatic nerve.

A sterilized 3D pelvic model, and a cup model could be used as guiding reference intraoperatively (Fig. 7.3). Acetabular pseudomembranes must be removed and a necrotic bone reamed according to the 3D model and the preoperative planning. If it is possible allograft must be used only in small quantities, to fill some remaining imperfections of contact with the construct, to achieve the best possible contact between the new cup and the supporting bone. The 3D trial models of the cup are available, and it is useful to check the bone-implant contact area and the correct position of the screw's holes and paths (Fig. 7.4). Cleaning of the bony bed for the new implant from remaining cement, screws, metal, is mandatory to achieve the same clean surface as planned by the CT reconstruction.

In the case of triflange model, the insertion of the cup usually is initiated with the position of the iliac flange, eased by translating the hip proximally with some flexion to relax the abductors. The ischial and pubic flanges are rotated into position while extending the hip. After the correct positioning of the custom cup, it has to be fixed with screws that have a diameter, direction, and length already defined (Fig. 7.5). The screws (insertion points, paths, screwing direction) must be planned and discussed with the engineers during the planning because not all insertion points can be intraoperatively reached.

The modularity of liners varies between companies and it is therefore important to know the available options preoperatively. Lateralized, elevated, and constrained options are typically available to aid in achieving appropriate hip length, soft-tissue tensioning, and stability [10].

7.5 PostOperative Rehabilitation Program

The postoperative rehabilitation includes immediate mobilization with protected weight-bearing using crutches for the first 30 to 60 days. Due to the absence or to the small quantity of bone grafting the weight-bearing is not contraindicated. If in doubt of the initial stability of the hip, and dislocation is considered possible, due to the number and severity of previous and actual surgeries, an orthesis can be adopted for 4 to 6 weeks to limit motion.

All kind of exercises, aiming to strengthen the muscles, (isometric initially, and assisted isotonic) and to restore an acceptable range of motion can be adopted, including pool rehab with deep-water bicycling (once the surgical wound has healed), if the compliance of the patient allows it. Availability in the literature of proven rehabilitation protocols for hip custom-made implants, is very poor.

7.6 PostOperative Evaluation

Radiological evaluation including AP pelvis x-rays and axial view of the affected hip should be done postoperatively at 6 weeks, 6 months, and 1 year, and, thereafter, at 1-year intervals. Postoperative CT scan may be requested to evaluate the congruence between the bone and the implant and the direction of the screws. Clinical evaluation could be performed by Harris Hip Score (HHS) which is still the most adopted evaluation tool. Other scores useful for evaluation are: Hip disability and Osteoarthritis Outcome Score (HOOS), Oxford Hip Score (OHS), modified Merle d'Aubigne and Postel scale, Western Ontario and McMaster Universities Arthritis Index (WOMAC), Short Form-36 (SF-36), and Visual Analogue Scale (VAS). No specifically designed scores for these peculiar and disabling situations have been produced so far.

7.7 Clinical Experience and Failures

In a recent review, Chiarlone et al. describe acetabular aseptic loosening (AL) like the main indication for revision total hip arthroplasty with a custom implant, followed by implant failure, osteolysis, PJI, multiple dislocations, instability, metallosis, dysplasia, Girdlestone, tumor and acetabular fractures [11]. Good results were shown by Fröschen et al. [12] at an average follow-up of 43 months in a series of 68 custom cups. Implant survival at last follow-up was 75% and Kaplan–Meier survival analysis, with explantation as the endpoint, revealed survival rates of 82.7% (3 years) and 77% (5 years). Christie et al. [13] reported no triflange cup removed and Harris hip scores improved from a preoperative mean of 33.3 points to a postoperative mean of 82.1 points in a series of 67 hips in 65 patients with an average follow-up of 53 months (range, 24–107 months). A series of 23 patients (24 hips) with Paprosky type IIIB defects treated with custom triflange acetabular components (CTAC) and mean follow-up of 57 months (minimum 2 years) reported no loosening or mechanical failure, with HHS improving from 42 (±16) to 65 (±18) [14]. According to the biomechanical parameter restoration compared to the preoperative planning, Weber et al. found deviations of the custom-made implant compared to the 3D-CT planning within 10° regarding inclination and anteversion and within 5 mm regarding center of rotation (COR) restoration in the majority of patients [15].

Recently, literature on the failures of the custom-made implants became available. The most common causes of revision are dislocation, aseptic loosening, infection, and mechanical failure. De Martino et al. [16] reported 11% of dislocation, 6% of deep infection, and 1.7% of aseptic loosening in a review enrolling 579 cases. In a single series of 95 complex acetabular reconstruction with custom triflange cup, Berend et al. [17] described that the implant was removed in seven hips (7.37%), and a further triflange implant was used in four and an excision arthroplasty was performed in three after the failure of reimplantation due to infection. If mechanical failure occurs, it is possible to provide a new custom system or an explantation. Wind et al. [18] reported in a series of 19 hips, that reoperations included 1 explantation for aseptic failure, 1 explantation for septic failure, 1 revision to constrained liner, 1 exchange of constrained liner due to locking ring failure, and 2 irrigations and debridement of postoperative wound infections.

Fröschen et al. [12] showed that 51 of the 68 cases treated (75%), reimplantation of a custom-made prosthetic hip component was considered clinically successful; there were 17 cases in which treatment failure occurred with a need for explantation of the custom-made implant. In these 17 cases, 15 patients needed explantation of the custom-made implant because of a PJI, and 2 patients needed explantation because of aseptic loosening of the implant [12].

Citak et al. [19] described that only 1 of 9 patients (11.1%) required revision surgery due to implant-associated failure after 13 months. Moreover, in terms of non-implant-associated revision rates, 5 patients (55.6%) required revision surgery due to hip dislocation ($n = 3$) and postoperative hematoma ($n = 2$). The authors affirm that they used in 2 cases a larger head, while in 1 case a neck adapter with a larger head to treat the instability [19]. Barlow et al. [20] reported that custom triflange acetabular components (CTAC) tend to lateralize the hip center by approximately 1 cm, and there is a trend toward nearly 2 cm of lateralization in the small subset of failed CTAC observed. They concluded that future efforts should focus on medializing the hip center in CTAC to improve ingrowth and survivorship.

Mechanical failure of custom system is also possible, and it could occur due to screws breakage, flange breakage, cement detachment, or cup breakage.

A small number of data are available in literature on the possibility to revise custom implants. In our opinion it is very important to prevent the possibility of custom implant failure using porous materials, good manufacturing system/technology, modularity, an adequate level of constraint associated to abductor repair/reconstruction if needed, and maniacal planning (to identify cup position, screws direction, good bone available if it is possible); the surgeons must be skilled and the surgery must not last long to reduce the risk of infection.

The acetabular custom-made implants represent a reliable solution in cases of unsuccessful multiple revisions in particular cases of bone loss classified as Paprosky Type IIIA-B, type III–IV according to American Academy of Orthopaedic Surgeons system, AIR IV, or a bone defect α2 and beyond considering our new classification, where the feature of the defect cannot be handled with standard implants. This strategy allows fitting the implant to the residual host bone, bypassing the bony deficiency, and restoring hip biomechanics (Fig. 7.6).

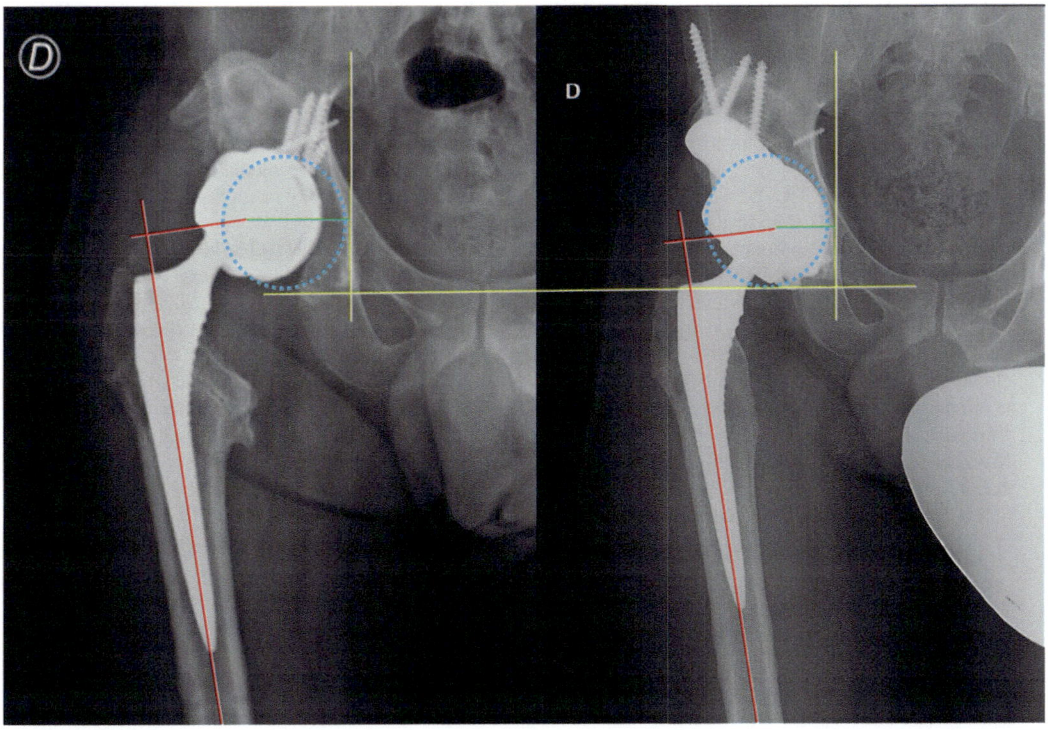

Fig. 7.6 Preoperative and 18 months follow-up X-rays of custom implant: biomechanical parameters are restored

Acknowledgments We thank the "Mario Boni Foundation" for the scientific support given to the paper and Mauro Andrenacci for the pictures on the proposed pelvic bone defects classification.

References

1. Lie SA, Havelin LI, Furnes ON, Engesæster LB, Vollset SE. Failure rates for 4762 revision total hip arthroplasties in the Norwegian arthroplasty register. J Bone Jt Surg Ser B. 2004;86(4):504–9.
2. Ong KL, Lau E, Suggs J, Kurtz SM, Manley MT. Risk of subsequent revision after primary and revision total joint arthroplasty. Clin Orthop Relat Res. 2010;468(11):3070–6.
3. Yu S, Saleh H, Bolz N, Buza J, Iorio R, Rathod PA, et al. Re-revision total hip arthroplasty: epidemiology and factors associated with outcomes. J Clin Orthop Trauma. 2020;11(1):43–6.
4. D'Antonio JA, Capello WN, Borden LS, Bargar WL, Bierbaum BF, Boettcher WG, et al. Classification and management of acetabular abnormalities in total hip arthroplasty. Clin Orthop Relat Res. 1989;243:126–37.
5. Paprosky WG, Perona PG, Lawrence JM. Acetabular defect classification and surgical reconstruction in revision arthroplasty. A 6-year follow-up evaluation. J Arthroplasty. 1994;9(1):33–44.
6. Meneghini R, Hanssen ADLD, Meneghini R, Hanssen AD, Lewallen DG. Uncemented hemispherical cups in extreme bone loss. In: Revision total hip and knee arthroplasty. London: Wolters Kluwer Health Adis (ESP); 2012. p. 163–78.
7. Amenabar T, Rahman WA, Hetaimish BM, Kuzyk PR, Safir OA, Gross AE. Promising mid-term results with a cup-cage construct for large acetabular defects and pelvic discontinuity. Clin Orthop Relat Res. 2016;474(2):408–14.
8. Taunton MJ, Fehring TK, Edwards P, Bernasek T, Holt GE, Christie MJ. Pelvic discontinuity treated with custom triflange component: a reliable option. Clin Orthop Relat Res. 2012;470(2):428–34.
9. Enneking WF, Dunham WK. Resection and reconstruction for primary neoplasms involving the innominate bone. J Bone Jt Surg Ser A. 1978;60A(6):731–46.
10. Goodman GP, Engh CA. The custom triflange cup build it and they will come. Bone Jt J. 2016;98B(1):68–72.
11. Chiarlone F, Zanirato A, Cavagnaro L, Alessio-Mazzola M, Felli L, Burastero G, et al. Acetabular custom-made implants for severe acetabular bone defect in revision total hip arthroplasty: a systematic review of the literature. Fakt Yang Berhubungan Dengan Minat Ibu Terhadap Pengguna Alat Kontrasepsi Implant Di Puskesmas Ome Kota Tidore Kepul. 2020;84(3):446–519. http://ir.obihiro.ac.jp/dspace/handle/10322/3933.
12. Fröschen FS, Randau TM, Hischebeth GTR, Gravius N, Gravius S, Walter SG. Mid-term results after revision total hip arthroplasty with custom-made acetabular implants in patients with Paprosky III acetabular bone loss. Arch Orthop Trauma Surg. 2020;140(2):263–73. https://doi.org/10.1007/s00402-019-03318-0.
13. Christie MJ, Barrington SA, Brinson MF, Ruhling ME, DeBoer DK. Bridging massive acetabular defects with the triflange cup: 2- to 9-year results. Clin Orthop Relat Res. 2001;393:216–27.
14. Berasi CC, Berend KR, Adams JB, Ruh EL, Lombardi AV. Are custom Triflange acetabular components effective for reconstruction of catastrophic bone loss? Clin Orthop Relat Res. 2014;473(2):528–35. https://doi.org/10.1007/s11999-014-3969-z.
15. Weber M, Witzmann L, Wieding J, Grifka J, Renkawitz T, Craiovan B. Customized implants for acetabular Paprosky III defects may be positioned with high accuracy in revision hip arthroplasty. Int Orthop. 2019;43(10):2235–43.
16. De Martino I, Strigelli V, Cacciola G, Gu A, Bostrom MP, Sculco PK. Survivorship and clinical outcomes of custom Triflange acetabular components in revision total hip arthroplasty: a systematic review. J Arthroplasty. 2019;34(10):2511–8. https://doi.org/10.1016/j.arth.2019.05.032.
17. Berend ME, Berend KR, Lombardi AV, Cates H, Faris P. The patient-specific Triflange acetabular implant for revision total hip arthroplasty in patients with severe acetabular defects: planning, implantation, and results. Bone Jt J. 2018;100B(1):50–4.
18. Wind MA, Swank ML, Sorger JI. Short-term results of a custom triflange acetabular component for massive acetabular bone loss in revision THA. Orthopedics. 2013;36(3):260–5.
19. Citak M, Kochsiek L, Gehrke T, Haasper C, Suero EM, Mau H. Preliminary results of a 3D-printed acetabular component in the management of extensive defects. Hip Int. 2018;28(3):266–71. https://doi.org/10.5301/hipint.5000561.
20. Barlow BT, Oi KK, Lee YY, Carli AV, Choi DS, Bostrom MP. Outcomes of custom flange acetabular components in revision total hip arthroplasty and predictors of failure. J Arthroplasty. 2016;31(5):1057–64. https://doi.org/10.1016/j.arth.2015.11.016.

3D Scapula/Shoulder Prosthesis

8

Alessandro Luzzati, Carmine Zoccali,
and Giovanni Beltrami

8.1 Introduction

Reconstruction after wide resection of skeletal tumors around the shoulder girdle is currently very important in order to try to assure the patients a better quality of life, since they can be long survivors more frequently than in the past. While modular prostheses assure good limb reconstruction in the majority of cases, no effective reconstruction systems are available for complex segments as the pelvis and the scapula, so the use of composite homograft prostheses is often considered the reference treatment.

Nevertheless, massive homografts present several problems related to long-term mechanical outcomes, which often result in failures [1, 2]; moreover, a consistent problem regards pediatric reconstruction in which homografts, harvested in adults, present important size mismatches.

3D-Printed Titanium Custom-Made Prostheses (3DPTCMP) appear to be a theoretically definitive, reliable, and effective solution, in terms of anatomical reconstruction and mechanical resistance. We present an overall consideration regarding shoulder girdle reconstruction, with particular regards to the titanium custom 3D-printed solution.

A. Luzzati (✉)
Oncological and Reconstructive Orthopaedic Department, IRCCS—Galeazzi Orthopaedic Institute, Milan, Italy

C. Zoccali
Department of Anatomical, Histological, Forensic Medicine and Orthopaedic Science, Sapienza University of Rome, Rome, Italy

Oncological Orthopedics, IFO - Regina Elena National Cancer Institute, Rome, Italy

G. Beltrami
Pediatric Oncological Orthopedic Department, Azienda Ospedaliero Universitaria Meyer, Florence, Italy
e-mail: beltramig@aou-careggi.toscana.it

Anatomical Considerations The shoulder girdle presents specific characteristics; in a restricted area the joint, composed by the humeral head, the glenoid cavity and the capsula, is closely in contact with the shoulder muscles, the brachial plexus and the axillary-humeral vessels.

The extrarotator muscles originate from the scapula and pass over the capsular joint, so the related tendons surround the humeral head, and insert themselves on the related apophysis.

These structures establish a barrier for the tumor, which may grow easier inside the joint, under the muscles, than outside them (Fig. 8.1).

Wittig et al., in 2001, codified the structures, introducing the concept of functional compartments according to the Enneking principles for tumor surgery [3].

In detail, the subscapularis muscle divides the shoulder girdle from the brachial plexus; when the tumor, onset from the humeral head, destroys

C. Zoccali et al. (eds.), *3D Printing in Bone Surgery*, https://doi.org/10.1007/978-3-030-91900-9_8

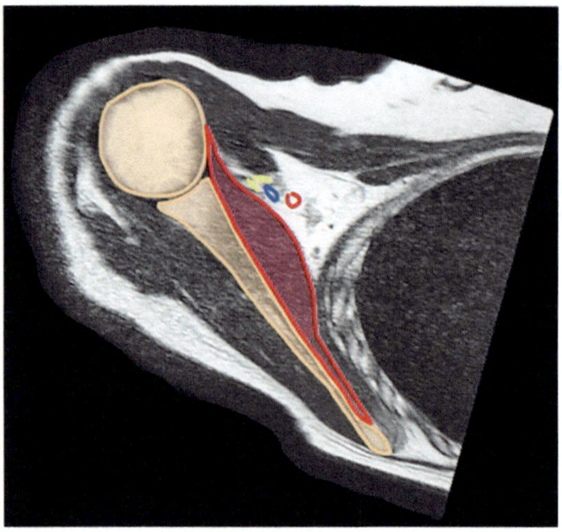

Fig. 8.1 Axial-MRI underlining the barrier action of the subscapularis muscle (red) for tumors arising in the scapula (orange) versus the neurovascular bundle

the cortical bone, it then grows posterior to the muscle toward the anterior surface of the scapula, often sparing the neurovascular structures [4].

Considering these concepts, several authors suggest extra-articular resections for primary tumors, usually possible because the neurovascular bundle is not involved. Moreover, a wide resection of a primary tumor located in the humeral head includes the joint and the extrarotator cuff, with a resulting instability that has to be taken into account for reconstruction.

The Primary Tumors in the Scapula Even if the shoulder girdle is considered the third most common site for bone tumors, primary tumors are quite rare in the scapula, while metastatic lesions are more common [5, 6]. In childhood, the most frequent primary tumor in the scapula is Ewing's Sarcoma. After adolescence, Chondrosarcoma becomes the most frequent primary tumor because there is a high incidence of malignant transformation of scapular exostoses [7, 8].

In the past, considering the shoulder's complex anatomy and biomechanics, wide excision without reconstruction was considered the best treatment.

Malware et al. were one of first to describe a classification of shoulder girdle resections in 1991 [5]. They identified six types of resections,

Table 8.1 Shoulder girdle resection classification

Malware et al. classification	Enneking et al. classification	Shehadeh et al. classification
Type I: Intra-articular proximal humerus resection **Type II**: Partial scapular resection **Type III**: Intra-articular total scapulectomy **Type IV**: Extra-articular total scapulectomy and humeral head resection **Type V**: Extra-articular humerus and glenoid resection **Type VI**: Extra-articular humeral and total scapular resection	**S1**: Scapular blade and spine **S2**: Glenoid, coracoid process and acromion **S3**: Humeral epiphysis (?) **S4**: Humeral metaphysis (?) **S5**: Humeral diaphysis (?)	*Humeral resections* **Type I**: Intra-articular proximal humerus resection **Type II**: Extra-articular proximal humerus resection **Type III**: Intra-articular total humerus resection; **Type IV**: Extra-articular total humerus resection *Scapular resections* **Type I**: Partial scapular resection, with preservation of the glenoid and the glenohumeral joint **Type II**: Intra-articular resection of the scapula **Type III**: Extra-articular resection of the scapula

based on the tumor site and the anatomic compartments (Table 8.1). Each type was then divided into two categories: A if the abduction system was spared or B if it was partially or completely resected.

A couple of years later, Enneking and colleagues, including Dunham and Malware, proposed a new classification of shoulder resections in which they identified five zones. This classification was successively adopted by the Musculoskeletal Tumor Society [9] (Table 8.1).

Recently, Shehadeh et al. have tried to give surgical indications based on the site of the disease, distinguishing tumors located in the humerus and tumors located in the scapula (Table 8.1) [10].

Humeral resections were differentiated in four types and A and B were specified for each one, based on the partial or complete resection of the deltoid excision, respectively; scapular resections were differentiated in three types.

They suggested modular prosthetic reconstruction for all humeral resections, with capsula reconstruction with a Goretex aortic graft positioned between the glenoid and the prosthesis for Type I and Type III resections, while the Dacron prosthesis is positioned between the acromion and the coracoid process for Type II and Type IV resections.

They suggested no reconstruction for scapular resections in pediatric patients and custom-made prostheses for adults, moreover for aesthetics because should function is only slightly increased.

Actually, all classifications are similar and suggest similar treatment.

When the tumor is located in the humerus, reconstruction in adults can be performed with available modular prostheses which can be standard or inverse, based on circumflex nerve sparing [11].

When the tumor is located in the scapula, there are three available options:

1. Humerus suspension: more indicated in elderly patients or in case of a high risk of infections; it was mostly used in the past decades. When muscles and soft tissues are partially spared, a sufficient function is present even in case the lateral third of the scapula is resected and not reconstructed (Fig. 8.2a, b) [6].
2. Homograft reconstruction: although still considered the reference treatment, the use of homograft reconstruction is today less frequent than in the past;

   We can distinguish reconstruction using homograft alone and reconstruction using homograft combined to a prosthesis (Composite Homograft Prosthesis).

   The first solution can be a valid alternative for little bone loss or in low-demanding patients because of the low osteointegration rate and related homograft resorption; Zhang et al., in 2009, published their experience in reconstruction after resection of scapular tumors using homografts; they report a MSTS score of 80% at median follow-up of 26 months. Although this could seem comforting, it is likely that the functional results decrease with a longer follow-up [12]; moreover, they verified a better function when the glenoid cavity is preserved.

   The use of a composite homograft prosthesis is associated to several problems related to the homograft; first of all, the availability: muscular-skeletal tissue banks are not widespread and it is not easy to find a homograft with compatible size and shape; moreover, the osteointegration is limited to the area in contact with the patient's bone and a process of resorption is common at long-term follow-up.
3. Custom-made Prosthesis: CMP represented a valid alternative in reconstruction after limb-sparing surgery. In 2007, Pritsch et al. published a comparison between humerus suspension and endoprosthesis reconstruction, they concluded that endoprostheses have better function and aesthetics for when rhomboids, latissimus dorsi, deltoid and trapezius muscles are spared [13].

Custom-Made Prosthesis CMP has two main objectives in the shoulder:

1. restoring connection between the spino-appendicular muscles or the remaining scapula and the humerus;
2. restoring/maintaining function.

Moreover, in pediatric patients, it plays an important role in restoring/maintaining anatomy where conventional prostheses are ineffective (oversize, diaphyseal stem, high mechanical request).

Restoring Connection: the type of connection between the scapular prosthesis and the humerus is quite debated in literature and no consensus is present.

In the first reported cases, the proximal humerus was not replaced, to reduce the invasiveness of the technique and to perform a "standard" reconstruction [14]. The problem was represented by possible progressive erosion of the

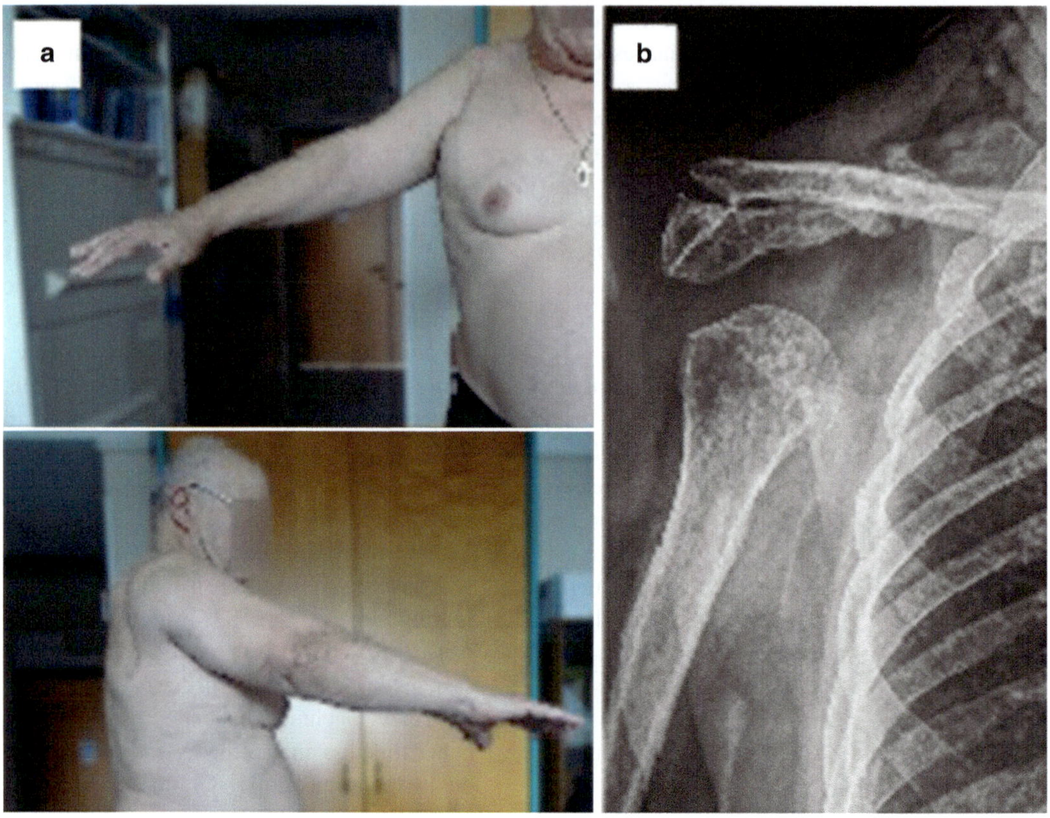

Fig. 8.2 (**a**) Abduction and anterior elevation after resection of the lateral aspect of the scapula: control at 6 months from surgery; (**b**) X-ray showing the glenoid resection; even though reconstruction was not performed, function can be considered sufficient

humeral head, due to mismatch and/or joint instability after muscle resection, as well as for the different wear of cartilage and titanium prosthetic surface. This can lead to persistent pain and limitation of the range of motion [15].

So, as today, many authors suggest the replacement of both the scapula and the humeral head. This with a view to reduce surface wear and to offer the implant greater stability.

Otherwise, when resection includes scapula, proximal humerus and muscles, joint stability is often precarious and constraining the glenohumeral joint is almost mandatory.

In 2018, Savvidou et all, published a series of 6 scapular reconstructions after tumor removals, with constrained reverse total shoulder arthroplasty [16].

They conclude, at 37 months of average follow-up, to have obtained a good pain control and a stable shoulder, but a limited function.

Nevertheless, in case of reconstruction with a constrained total shoulder arthroplasty, the weight of the entire arm is directly conveyed on the scapula prosthesis and, in case of partial scapula resection, on the prosthesis-scapular bone interface.

This could be responsible for mobilization of the scapular prosthesis or distal migration of the entire shoulder, because of the weight of the arm.

These possible events absolutely contraindicate the use of constrained implants in pediatric age, even if an extra-articular resection of the shoulder girdle is performed.

In general, a non-constrained glenohumeral joint is suggested, when it is possible to spare muscles/capsule and nerves, maintaining a residual shoulder.

Always considering the resurface of both humerus and scapula, in case of resection of capsule and rotator cuff, inverse shoulder prostheses have been utilized to maintain abduction. This surgical solution, linked to the salvage of the axillary nerve and deltoid, offers an excellent range of motion. Nevertheless, a consistent high failure rate, in the short, middle, and long term, has to be taken into account. Barco et al. (2016) reported an overall revision rate from 9.5 to 47%, with several possible complications (instability, infection, notching, mechanical failure, nerve injury, acromial/ spine fracture, intraoperative fracture, component disassembly). For this reason, after an oncological resection around the shoulder girdle, an accurate balance between functional improvement and long-term complications has to be performed, especially in the pediatric population.

If a standard humeral prosthesis is chosen, the connection between the humeral prosthesis and the scapula can be guaranteed by the use of an artificial cuff as the trevira tube however, a possible increase of the infection rate has to be taken into account [17, 18]. Nevertheless, functional flaps are necessary to restore motion.

Puchner et al., in 2014, published a series of 29 scapular resections whereof two patients underwent reconstruction with standard shoulder CMP; they obtained acceptable functional results with a MSTS score of 83% and 77% [6].

Restoring/maintaining function: we can identify three key points

- Muscle sparing: obviously, maintaining muscles is important for function but, unfortunately, it is often impossible because they have to be sacrificed to guarantee a good margin. When extrarotator muscles are sacrificed, shoulder cinematic during abduction is severely compromised so an inverse prosthesis, **with the previously described limitations**, has to be taken into account; in case of partial damage of the deltoid muscle, the serratus anterior muscle can partially compensate, activating the scapular-thoracic joint.
- Nerve sparing: the *circumflex nerve* considerably influences shoulder function; it originates from the posterior cord of the brachial plexus, travels through the quadrangular space, surrounds the humeral metaphysis, and innerves the deltoid and teres minor. It is important to spare it during resection when possible because it is fundamental to maintain some level of abduction of the shoulder. Unfortunately, it is often involved in tumors of the proximal humerus but it is often not involved in scapular tumors. The *suprascapular nerve* originates from the upper trunk of the brachial plexus; it then runs along the superior border of the scapula, passes through the suprascapular notch inferior to the superior transverse scapular ligament and enters the supraspinous fossa where it innerves the supraspinatus muscle, and then it passes through the spinoglenoid notch toward the infraspinatus fossa where it innerves the infraspinatus muscle [19]. During its path, it is in close contact with the scapular bone, so tumors originating in the lateral third of the scapula frequently involve it; the *subscapular nerves* (upper, middle, and lower) originate from the posterior cord of the brachial plexus; the upper nerve immediately innervates the subscapularis muscle, the middle (thoracodorsal) nerve innervates the latissimus dorsi muscle and the lower nerve innervates the lower part of the subscapularis muscle and the teres major muscle. The middle and lower subscapularis nerves travel ventrally to the subscapularis muscle belly which protects them from tumor infiltration.
- Function restoring using functional flaps: after wide resection of bone, muscle, and nerves, the only way to restore function is to use a motor unit transfer. With the largest surface area of any extremity-related muscle in the body, the latissimus dorsi (LD) flap is the most widely used, as it can cover most large defects of the shoulder [20, 21].

Moreover, the vascular pedicle, which utilizes the thoracodorsal artery and nerve, allows extensive mobilization. It can be used as a pure muscle flap or with a skin paddle, and when the innervation is properly spared, it can be used to restore some movement of the shoulder. The latissimus dorsi has been widely employed around the shoulder girdle, for rotator cuff, deltoid, or tricep "functional muscle" reconstruction. Furthermore, the rotational LD may act as a scapular stabilizer, suspender and as a subscapular plane reconstruction option, offering an efficient surgical solution, even in pediatric age [22].

The role of the acromion: the acromion plays a key role in shoulder motion, for arm abduction and anterior elevation. When resection includes it, the action of the deltoid can be not effective, even if the muscle is spared.

So, if possible, the designed prosthesis should also include its reconstruction, with particular attention to decrease the size of implants respect to normal anatomy, this in order to reduce potential skin suffering and guarantee deltoid reinsertion.

8.2 3D-Printed Titanium Custom-Made Prosthesis

The diffusion of additive manufacturing using titanium powder gives an important impulse to its application in CMP production.

Additive manufacturing has allowed to decrease costs and to simplify the production process which is now possible in small factories.

Shoulder prosthesis production obtained several advantages from this technology, allowing to reconstruct entire segment as the scapula or just little sections as the glenoid cavity.

The total scapula prosthesis can reproduce normal scapula anatomy or just the wedges. During projection, it needs to have peripheral holes and loops to allow muscle attachment; acromion reconstruction is quite important to fix the deltoid muscle, moreover if the circumflex nerve is spared.

When it is possible to spare part of the scapula with its muscular attachments, the functional results can be better. Otherwise, it is not easy to find the best way to fix the prosthesis to the remaining scapular bone.

A possible system is to furnish the prosthesis with a plate with holes, which adheres to the scapular blade and is screwed to a smaller plate on the other side of the scapular blade; this system allows a good primary stability, but in the long-term, the bone included between the two plates can become ischemic and can go toward necrosis and consequent prosthetic mobilization.

An alternative method uses screws which go through the prosthesis inside the lateral margin and the superior border as showed by Biazzo in 2018, for resections of the glenoid cavity and the lateral third of the scapula [15]. When the resection also includes the supraspinatus fossae, the medial border of the scapula can be used as well.

The scapular prosthesis should have holes along its entire body to allow the fixation of the surrounding muscles and/or eventually of the muscular flaps (Fig. 8.3).

Pediatric Reconstruction After bone tumor resection around the shoulder girdle, "pediatric age" represent a specific reconstructive chapter, with particular rules [23, 24].

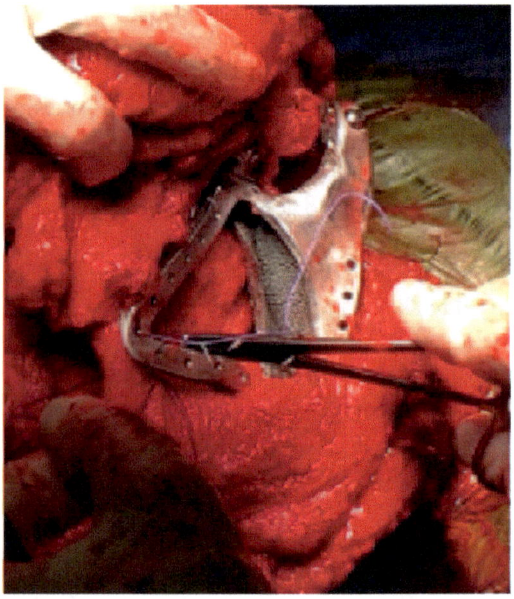

Fig. 8.3 An intraoperative picture showing the reattachment of the surrounding muscles to the 3DPCMP to cover it and restore function. This procedure is also helpful to suspend the prosthesis in a correct position after total scapulectomy

This for several reasons:

1. The term "pediatric age" includes several classes of different patients, from infancy to childhood.
2. Immature bone has its own healing capability, remodeling, and growth characteristics.
3. The "conventional" prosthetic reconstructions are often discouraged, for stem stress shielding, growth plate violation, and early failure.
4. The constrained prosthesis tends to fail for several mechanical or biological long-term complications. On the contrary, a theoretical "unstable reconstruction" in pediatric age has more chances of long-term durability and efficacy.
5. "Esthetical" reconstructions are unnecessary, for the amazing functional recovery and balance capability.

For the overall analysis, including specific surgical difficulties, after an oncological resection around the shoulder girdle, children are often treated either by a "non-reconstruction" or by a "biological reconstruction." In particular, after scapular resection, "non-reconstruction" means an efficient elbow and wrist function, while the active movement of the shoulder is achieved with momentum, and never against resistance. In case of extra-articular resections, the proximal humerus may be reconstructed with massive homografts or APCs suspended to the clavicle, with minimal active range of motion of the shoulder.

In order to improve shoulder motion, a scapular reconstruction may be attempted by massive homograft reconstruction. The difficulties are represented by mismatch (adult donor) and middle- or long-term mechanical failure. For this reason, this option is discouraged [25, 26].

Recycled bone may be an option for "perfect anatomical fitting," but long-term results undermine the efficacy (massive resorptions, infections, fractures, etc.) [27].

The introduction of 3DTCMP in clinical practice, has offered new perspective options of reconstruction, also in the pediatric age.

In this group, the main advantages are:

- The chance to perfectly establish the size of the reconstruction in a 3D view, including wedges, apophysis, articular surface etc. This allows to exactly plan the size of implants, deciding where it is necessary to be "anatomic, over-sized and under-sized."
- The chance to establish the "best" osteosynthesis device, planning the anatomical plate, pins and screws with different sizes.
- The chance of a solid, strong reconstruction, completed by the presence of holes and loops for muscle attachment.
- The chance to use the custom prosthesis as a biological spacer, able to guarantee function until the end of growth, before definitive, "adult type" reconstruction.

Nevertheless, possible complications also have to be taken into account:

- mechanical erosion of the counter-lateral articular surface,
- mechanical wear of the thoracic wall and ribs in scapular reconstruction,
- possible migration and instability of the implant, due to elevated functional requests and scarce cooperation.
- no previous literature reports, with difficult projects.

All considering, in pediatric age, a possible way to take advantage of the benefits of titanium 3D-printed technology for shoulder girdle reconstruction, is to "add biology" to the mechanical implants. In particular, the association of rotational LD motor unit transfer to a scapular titanium 3D implant, offers the chance of a potentially definitive and effective reconstruction. The scapular prosthesis is anatomical and resistant; the rotational and functional LD flap offers scapular stability, a safe subscapularis plane and improves the range of motion [28].

The same considerations can also be useful in custom 3D proximal humerus reconstruction, where the LD rotational flap may reconstruct deltoid function, if necessary.

As stated before, constrained implants are discouraged in infancy, as well as reverse shoulder prostheses. So, for recovering and lowering the wear of the counter-lateral articular surface, an interposition arthroplasty by autologous and/or homologous fascia may be helpful.

The same for reconstruction of capsule and ligament, in order to limit synthetic mesh in pediatric age (Fig. 8.4).

That said, the use of custom-made prostheses in pediatric age must absolutely be limited to selected cases in which it appears indispensable for functional recovery, and mainly associated to muscular transfer.

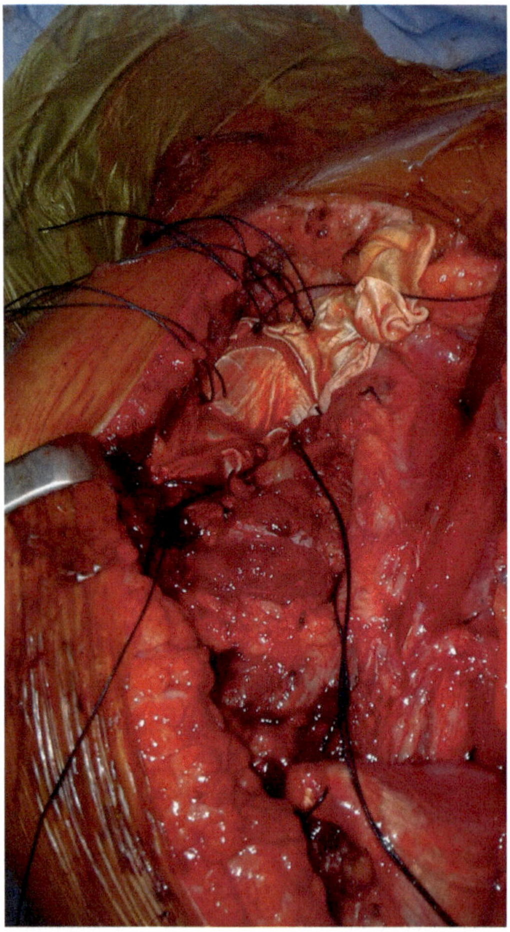

Fig. 8.4 An intraoperative picture showing the use of a homoplastic fascia lata to reconstruct capsular ligaments

Exemplificative Case Female patient, 36 years old, presented at observation of her general practitioner complaining pain in her right shoulder. After performing an X-ray (Fig. 8.5a), the patient was addressed to orthopedic consultation. The orthopedic surgeon prescribed NSAIDs and rehabilitation. After 3 months, considering the absence of significant results, an MRI was done (Fig. 8.5b) showing a tumor mass onset in the glenoid cavity and growing anteriorly through the coracoid process. The patient was addressed to a specialized oncological center where a total-body CT scan was performed revealing the absence of distant metastases and the presence of calcifications in the mass, suggestive of a tumor of chondroid nature (Fig. 8.5c). The successive CT-guided trocar biopsy evidenced a grade 2 Chondrosarcoma and the patient was addressed to surgery.

Considering the specific anatomy, wide resection and reconstruction with a custom-made prosthesis was indicated.

Prosthesis design: the tumor involved the glenoid cavity, the coracoid process and the surrounding soft tissues. The resection was planned to obtain a wide margin and patient specific cutting guides were produced to facilitate the correct osteotomies (Fig. 8.6a). The prosthesis was built to reproduce the anatomy of the resected part without the coracoid process because its tendon attachments were considered compromised. Fixation was ideated with a plate with screws (Fig. 8.6b).

Surgery: performed with the patient in left-lateral position. A dissection was performed anteriorly to isolate the neurovascular bundle (Fig. 8.7a); posteriorly, considering the disease was intraosseous, the supraspinatus and infraspinatus muscles were isolated and spared (Fig. 8.7b). The osteotomies were performed using the cutting guides and the tumor was extirpated with wide margins.

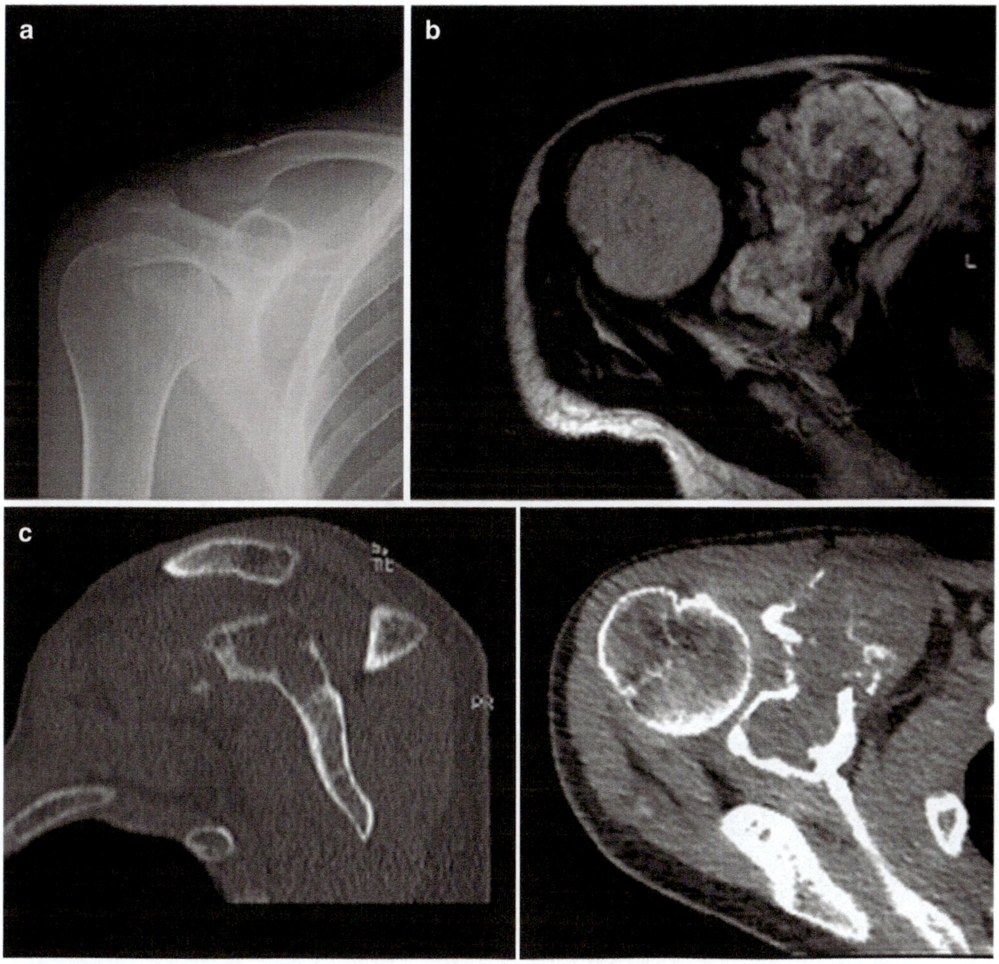

Fig. 8.5 (**a**) The X-ray was quite normal; (**b**) axial-MRI showing a tumor probably onset in the glenoid cavity and grown through the coracoid process. (**c**) CT sagittal view (left side) and axial view (right side) showing the tumor with calcification in the matrix compatible with a chondroid tumor

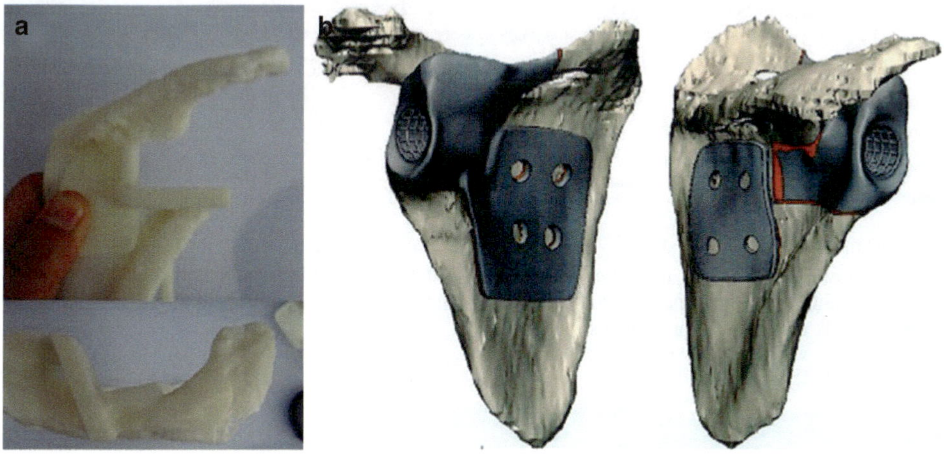

Fig. 8.6 (**a**) The cutting guides projected to perform the osteotomies; (**b**) a rendering of the 3DPTCMP

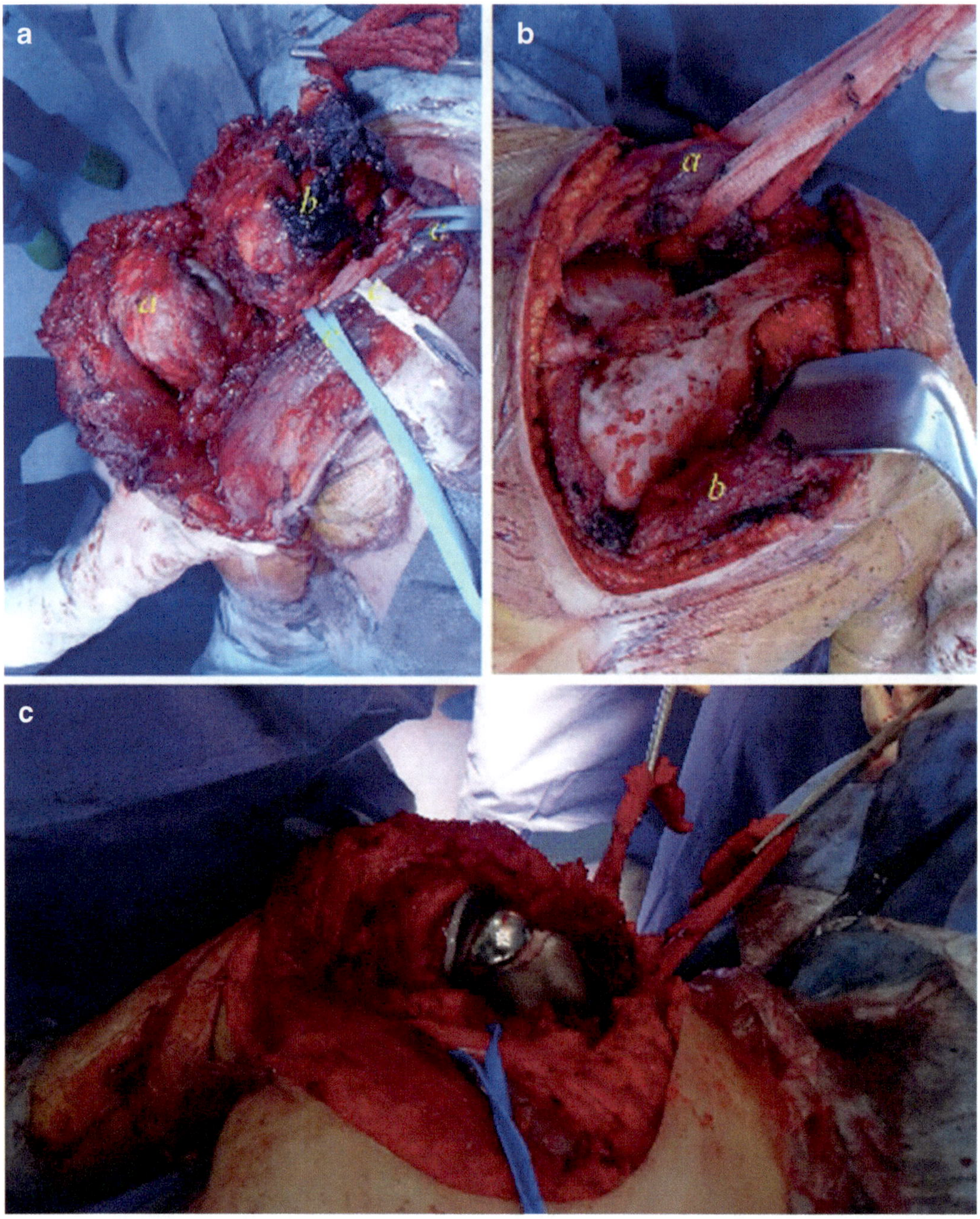

Fig. 8.7 (**a**) Intraoperative picture showing the anterior dissection with the humeral head (a), the tumor (b) and the neurovascular bundle (c); (**b**) intraoperative picture showing the posterior dissection; the supraspinatus muscle (a) and the infraspinatus muscle (b) were isolated and elevated; (**c**) the reconstruction with a scapular 3DPCMP and an inverse shoulder prosthesis

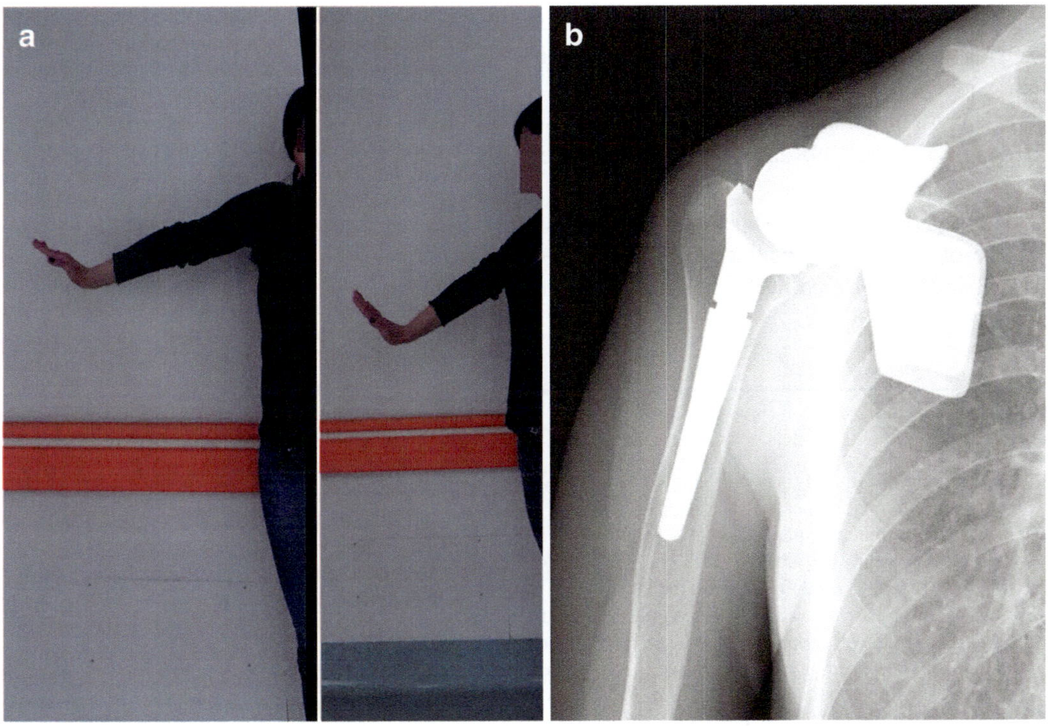

Fig. 8.8 (**a**) Function at 5 years pf follow-up; (**b**) X-ray showing the absence of signs of prosthesis mobilization

Reconstruction was performed using the 3DPTCMP for the scapula and a reverse shoulder prosthesis for the proximal humerus (Fig. 8.7c).

The final histology revealed a G3—central Chondrosarcoma.

Results: At 5 years of follow-up the patient is apparently free of disease, with a painless shoulder, and a satisfying function (active abduction: 70°, anterior active elevation: 60°) (Fig. 8.8a), no signs of prosthesis mobilization at X-ray (Fig. 8.8b).

8.3 Conclusion

For malignant tumors of the scapular region, limb salvage surgery has become, in the past years, the consensus procedure for most patients. Different types of wide shoulder girdle resections are often necessary, implying complex shoulder defects. Surgical reconstructive options and residual function depend on general status, age, type of resection, surgical experience. After extra-articular resection with important sacrifice of muscles and soft tissues, adult patients need standard or constrained implants, with generally poor functional results. In selected cases, inverse prostheses may offer an extremely effective range of motion, but the many possible complications have to be considered. Conventional megaprostheses in proximal humerus reconstruction, associated to synthetic mesh, are well proven options, with uncertain functional recovery.

In pediatric age, biological reconstruction of the proximal humerus (massive homograft, APC, vascularized fibular graft), achieve satisfactory bone stock recovery, with possible difficulties in the long term. Scapular homografts and recycled bone present many limitations and long-term difficulties.

The introduction of 3D-printed technology both in adults and in children seems to be useful and effective in trying to resolve the ancient problems: anatomical reconstructions, durable solutions and no limitation in term of size and site (partial or total resection), stressed this type of surgical options.

Despite this, after wide bone and soft tissue excision around the shoulder girdle, functional improvement is sometimes possible only associating a motor unit transfer. LD free- or rotational-flap seems to be reliable and effective, due to the inner anatomical structure.

This is particularly true in pediatric age, where the use of a titanium scapular 3D-printed prosthesis has to be covered by healthy and efficient muscles.

References

1. El Beaino M, Liu J, Lewis VO, Lin PP. Do early results of proximal humeral allograft-prosthetic composite reconstructions persist at 5-year follow-up? Clin Orthop Relat Res. 2019;477(4):758–65. https://doi.org/10.1097/CORR.0000000000000354.
2. Aponte-Tinao LA, Ayerza MA, Albergo JI, Farfalli GL. Do massive allograft reconstructions for tumors of the femur and tibia survive 10 or more years after implantation? Clin Orthop Relat Res. 2020;478(3):517–24. https://doi.org/10.1097/CORR.0000000000000806.
3. Enneking WF. General principles of musculoskeletal tumorsurgery. In: Enneking WF, editor. Musculoskeletal tumor surgery, vol. 1. New York: Churchill Livingstone; 1983. p. 3–68.
4. Wittig JC, Kellar-Graney KL, Malawer MM, Bickels J, Meller I. Limb-sparing surgery for high-grade sarcomas of the proximal humerus. Tech Shoulder Elbow Surg. 2001;2:54–69.
5. Malawer MM, Meller I, Dunham WK. A new surgical classification system for shoulder-girdle resections. Analysis of 38 patients. Clin Orthop Relat Res. 1991;(267):33–44.
6. Puchner SE, Panotopoulos J, Puchner R, Schuh R, Windhager R, Funovics PT. Primary malignant tumours of the scapula—a review of 29 cases. Int Orthop. 2014;38(10):2155–62. https://doi.org/10.1007/s00264-014-2417-8.
7. Hayashi K, Karita M, Yamamoto N, Shirai T, Nishida H, Takeuchi A, Kimura H, Miwa S, Tsuchiya H. Functional outcomes after total scapulectomy for malignant bone or soft tissue tumors in the shoulder girdle. Int J Clin Oncol. 2011;16(5):568–73. https://doi.org/10.1007/s10147-011-0229-z.
8. Malawer MM. Tumors of the shoulder girdle. Technique of resection and description of a surgical classification. Orthop Clin North Am. 1991;22(1):7–35.
9. Enneking WF, Dunham W, Gebhardt MC, Malawar M, Pritchard DJ. A system for the functional evaluation of reconstructive procedures after surgical treatment of tumors of the musculoskeletal system. Clin Orthop Relat Res. 1993;286:241–6.
10. Shehadeh A, Ja'afar A, Isleem U, Hamad A, Salem A. Shoulder girdle resection: surgical technique modification and introduction of a new classification system. World J Surg Oncol. 2019;17(1):107.
11. Guven MF, Aslan L, Botanlioglu H, Kaynak G, Kesmezacar H, Babacan M. Functional outcome of reverse shoulder tumor prosthesis in the treatment of proximal humerus tumors. J Shoulder Elbow Surg. 2016;25(1):e1–6. https://doi.org/10.1016/j.jse.2015.06.012.
12. Zhang K, Duan H, Xiang Z, Tu C. Surgical technique and clinical results for scapular allograft reconstruction following resection of scapular tumors. J Exp Clin Cancer Res. 2009;28:45.
13. Pritsch T, Bickels J, Wu CC, Squires MH, Malawer MM. Is scapular endoprosthesis functionally superior to humeral suspension? Clin Orthop Relat Res. 2007;456:188–95.
14. Fan H, Fu J, Li X, Pei Y, Li X, Pei G, Guo Z. Implantation of customized 3-D printed titanium prosthesis in limb salvage surgery: a case series and review of the literature. World J Surg Oncol. 2015;13:308.
15. Biazzo A, De Paolis M, Donati DM. Scapular reconstructions after resection for bone tumors: a single-institution experience and review of the literature. Acta Biomed. 2018;89(3):415–22.
16. Savvidou OD, Zampeli F, Georgopoulos G, Dimopoulos L, Antoniadou T, Papanastassiou I, Papagelopoulos PJ. Total scapulectomy and shoulder reconstruction using a scapular prosthesis and constrained reverse shoulder arthroplasty. Orthopedics. 2018;41(6):e888–93.
17. Bickels J, Wittig JC, Kollender Y, Kellar-Graney K, Meller I, Malawer MM. Limb-sparing resections of the shoulder girdle. J Am Coll Surg. 2002;194(4):422–35.
18. Schmolders J, Koob S, Schepers P, Kehrer M, Frey SP, Wirtz DC, Pennekamp PH, Strauss AC. Silver-coated endoprosthetic replacement of the proximal humerus in case of tumour-is there an increased risk of periprosthetic infection by using a trevira tube? Int Orthop. 2017;41(2):423–8. https://doi.org/10.1007/s00264-016-3329-6.
19. Avery BW, Pilon FM, Barclay JK. Anterior coracoscapular ligament and suprascapular nerve entrapment. Clin Anat. 2002 Nov;15(6):383–6.
20. Barco R, Savvidou OD, Sperling JW, Sanchez-Sotelo J, Cofield RH. Complications in reverse shoulder arthroplasty. EFORT Open Rev. 2016;1.
21. Pescador D, Blanco J, Corchado C, Jiménez M, Varela G, Borobio G, et al. Chondrosarcoma of the scapula secondary to radiodermatitis. Int J Surg Case Rep. 2012;3(4):134–6.
22. Pierce TD, Tomaino MM. Use of the pedicled latissimus muscle flap for upper-extremity reconstruction. J Am Acad Orthop Surg. 2000;8(5):324–31.
23. Sorger JI, Scharschmidt T, Rajani R, Randall RL. Bone tumors and reconstructive options in pediatric and young adult patients. Instr Course Lect. 2019;68:613–26.

24. Groundland JS, Binitie O. Reconstruction after tumor resection in the growing child. Orthop Clin North Am. 2016;47(1):265–81. https://doi.org/10.1016/j.ocl.2015.08.027.
25. Ogink PT, Teunissen FR, Massier JR, Raskin KA, Schwab JH, Lozano-Calderon SA. Allograft reconstruction of the humerus: complications and revision surgery. J Surg Oncol. 2019;119(3):329–35. https://doi.org/10.1002/jso.25309.
26. Lozano-Calderón SA. Outcome after reconstruction of the proximal humerus for tumor resection: a systematic review. Clin Orthop Relat Res. 2014;472(7):2245–53. https://doi.org/10.1007/s11999-014-3474-4.
27. Nishida J, Shimamura T. Methods of reconstruction for bone defect after tumor excision: a review of alternatives. Med Sci Monit. 2008;14(8):RA107–13.
28. Beltrami G, Ristori G, Scoccianti G, Tamburini A, Capanna R, Campanacci D, Innocenti M. Latissimus dorsi rotational flap combined with a custom-made scapular prosthesis after oncological surgical resection: a report of two patients. BMC Cancer. 2018;18(1):1003. https://doi.org/10.1186/s12885-018-4883-7.

9 3D Vertebral Prosthesis

Marco Girolami, Maria Sartori, Stefano Bandiera, Giovanni Barbanti-Brodano, Gisberto Evangelisti, Riccardo Ghermandi, Valerio Pipola, Giuseppe Tedesco, Silvia Terzi, Emanuela Asunis, Luigi Falzetti, Giovanni Tosini, Eleonora Pesce, Federica Trentin, Cristiana Griffoni, Donato Monopoli, Milena Fini, and Alessandro Gasbarrini

9.1 Introduction

In the last three decades there have been tremendous technical and technological advances that profoundly changed spine surgery, allowing what seemed to be impossible before. The spread of transpedicular segmental fixation paved the way for more complex reconstructions, thus allowing more aggressive approaches with emerging, in the spinal oncology community, of the role of en bloc resection with oncologically appropriate margins in the treatment of primary bone tumors. Given the encouraging results achieved in terms of local control and overall survival, increasing interest grew toward more refined reconstructions of the spine.

The advent of additive manufacturing techniques with their unparalleled versatility, have offered a very attractive prospect in the reconstruction of substance losses, such as those produced by the resection of musculoskeletal neoplasms.

9.2 3D-Printing in Spine: Review

3D-printing found several applications in the field of spine surgery. Several Authors asserted the value of preoperative modeling [1] that would be useful to ease understanding of patient anatomy, particularly in those cases where this is such altered by the underlying pathology that standard landmarks cannot be considered reliable. This includes complex spinal deformities such as severe kyphoscoliosis [1, 2], craniovertebral junction anomalies [1, 3], or spinal tumors [4, 5].

M. Girolami (✉) · S. Bandiera · G. Barbanti-Brodano
G. Evangelisti · R. Ghermandi · V. Pipola
G. Tedesco · S. Terzi · E. Asunis · L. Falzetti
G. Tosini · E. Pesce · F. Trentin · C. Griffoni
A. Gasbarrini
Department of Oncologic and Degenerative Spine Surgery, IRCCS Istituto Ortopedico Rizzoli, Bologna, Italy
e-mail: marco.girolami@ior.it; giovanni@barbantibrodano.com; gisberto.evangelisti@ior.it; riccardo.ghermandi@ior.it; giuseppe.tedesco@ior.it; silvia.terzi@ior.it; giovanni.tosini@ior.it; cristiana.griffoni@ior.it; gasbarrini@me.com

M. Sartori · M. Fini
Complex Structure of Surgical Sciences and Technologies, IRCCS Istituto Ortopedico Rizzoli, Bologna, Italy
e-mail: maria.sartori@ior.it; milena.fini@ior.it

D. Monopoli
Instituto Tecnológico de Canarias (ITC), Canary Island, Spain
e-mail: dmonopoli@itccanarias.org

C. Zoccali et al. (eds.), *3D Printing in Bone Surgery*, https://doi.org/10.1007/978-3-030-91900-9_9

Such models can be used for training purposes prior to surgery [3, 6, 7] (or interventional procedures [8]) and prepare the sizes of the implants that may be necessary. Moreover, they can even be sterilized to make them available on the surgical field [1] to work as an additional reference tool to enhance safety of otherwise standard procedures, such as free-hand pedicle screw placement [1, 9]. Moreover, the use of printed models has been advocated as a teaching tool with patient to further aid in their education and counseling.

Further advance of the application of 3D-printing into clinical practice has been production of patient-specific tools to guide execution of procedures (mainly complex spinal three-column osteotomies [9] or screw placement [10–13]) in such challenging scenarios.

The ultimate frontier has been application of 3D-printing technology to production of implants and prosthetic devices. Although this technology perfectly fits with the demanding needs of personalized reconstruction after tumor resection [14–19], it has been nowadays widely applied by several companies on large-scale production of standard off-the-shelf devices, mainly interbody cages (i.e., Tritanium® Stryker, Conduit™ DePuy Synthes/Johnson&Johnson, etc).

9.3 En Bloc Resection

En bloc resection is a complex surgical procedure aiming at removal of a tumor in single piece (Fig. 9.1). It is indicated in:

- benign aggressive [20, 21] (Enneking stage 3, i.e., giant cell tumors, osteoblastoma);
- malignant primary bone tumors [22–24] (i.e., chordoma, chondrosarcoma, osteosarcoma, Ewing sarcoma);
- highly selected cases of spinal metastases [25] (i.e., solitary metastasis from clear cell renal carcinoma).

According to where dissection is carried out, resection will be:

- *marginal*, when it is carried out along the capsule (or through the reactive peritumoral pseudocapsule),
- *wide*, when a thick layer of peripheral healthy tissue, or an anatomic barrier not yet infiltrated by the tumor (i.e., pleura of fascia) fully covers the tumor.

If the tumor is violated by planned (in order to save important neurovascular structures) or unplanned transgression, then resection is en bloc *intralesional*.

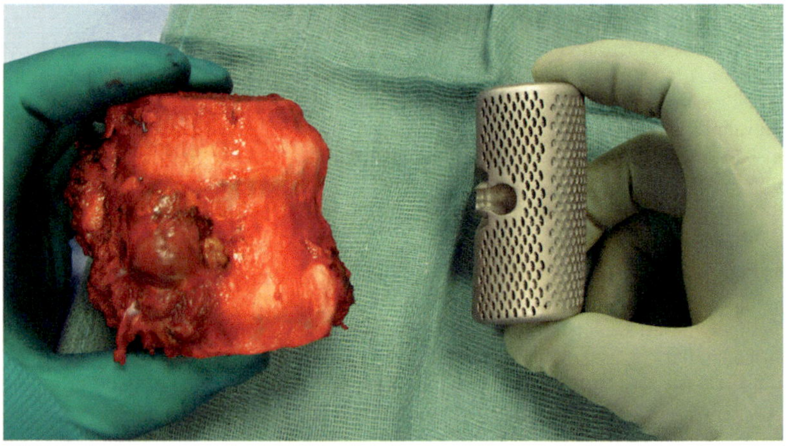

Fig. 9.1 En bloc resection is a complex surgical procedure aiming at removal of a tumor in single piece

Oncological appropriateness of a resection is assessed by the pathologist after evaluation of the margins [26, 27] of the surgical specimen with respect to the diagnosis.

According to the Weinstein-Boriani-Biagini (WBB) surgical staging system [28], 7 types of en bloc resections in the spine have been described.

9.4 Anterior Column Reconstruction: Goals and Options

The multiple options that have been described for anterior column reconstruction can be roughly split into two groups: biological and prosthetic options.

Nevertheless, goals of reconstruction are: (1) restoration the load-bearing capacity of the anterior column, (2) fill the bone loss with appropriate segmental alignment.

9.4.1 Biological Options (Bone Grafts)

Bone grafts are cheap, very versatile, and have great potential for osteointegration. Use of bone grafts from the same patient (autograft) is restricted by the limited amount of bone that can be harvested (especially for structural grafts). Moreover, painful sequelae at the donor site are exceedingly common. For these reasons this option is not recommended nowadays for routine use.

Use of bone grafts from donors (allograft) is preferred because allows to overcome these limitations. They are stored in muscoloskeletal tissue banks, thus available in any amount without sequelae for the patient except for a negligible (but unavoidable) risk of disease transmission.

The major drawback of the use of structural bone grafts is that connection to the posterior instrumentation might be challenging, so protection with anterior plating is advisable to avoid segmental kyphosis during the creeping substitution phase.

Vascularized bone grafts (i.e., rib or fibular flaps) have been used successfully but mostly as a biological adjunct in order to enhance potential for osseointegration of large allografts, rather than as structural bone grafts itself.

9.4.2 Prosthetic Options

This group includes very different devices that were created in order to overcome the limitations of the use of bone grafts, and whose design progressively evolved from one another. None of these options has been proven to be overall better than the others, but each of these has a specific profile of pros and cons.

Titanium mesh cages are the classical options that have been successfully used to span deficiencies in the anterior column in a wide variety of pathologies (trauma, tumors, infections, or deformities). These cages are available in long segments that can be cut intraoperatively to the size of the actual bone loss, from simple discectomies for interbody fusion to resection of several vertebral bodies. They allow immediate weight-bearing and potential for osteointegration since can be packed with cancellous bone graft.

Carbon fiber modular cages represent another commonly used option, especially in oncology cases, because allows optimal adjuvant radiation therapy protocols since scattering in the postoperative imaging is minimal (given the low atomic number of the carbon). Moreover, carbon fiber proved to enhance fusion on long-term follow-up. The main drawback that limits its use is the high cost of the implants.

Expandable cages emerged with the rise of minimally invasive approaches in the last decade. Their main advantage is represented by the possibility to place them through minimally invasive approaches and to expand them in situ to the final size. However, limitations are represented by the small amount of bone graft that can be packed around the cage for anterior fusion, and by high costs.

Polymethyl-methacrylate (PMMA) is another classic option reported as suitable for short life expectancy patients, because of good resistance to compression and low costs without any potential for osteointegration.

9.5 Preoperative Planning and Implant Design

Design of the prosthesis starts from a preoperative thin-cut (1–1.5 mm) computed tomography (CT) that allows evaluation of the patient-specific anatomy such as shape, width, and length of the endplates, so as the extent of the planned resection. Based on these data, a computer-aided design (CAD) model of the spine is generated and a virtual implant is designed (Fig. 9.2). Opportunity to visualize a virtual model prior to realization allows further refinements (i.e., fixation technique) until the final version can be produced. Finally, the approved model can be fabricated by successive layering of melted Ti_6Al_4V powder (Arcam AB, Mölndal, Sweden).

9.6 3D-Printed Reconstruction After Surgery for Spinal Tumors

Authors already reported on their preliminary results on the use of 3D-printed implants for anterior column reconstruction after en bloc resection for spinal tumors in the thoracolumbar

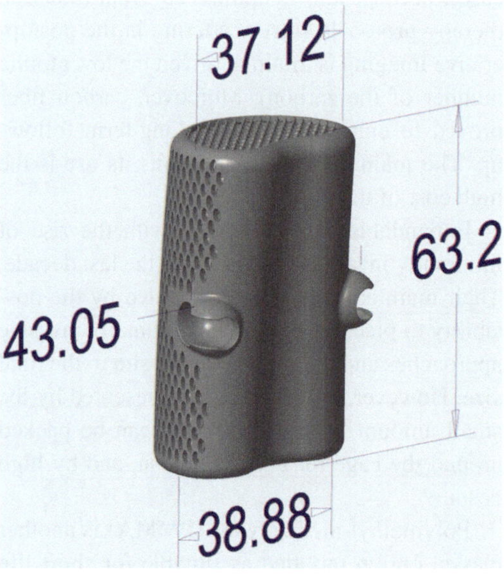

Fig. 9.2 A virtual implant is designed on a computer-aided design (CAD) model of the spine

from November 2015 to June 2017 [29]. Since then, reconstruction with 3D-printed implants has been performed in 11 more patients treated for spinal tumors: in 9 of these it was following en bloc resection (8 in the thoracolumbar spine—Figs. 9.3, 9.4, 9.5, and 9.6 and following—and 1 in the sacrum), and in the remaining 2 after extracapsular debulkings in the upper cervical spine (C2 in both cases).

9.6.1 3D-Printed Vertebral Prosthesis: Pros

- Immediate availability of custom-made implant of the proper size, that exactly reflects the dimension and shape of the resected specimen makes reconstruction quicker;
- 3D-printing allows design of the fine details that are expected to promote bone ingrowth such as size and shape of fenestrations and porosity of the metal; these features can be replicated all along the inner- and outermost surfaces of the implant;
- progressive layering process allows production of a lattice structure of such regularity that only a minimal percentage (up to <10%) of the actual volume of the implant is occupied by titanium, leaving a high potential for bone ingrowth;
- opportunity to design custom-made fixation strategies, especially at the lumbosacral junction or the upper cervical spine.

9.6.2 3D-Printed Vertebral Prosthesis: Cons

- preoperative planning must be meticulously respected in order not to have mismatch between the resected specimen and the prosthesis (availability of an alternative reconstructive option is strongly suggested in case an unpredictable situation forces to an intraoperative change of the surgical plan);
- timing of production must be taken into account when reconstruction is planned for oncologic disease, since biology of the tumor

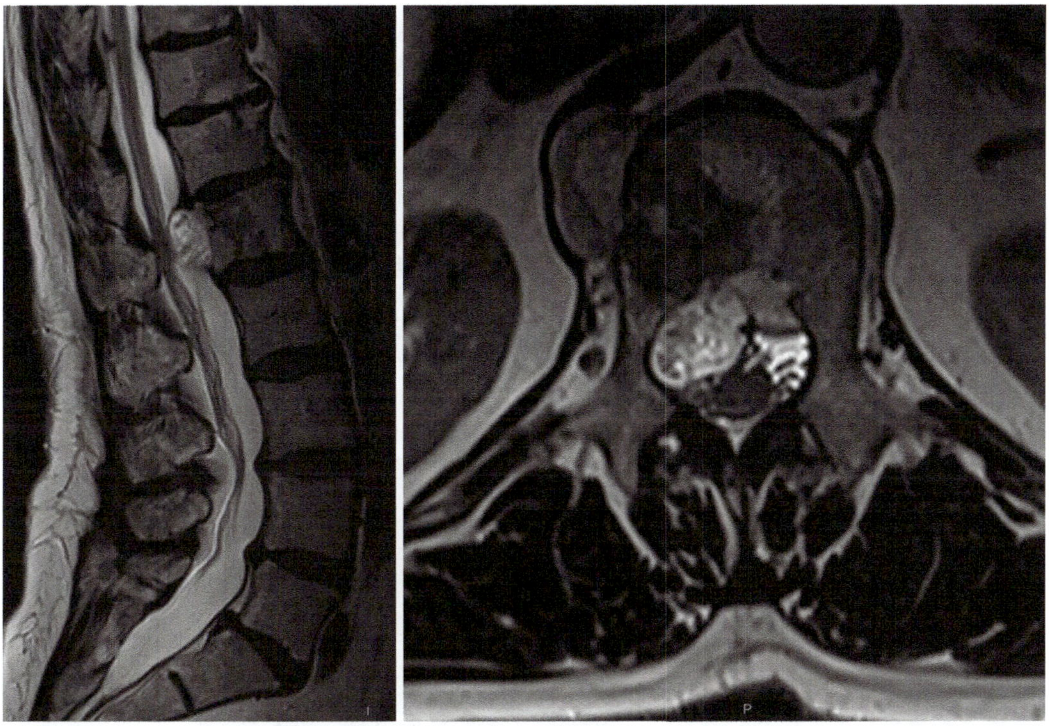

Fig. 9.3 73-years-old female patient affected by L1 chordoma. Preoperative magnetic resonance imaging (MRI) showing prevertebral (layer A) and epidural (layer D) extracompartmental extensions of the tumor

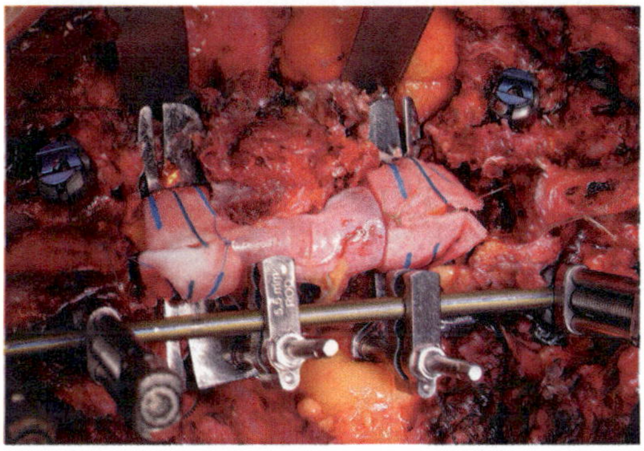

Fig. 9.4 Surgery was performed as one stage posterior-only procedure (type 2B)

progresses in the meanwhile of realization of the prosthesis.

It is Authors' belief that resection technique itself plays a significant role even in the reconstruction. In fact, ability to achieve smooth surfaces where to reconstruct on allows maximization of the contact area between host bone and prosthesis, decreasing stress concentration, thus impacting on possibility to achieve a solid primary stability. Therefore, in Authors' practice, all the osteotomies are performed using thread-wire saws with a dedicated device for spinal cord protection (except for the vertical osteotomy in sagittal resections).

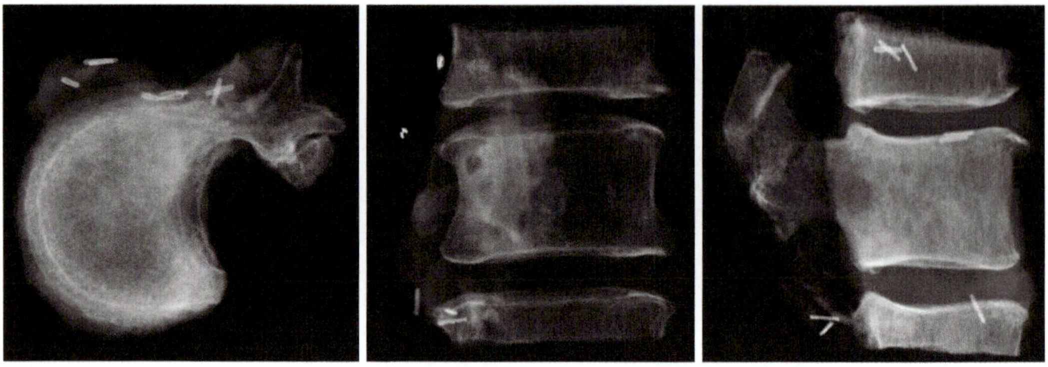

Fig. 9.5 Pathologic examination on the surgical specimen reported wide margins

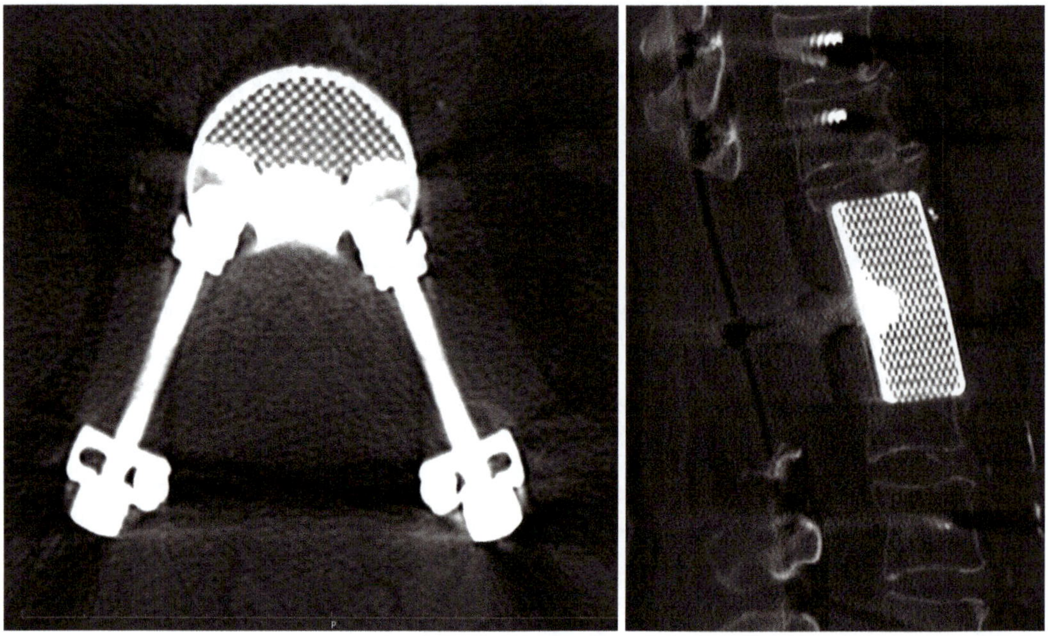

Fig. 9.6 Postoperative CT scan

Acknowledgments The Authors acknowledge the invaluable contribution of Carlo Piovani for patient storage and data collection.

Conflicts of Interest Donato Monopoli-Forleo is employed as a researcher at Instituto Tecnológico de Canarias (ITC), Canary Island, Spain.

Disclosure of Funding This study was partly funded by National Funding Organisations (Ministero della Salute – IMH) under the frame of EuroNanoMed III Project "Next generation antibacterial nanostructured osseointegrated customized vertebral replacement – NANOVERTEBRA" Joint Transnational call for proposals (JTC 2018).

References

1. Galvez M, Asahi T, Baar A, et al. Use of three-dimensional printing in Orthopaedic surgical planning. J Am Acad Orthop Surg Glob Res Rev. 2018;2(5):e071. https://doi.org/10.5435/JAAOSGlobal-D-17-00071.
2. Tan LA, Yerneni K, Tuchman A, et al. Utilization of the 3D-printed spine model for freehand pedicle screw placement in complex spinal deformity correction. J Spine Surg. 2018;4(2):319–27. https://doi.org/10.21037/jss.2018.05.16.
3. Gao F, Wang Q, Liu C, Xiong B, Luo T. Individualized 3D printed model-assisted posterior screw fixation

for the treatment of craniovertebral junction abnormality: a retrospective study. J Neurosurg Spine. 2017;27(1):29–34. https://doi.org/10.3171/2016.11.SPINE16713.

4. Xiao JR, Huang WD, Yang XH, et al. En bloc resection of primary malignant bone tumor in the cervical spine based on 3-dimensional printing technology. Orthop Surg. 2016;8(2):171–8. https://doi.org/10.1111/os.12234.
5. Parr WCH, Burnard JL, Singh T, McEvoy A, Walsh WR, Mobbs RJ. C3-C5 Chordoma resection and reconstruction with a three-dimensional printed titanium patient-specific implant. World Neurosurg. 2020;136:226–33. https://doi.org/10.1016/j.wneu.2019.11.167.
6. Park HJ, Wang C, Choi KH, Kim HN. Use of a life-size three-dimensional-printed spine model for pedicle screw instrumentation training [published correction appears in J Orthop Surg Res. 2021 May 8;16(1):303]. J Orthop Surg Res. 2018;13(1):86. https://doi.org/10.1186/s13018-018-0788-z.
7. Ling Q, He E, Ouyang H, Guo J, Yin Z, Huang W. Design of mulitlevel OLF approach ("V"-shaped decompressive laminoplasty) based on 3D printing technology. Eur Spine J. 2018;27(Suppl 3):323–9. https://doi.org/10.1007/s00586-017-5234-0.
8. Taverner MG, Monagle JP. Three-dimensional printing: an aid to epidural access for neuromodulation. Neuromodulation. 2017;20(6):622–6. https://doi.org/10.1111/ner.12600.
9. Pijpker PAJ, Kuijlen JMA, Kraeima J, Faber C. Three-dimensional planning and use of individualized osteotomy-guiding templates for surgical correction of kyphoscoliosis: a technical case report. World Neurosurg. 2018;119:113–7. https://doi.org/10.1016/j.wneu.2018.07.219.
10. Wang D, Wang Y, Wang J, et al. Design and fabrication of a precision template for spine surgery using selective laser melting (SLM). Materials (Basel). 2016;9(7):608. https://doi.org/10.3390/ma9070608.
11. Liu K, Zhang Q, Li X, et al. Preliminary application of a multi-level 3D printing drill guide template for pedicle screw placement in severe and rigid scoliosis. Eur Spine J. 2017;26(6):1684–9. https://doi.org/10.1007/s00586-016-4926-1.
12. Mobbs RJ, Choy WJ, Singh T, et al. Three-dimensional planning and patient-specific drill guides for repair of spondylolysis/L5 pars defect. World Neurosurg. 2019;132:75–80. https://doi.org/10.1016/j.wneu.2019.08.112.
13. Kim J, Rajadurai J, Choy WJ, et al. Three-dimensional patient-specific guides for intraoperative navigation for cortical screw trajectory pedicle fixation. World Neurosurg. 2019;122:674–9. https://doi.org/10.1016/j.wneu.2018.11.159.
14. Xu N, Wei F, Liu X, et al. Reconstruction of the upper cervical spine using a personalized 3D-printed vertebral body in an adolescent with Ewing sarcoma. Spine (Phila Pa 1976). 2016;41(1):E50–4. https://doi.org/10.1097/BRS.0000000000001179.
15. Li X, Wang Y, Zhao Y, Liu J, Xiao S, Mao K. Multilevel 3D printing implant for reconstructing cervical spine with metastatic papillary thyroid carcinoma. Spine (Phila Pa 1976). 2017;42(22):E1326–30. https://doi.org/10.1097/BRS.0000000000002229.
16. Mobbs RJ, Coughlan M, Thompson R, Sutterlin CE III, Phan K. The utility of 3D printing for surgical planning and patient-specific implant design for complex spinal pathologies: case report. J Neurosurg Spine. 2017;26(4):513–8. https://doi.org/10.3171/2016.9.SPINE16371.
17. Choy WJ, Mobbs RJ, Wilcox B, Phan S, Phan K, Sutterlin CE 3rd. Reconstruction of thoracic spine using a personalized 3D-printed vertebral body in adolescent with T9 primary bone tumor. World Neurosurg. 2017;105:1032.e13–7. https://doi.org/10.1016/j.wneu.2017.05.133.
18. Wei R, Guo W, Ji T, Zhang Y, Liang H. One-step reconstruction with a 3D-printed, custom-made prosthesis after total en bloc sacrectomy: a technical note. Eur Spine J. 2017;26(7):1902–9. https://doi.org/10.1007/s00586-016-4871-z.
19. Kim D, Lim JY, Shim KW, et al. Sacral reconstruction with a 3D-printed implant after Hemisacrectomy in a patient with sacral osteosarcoma: 1-year follow-up result. Yonsei Med J. 2017;58(2):453–7. https://doi.org/10.3349/ymj.2017.58.2.453.
20. Charest-Morin R, Fisher CG, Varga PP, et al. En bloc resection versus Intralesional surgery in the treatment of Giant cell tumor of the spine. Spine (Phila Pa 1976). 2017;42(18):1383–90. https://doi.org/10.1097/BRS.0000000000002094.
21. Versteeg AL, Dea N, Boriani S, et al. Surgical management of spinal osteoblastomas. J Neurosurg Spine. 2017;27(3):321–7. https://doi.org/10.3171/2017.1.SPINE16788.
22. Dekutoski MB, Clarke MJ, Rose P, et al. Osteosarcoma of the spine: prognostic variables for local recurrence and overall survival, a multicenter ambispective study. J Neurosurg Spine. 2016;25(1):59–68. https://doi.org/10.3171/2015.11.SPINE15870.
23. Fisher CG, Versteeg AL, Dea N, et al. Surgical management of spinal chondrosarcomas. Spine (Phila Pa 1976). 2016;41(8):678–85. https://doi.org/10.1097/BRS.0000000000001485.
24. Gokaslan ZL, Zadnik PL, Sciubba DM, et al. Mobile spine chordoma: results of 166 patients from the AOSpine knowledge forum tumor database. J Neurosurg Spine. 2016;24(4):644–51. https://doi.org/10.3171/2015.7.SPINE15201.
25. Tomita K, Toribatake Y, Kawahara N, Ohnari H, Kose H. Total en bloc spondylectomy and circumspinal decompression for solitary spinal metastasis. Paraplegia. 1994;32(1):36–46. https://doi.org/10.1038/sc.1994.7.
26. Enneking WF, Spanier SS, Goodman MA. A system for the surgical staging of musculoskeletal sarcoma. Clin Orthop Relat Res. 1980;(153):106–20.
27. Boriani S, Weinstein JN, Biagini R. Primary bone tumors of the spine. Terminology and surgical stag-

ing. Spine (Phila Pa 1976). 1997;22(9):1036–44. https://doi.org/10.1097/00007632-199705010-00020.
28. Boriani S. *En bloc* resection in the spine: a procedure of surgical oncology. J Spine Surg. 2018;4(3):668–76. https://doi.org/10.21037/jss.2018.09.02.
29. Girolami M, Boriani S, Bandiera S, et al. Biomimetic 3D-printed custom-made prosthesis for anterior column reconstruction in the thoracolumbar spine: a tailored option following en bloc resection for spinal tumors: preliminary results on a case-series of 13 patients. Eur Spine J. 2018;27(12):3073–83. https://doi.org/10.1007/s00586-018-5708-8.

3D Skull Prosthesis 10

Riccardo Boccaletti and Domenico Policicchio

Abbreviations

CAD/CAM	Computer aided design/computer aided manufacturing
HA	Hydroxyapatite
PEEK	Poly ether ether ketone
PMMA	Polymethylmethacrylate
VASC	Visual analog scale for cosmesis

10.1 Introduction

Over the past three decades, management of patients with cranial defects (cranio-lacunia) has become a very common problem in neurosurgery. The "historical" clinical indications for patients with primary and secondary neoplasms of the skull, trauma or infection whether primary or post-surgical, are nowadays associated with increased indications of decompressive craniotomy for the treatment of malignant endocranial hypertension of various origins (severe head injuries, ischemic and haemorrhagic strokes, cerebral venous thrombosis, subarachnoid haemorrhages, infectious meningo-encephalic processes) [1–5]. Numbers of patients with bone defects have also increased as a result of improvements in the neuro-resuscitation management of serious pathologies in which decompressive craniectomy has, along with advanced intensive medical methods, brought about a higher survival rate of patients with extremely serious acute cerebral pathological events. This has determined the need for neurosurgical treatment for reconstruction of the cranial defect (delayed cranioplasty). In cases of elective pathologies, in the preoperative phase, it is possible to define the extent of the bone defect and prepare the artificial prosthesis before surgery in order to perform the resection and reconstruction treatment in a single surgical procedure (single step surgery: resection-reconstruction).

The reconstruction of the cranial defect has two main purposes: to ensure adequate protection of the encephalic structures and to restore the aesthetic aspect. However, it is nonetheless important to take into account the restoration of the physical conditions of the contents of the skull. From the literature data it emerges that reconstruction of the cranial defect determines an improvement in the neurological and neuropsychological outcome of the patient, in both the short term and the long term after the traumatic event ("Trephined Syndrome") [1, 6–8]. This clinical improvement is due to the restoration of normal intracranial pressure, with recovery of self-regulation of cerebral blood flow and its normal circulation.

R. Boccaletti · D. Policicchio (✉)
Department of Neurosurgery, Azienda Ospedaliero Universitaria di Sassari, Sassari, Italy
e-mail: riccardo.boccaletti@aousassari.it; domenico.policicchio@aousassari.it

C. Zoccali et al. (eds.), *3D Printing in Bone Surgery*, https://doi.org/10.1007/978-3-030-91900-9_10

Both clinical experience and plentiful literature data show that the operation of cranial reconstruction, or cranioplasty, may appear to be considered a technically simple surgery with low risk of complications. On the contrary, it is clearly burdened by a higher complication rate than the simple elective craniotomy: 10–20% and 5–7% respectively [1, 2, 4, 5, 9–11]. The reason for this greater morbidity (variable according to the case studies considered) is largely due to the different clinical conditions of the patients undergoing cranial reconstruction. Normally, in fact, they present outcomes of serious encephalic pathologies (severe head injuries, haemorrhages or cerebral ischemia), with long periods of hospitalization in Intensive Care, high incidence of systemic infections and metabolic alterations, frequent local chronic inflammatory phenomena that compromise the local skin trophism (lacerated-contusive wounds, incisions for ventriculostomy and/or ICP monitoring, previous major intervention, subgaleal hematomas, CSF fistula, etc.).

Besides the inadequate aesthetic result, the main complications of cranioplasty include the far more serious postsurgical haematomas, infections and reabsorption of the dural graft with CSF fistola, and ischemic skin changes with delayed healing. All of these frequently require surgical revision with the eventual removal of the artificial operculum (Fig. 10.1) and the need for a reconstruction intervention.

At the present time management of patients with cranial bone defect requires considerable attention as there is still no agreement on surgical timing, nor on the operating technique or the materials to be used for cranioplasty. Clinical and engineering studies are needed in order to determine the most suitable techniques and materials to optimize results.

Theoretically, the success of cranioplastic surgery necessitates careful selection of the prosthesis: it should be tailored to the patient's clinical scenario, made with a material ideally malleable, sterilizable, non-magnetic, radiolucent, light but resistant and easy to fix stably to the skull bone.

On the market at present there is a wide range of prostheses suitable for use in cranioplastic surgery.

These may be divided into two general categories: autograft (autologous grafts) and allograft (heterologous grafts), that is, bone substitutes comprising a heterogeneous group of biomaterials (PMMA: polymethyl methacrylate, HA hydroxyapatite, titanium). Autologous grafts (autograft) are portions of autologous bone tissue taken from different areas of the skeleton at the same time as the reconstructive surgery. Depending on the size, shape and location of the bone defect, it is possible to use the bone operculum made at the time of the decompressive craniectomy, or portions of calvaria taken from areas adjacent to the craniectomy site, or bone portions taken from the ribs or from long bones of the inferior limbs (usually the tibia). In the case of large superficial cranial defects the use of the cranial operculum, or parts of the calvaria, enables closure of the skull and gives relatively qualitative cosmetic results. On the other hand, smaller deeper defects resulting in minor aesthetic impact may be closed by taking bone portions from other skeletal sites.

Theoretically, the autologous bone flap, obtained during the first surgery (clean craniectomies), is the ideal "prosthesis" for cranial reconstruction due to the fact that it does not present biological incompatibility, its shape is perfect for restoring normal cosmetics, and it ensures immediate and adequate protection for intracranial structures. Since the new guidelines for biological material conservation, autologous bone flap have been stored in the abdominal wall of the patient's subcutaneous pocketing. Having become obsolete as a method at least in Western countries, the autologous bone flaps are now cryopreserved in certified bone storage banks. Despite strict methodological and organizational procedures, many difficulties still arise in adequately storing the bone flaps. Infact, it has been reported that autografts have rather high failure rates related to infection or reabsorption [3, 4, 10–13]. In both cases, many patients must be reoperated for the removal of the infected or

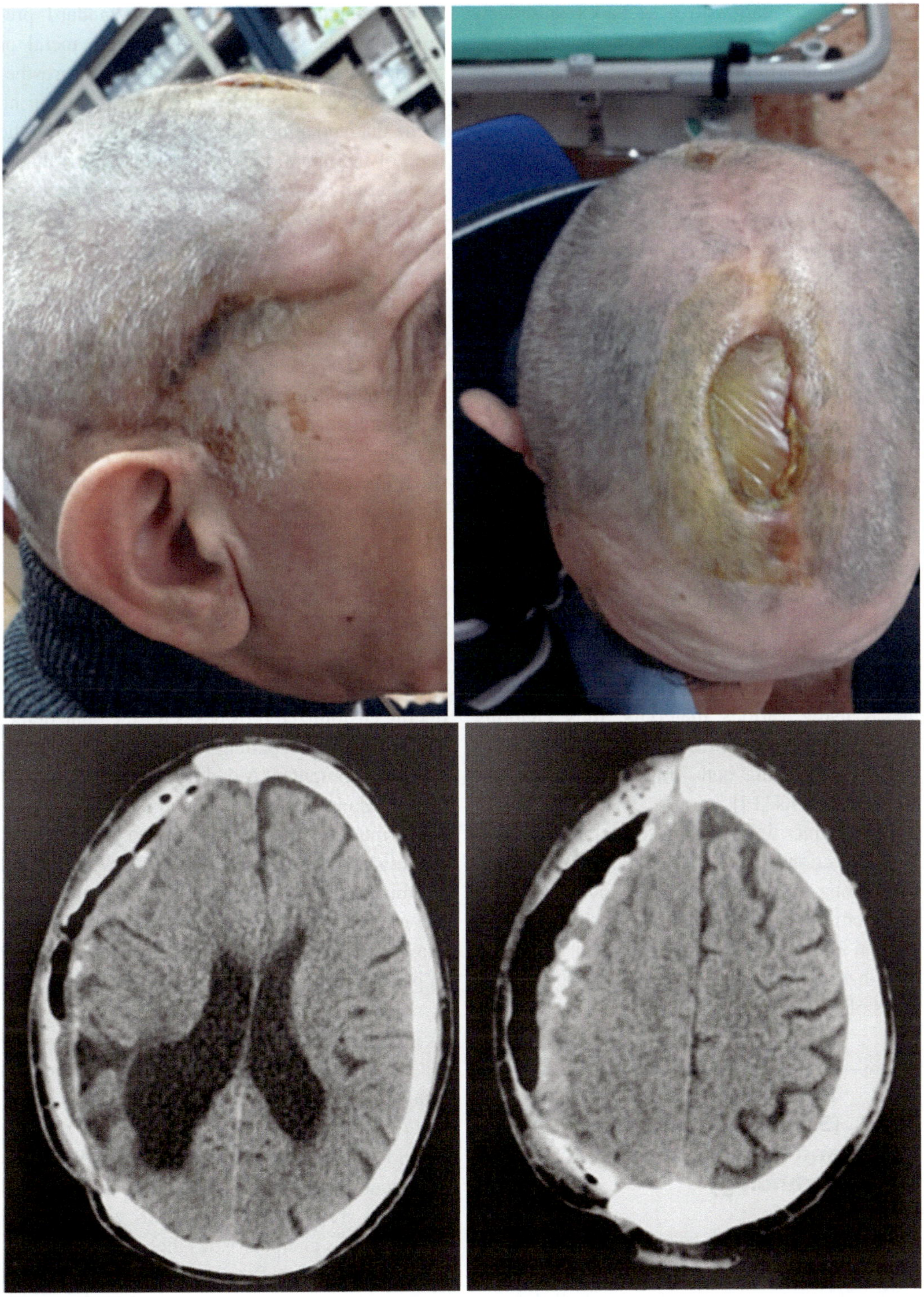

Fig. 10.1 Example of delayed complications (3 years after surgery): wound dehiscence with exposure of underlying PMMA prosthesis, CT scan reveal subdural air and fluid collection secondary to infection

resorped bone flap with a second cranioplasty procedure, with its related problems. For these reasons, many biomaterials have been used for cranial reconstruction over the years. The most common are hydroxyapatite (HA), polymethylmethacrylate (PMMA), PEEK and titanium [1, 3–5, 8, 13]. Each of these has its own advantages and disadvantages in terms of clinical results, manufacturing feasibility, costs, and ease of use in the operating room. The choice of the prosthesis would mainly depend on the patient's clinical status, the experience and preference of the surgeon, clinical-based evidence, as well as on hospital financial resources and availability. Regardless of the type of construction material, allograft scan be constructed using two different techniques: malleable standard pre-curved mesh prostheses that are manually shaped and adapted to the patient's bone defect and 3D-printed custom-made prostheses. The two types of prosthesis can be used in various ways and with different indications, and differ in costs and results. The use of 3D printing technology has recently facilitated the construction of customized prostheses using various materials, thus enabling more patients to benefit from this technology as well as optimizing both clinical-functional and aesthetic results [14].

The chapter will consider technical aspects of the production of customized cranial prostheses, indications for their use, the surgical implantation technique and results in terms of cosmetics, clinical complications and costs, and will compare these results with those relating to the other types of cranioplastics.

10.2 Types of Cranial Prosthesis (Standard Pre-Curved and Custom-Made). 3D Technology

Today, apart from autograft, there are different kinds of cranial prosthesis available on the market for the reconstruction of bone skull defects. Regardless of the production material, the construction methods fall into two categories: (a) manually moldable and standard pre-curved meshes and (b) custom-made prostheses.

The manually moldable and standard pre-curved meshes are standard laminar, metal or plastic, quadrangular, flat or pre-curved prostheses, which are adapted to the patient by cutting them out and modelling them manually at the time of implantation so as to make them adhere to the cranial surface and match the bone defect as best as possible. The pre-curved meshes are similar to the standard flat titanium mashes, but produced in various standard pre-cut shapes suitable for covering standard bone defects in the front-temporal, parietal, occipital and frontal region and whose curvature is created on the reference of a standard skull. Likewise, in this case, it is usually necessary to model the mesh in order to adapt it as best as possible to the bone defect. Such prostheses obviously have advantages and disadvantages which will be discussed in detail in the next sections. In general, the most obvious feature is that, in the reconstruction procedures of complex cranial and craniofacial defects with irregular shapes, it is very difficult to adapt these implants to the cranial surface. For this reason, production of allograft prostheses turned to producing customized prostheses for the bone defect of each individual patient using CAD/CAM techniques (Computer Aided Design / Computer Aided Manufacturing). Many techniques have been introduced for customized cranioplasty manufacturing. One of the most widely used combines medical imaging and three-dimensional bio-modelling (3D printing customized titanium prosthesis), permitting the development of a sort of personalized cranioplastic surgery. With three-dimensional (3D) printing it has become possible to produce customized, precisely fitting cranioplastic implants. They derive from 3D medical images (CT or MRI) feeding 3D printers.

Over the past few years, the use of 3D printing technology for customized cranial prostheses has significantly increased. The most widely used materials are HA, PMMA, PEEK and titanium. The latter has characteristics that make it particularly suitable for the needs of neurosurgical patients: low rate of infection, high and immediate biomechanical resistance creating a good protection for the brain in the case of trauma, and suitability for postoperative imaging studies [3, 5, 9, 15].

Custom-made titanium prostheses are made using Additive Manufacturing and titanium alloy powder (Ti6Al4V—ELI) as raw material. The technology uses the EBM (Electron Beam Melting) process resulting in prostheses with excellent mechanical and biological osteo-integrating properties. EBM is the acronym for Electron Beam Melting, i.e. electron beam fusion, and indicates a 3D printing technique in which a suitably concentrated high energy electron beam hits a bed of titanium powder, causing it to melt. This technology offers a wide scope for design in terms of both spatial conformation and structure, allowing not only the shape but also the structure to be customized to the needs of each patient. In this way the constraints and limits imposed by traditional construction technologies can be easily overcome. Furthermore it has been shown that by varying the geometric parameters of the trabeculae, i.e. by creating differential porosity, osteo-integration of the prosthesis is optimized. This occurs because cell migration and tissue colonization of the same is facilitated, as well as a more efficient neo-vascularization with consequent improvements in oxygenation, the diffusion of nutrients and growth factors all of which stimulate the bone neo-formation process and weight reduction, all the while maintaining an important primary resistance and stability. It should be remembered that in addition to its excellent proven bio-integrative properties, titanium has a characteristically high mechanical resistance and flexibility, is resistant to bacterial colonization, and its radio-transparency makes it compatible with CT and MRI which are the most widely used radiological methods today in the follow up of neurosurgical patients.

The production process of customized prostheses involves various steps. Firstly, the patient with craniolacunia undergoes a CT scan of the skull obtained with a thin layer volumetric technique including the whole skull. The examination can be performed at any time during the patient's clinical course since the state of the parenchyma (brain swelling, oedema, bleeding, infection, etc.) does not affect the process of defining the three-dimensional geometric definition of the craniolacunia. The CT scan study is stored in DICOM format (Digital Images and Communications in Medicine) which generates an interface between the medical equipment and any other device to visualize the images. Images are processed using a bone filter so as to observe only the bone structure. The next phase involves the development of a three-dimensional reconstruction of the patient's skull that highlights the area of bone defect. The initial imaging of the prosthesis is then generated by a digital subtraction mirror-imaging process, based on the "normal" feature of the patient's cranium. The shape and dimension of the "ideal" prosthesis is processed step by step. This virtual model will be used as a framework for the manufacturing of the titanium model. The third phase involves the technicians responsible for the design of the prosthesis who, working remotely and in collaboration with the surgeon, carry out the definitive project, if necessary redefining the shape and porosity of the prosthesis, identifying the seat, the number and the length of the anchoring flaps. The definitive project is contextually reevaluated, and if correct, approved and then sent to production [14]. The titanium prosthesis will therefore have a variably porous and perforated structure (10 perforations per cm^2); it will guarantee a perfect fitting in the bone defect, with high congruence precision along the contours, so no intraoperative modification will be necessary; it will be equipped with small pre-perforated 1 mm thick tabs/flaps (4–6 anchoring points) with holes to accommodate the titanium fixing screws which are self-perforating and self-tapping, with a diameter of 1,5mm and 3mm long. Finally, the prosthesis will be delivered in a non-sterile package which is autoclavable at 134° and which indicates a unique identification code relating to the patient. The average production time from the acquisition of the CT scan to delivery to the hospital is about 15–20 days.

10.3 Indications for Use

The optimal cranial prosthesis must guarantee the following objectives: protection of the brain and restoration of the aesthetic aspect. Given the high rate of complications in cranial reconstructive surgery, both in the short and long term, it is essential to use surgical materials and techniques that guarantee good results even after some time.

Two types of patients should be considered: (a) patients undergoing decompression craniotomy (who will need "late" reconstruction of the cranial bone defect (delayed cranioplasty); (b) patients undergoing cranial bone resection surgery for primary or secondary neoplastic disease, whether infectious or traumatic, in which the cranial reconstruction may be performed during the same surgery (single step resection-reconstruction).

Theoretically, in patients with cranial defect secondary to decompressive craniotomy, the autologous bone flap is recommendable for cranial reconstruction as it does not present problems of rejection, its shape and dimensions are ideal to restore aesthetics and its adequate plating provides immediate protection of the brain, making reconstructive surgery quick and simple. For a long time this method has been considered the gold standard. Initially the bone operculum taken during the decompression operation was preserved in a subcutaneous pocket at the abdominal level. Subsequently, in line with the new directives on the conservation of biological tissues, this method was replaced with cryo-conservation in special certified bio-banks.

Although both procedures have been widely used, and there are several reports in literature that document their relative efficacy and safety [15–18], the accumulation of experiences in the various territorial conditions and the progressive increase in the duration of the follow-up have made it clear that use of the autologous bone flap has a fairly high failure rate in the long term. These failures are mainly due to infections (osteomyelitis) and bone reabsorption which obviously require re-intervention for removal of the operculum and subsequent cranial reconstruction. It has been hypothesized that the operculum could become contaminated in all stages of the process (decompressive surgery, Initial packaging or transfer-storage at the bio-bank). Recently, in 2017, Chan DYC et al. carried out a study on cranial bone flap viability and microbial contamination after deep-frozen storage (at −80 °C). They found that cryo-stored skull bone flaps beyond 4 months showed no viable osteoblasts, and bacterial contamination rate of bone flaps was 27.8% [19]. These laboratory data can in part justify, respectively, both infectious complications and the high resorption rate of (the) autologous bone operculum. On the other hand, literature data and clinical experiences seem to suggest that cranial prostheses produced with bone substitutes (allografts) present better long-term outcomes [4]. Van de Vijfeijken et al. published the results of a systematic review of the literature in which they suggest that autologous bone is dissuaded for cranioplasty after decompressive craniectomy. The aim of this work was to evaluate the safety, in terms of rate of infection, resorption and removal (reoperation) of different materials used for cranioplasty for any indication. The authors included 228 articles, for a total of 10,346 cranioplasty procedures; infection was the most common complication (about 6% of the total), followed by postoperative haematoma (1.9%) and wound problems (1.1%). In their review, autologous bone flap and PMMA had the highest rate of infection (6.9% and 7.8%, respectively) compared to hydroxyapatite (3.3%) and titanium (5.4%). Overall, based on the results, it appears that autografts carry a greater failure risk than allografts [4]. These data were also confirmed by a randomized clinical trial published by Honeybul et al. [3], in which the authors compared cranioplasty performed using autologous bone flap versus custom-made titanium prostheses. This randomized controlled study showed that primary titanium cranioplasty after decompressive craniectomy was associated with better cosmetic and functional outcomes than primary autologous cranioplasty without increasing overall health care costs. Bone resorption appeared to be more common in young patients who had autologous cranioplasty. Primary titanium cranioplasty should be seriously considered for young patients who require reconstruction of the skull vault following decompressive craniectomy [3]. Titanium's low infection rate compared to autologous bone is confirmed by Matsuno's work in which titanium prostheses showed significantly lower infection rates than autologous bone, PMMA and ceramic [11]. These works confirm the evidence that allografts guarantee better results than autologous bone flap. The choice of using allogenic cranial prostheses solve the problems related to adequate storing of the autologous bone flap, eliminating surgical times and any complications of the abdomen pocket as well as the costs and logistic difficulties related to cryopreservation.

Allografts, as already mentioned above, can be of three types: manually shaped, pre-curved standard and custom-made. They have different characteristics that must be considered when choosing one over the other and for individual patients.

Manually shaped prostheses are made up of standard-shaped implants (metal or plastic sheets) that are adapted to the patient's defect by cutting and modelling them at the time of implantation. Once the three-dimensional shape has been defined, they are locked in position by means of a tailored plating with the aim of limiting as much as possible ragged-edged distortions of the prosthesis which can lead to erosion of the skin and subsequent failure of the implant due to infection or failure of the skin to scar. Due to the intrinsic difficulty of modelling, these systems should be used in case of cranial defect which are as flat as possible, simple shape and small size: for example, lateral parietal bone defects or small posterior cranial defect (such as retro mastoid craniectomy). Indeed, anterior craniectomies with large defects including the region of sphenoid wings and/or orbit lateral wall always require a fairly long moulding time in order to perfectly adapt the surface of the prosthesis to the surrounding bone surface, often resulting in a not so well aesthetic and functional result. These prostheses nevertheless have the advantage of being able to be used during the resection surgery (single step resection-reconstruction). The patients who are usually selected for this type of prosthesis are those who will undergo closure of the skull in the same session: patients with primary or secondary neoplastic pathology involving small bone portions of the skull (intradiploic meningioma, brainmetastasis with involvement of the dura mater and the skull vault), traumatic brain injuries with closed fractures that are comminuted or marginally open with minimal local infectious risk. They are also used in the case of craniectomy closure, for example retro-mastoid or spheno-orbital, to fill small bone defects with the aim, only minimally aesthetic, of reducing the risk of CSF fistula and diplopia for pulsating enophthalmos. Also, in the case of cancer patients the use of this type of prosthesis has great advantages, especially in reducing the waiting time to perform radiotherapy or for those cases where it is necessary to limit as much as possible the time spent in an intensive hospital environment. From a surgical point of view, the need to package the prosthesis certainly results in an increase in operating times and consequently in a greater risk of infection. Without doubt, the better the remodelling of the metal sheet, the better the result at a distance as the risks of an internal decubitus skin lesion are reduced.

The standard pre-curved prostheses, on the other hand, are produced in various standard shape suitable for covering relatively large bone defects in the front-temporal, parietal, occipital and frontal region whose curvature is created on the basis of a skull of standard shape and size. They are constructed with malleable perforated titanium nets which must be applied on the skull vault and adapted so as to adhere perfectly to the edges of the bone defect. In specific cases, the relative malleability of the prosthesis and the possibility of trimming the margins ensures optimal positioning of the prosthesis by fixing it to the cranial casing with a plating or by inserting the screws directly into the mesh of the metal sheet. Adherence to the cranial surface, however, is not always easy. Nevertheless it is recommended that a sufficient number of flaps or screws be used in such a way as to make the surface of the edges of the prosthesis as smooth as possible. Similarly to the previous types, this prosthesis has the advantage of being able to be used in single step resection-reconstruction and consequently in those patients who benefit from a single surgical intervention: patients with primary or secondary neoplastic lesions of the cranial theca, head injuries with unopened extensive comminuted fractures or with minimal risk of local infection. Unlike malleable prostheses, to their advantage these allow a moderate/ minimal aesthetic reconstruction since the three-dimensional pre-curvature provides limited reconstruction of the sphericity of the skull. Naturally, the aesthetic reconstructive aspect is far secondary to the protective and functional aspect that this type of prosthesis allows. In particular cases, such as patients suffering from local infectious outcomes or with trophic alterations of the skin ranging from secondary to large lacerated-contusive traumas, being able to minimize the curvature of the prosthesis can avoid excessive skin stress and reduce the risk of the skin not scarring. As for the surgery, because these require minimal intraoperative packaging, operating times are slightly longer than normal with minimal increase in short- and long-term complications.

Custom-made prostheses produced with 3D technology have an average production time of 10–20 days (variable depending on the material and the manufacturer). Their average cost ranges between 4500–6000 euros. Pre-curved prostheses (usually in titanium), have an average cost of 1000–1500 euros and are readily available in the hospital in case of need.

The choice whether to implant custom made prostheses produced with 3D printing technology must take the following points into consideration: firstly, the clinical aspect based on the particular needs of the individual patient, balancing the advantages and disadvantages of these compared to the other types of prosthesis (manually shaped or pre-curved); secondly, the economic aspect, that is, the relationship between costs and benefits, especially in the long term. These could be employed in patients with large areas of the craniolacunia of the vault, possibly including lateral portions of the base or orbit, who will undergo reconstructive surgery at a later time from the decompression intervention (delayed cranioplasty). In these cases the prescription, design and manufacturing times of the prosthesis are compatible with the clinical needs of the patient. In most patients with craniolacunia as a result of decompressive craniotomy, the cranial reconstruction intervention is scheduled some time (3–4 weeks) after decompression and, consequently, the realization and delivery of the product can be safely scheduled allowing surgery to be performed in the best possible conditions for the patient. Production and delivery time can be problematic and requiring careful consideration only in those particular cases when it is necessary, for various clinical or organizational reasons, to proceed with the surgery sooner (<2 weeks), for example, in patients with secondary sinking skin flap syndrome (SSFS) [20], i.e. decompressed and subjected to external ventricular drainage, In these cases, the difficulty in setting the CSF derivation can lead to hyperdrainage, with hypotensive CSF syndrome, deviation of the median structures and sinking skin flap syndrome. A second group is that of decompressed patients with an external ventricular derivation to be replaced in a few days with a ventricolo-peritoneal shunt. The absence of cranial closure makes the setting of the valve troublesome with difficult control of hydrocephalus. Furthermore, the alteration of the CSF dynamics can determine the formation of CSF or sub-dural blood collection at the decompressive craniectomy with the formation of hygroma or subdural haematoma. A final group comprises those who must undergo encephalic radiation therapy. In such cases, any radiation, in the presence of a bone defect, can increase the risk of brain radionecrosis and post-actinic trophic cutaneous changes that can jeopardize the success of the intervention. Overall, these cases are few: cases in which, however, waiting longer than 2 weeks is not recommended.

10.4 Surgical Procedures

As mentioned, reconstructive surgery of cranial defects is burdened by a relatively high rate of infectious and local complications. Therefore, it must be carried out by observing strict rules of behaviour and techniques aimed at reducing the risk of contamination of the prosthesis and curtailing skin lesions from internal decubitus. The operation is performed under general anaesthesia in the supine position. A first dose of a broad-spectrum antibiotic agent is given intravenously at induction of anaesthesia, then a repeat dose every 4 h for the next 24 h. The patient's hair is completely removed using hair clippers. Great care is taken to avoid skin damage. The skin is thoroughly washed and then disinfected. An iodine-impregnated incision-drape is placed over the exposed skin, and care is taken to ensure that all surfaces are completely covered. In the case of delayed cranioplasty the previous incision made during the craniectomy operation is reopened; this strategy ensures the best vascularization for the skin flap (avoiding overlapping or crossed incisions) and allows adequate exposure of the cranial defect. The wound is then opened using a scalpel and sharp dissection, and the skull defect is progressively exposed in sub-periosteal plane. Once the scalp flap is reflected, the temporal muscle is usually dissected from the dura and reflected laterally. However, if the muscle appears densely adherent to the dura mater, we prefer to leave it attached to the dura, reducing the risk of dura and brain lacerations, and the cranioplasty is placed on top of both structures (muscle and dura mater). Great care is taken to avoid opening of the dura in order to reduce the risk of CSF leakage and or subdural haemorrhage. Once the dissection along the dural plane is completed, all the edges of the craniolacunia are exposed, cleaning the bone with the dissector. Once exposure is completed, scrupulous washing and haemostasis are carried out. The prosthesis must be handled only with clean gloves. At this point the prosthesis is positioned on the bone defect. For malleable and pre-curved standard mesh it is necessary to adapt the prosthesis as best as possible by cutting and molding the mesh to modify the curvature and obtain the best fitting on the bone defect. Any sharp edges along the surface of the prosthesis must be avoided as they can induce skin laceration and post-op local pain. For the custom-made 3D-printed prosthesis no molding or lengthy manipulation is necessary as it fits perfectly on the bone defect. Usually it is only necessary to adjust the angle of the small fixing plates along the margin. The prosthesis is secured to the bone skull with titanium screws (Fig. 10.2).

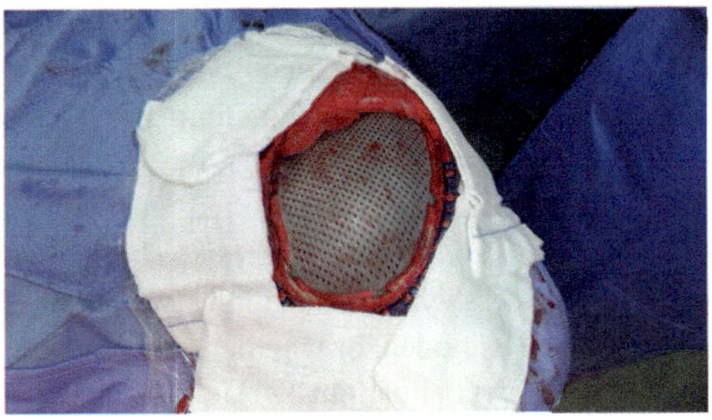

Fig. 10.2 Intraoperative picture; 3D-printed custom made prosthesis fixed in place

Central dural tenting sutures are placed routinely. A wound suction drainage is placed under the skin. A post-op CT scan is obtained the following day and the drainage removed.

10.5 Comparison Between Custom-Made 3D-Printed Prostheses and Standard Pre-Curved Prostheses

A thorough evaluation and comparison of different biomaterial available for cranioplasty is beyond the scope of this chapter. Our goal is, rather, to compare malleable-standard pre-curved and 3D-printed custom-made prostheses. Our Department has chosen to use titanium prostheses because, in our opinion and on the basis of the evidence from literature, this material is superior compared to the others available on the market [3, 5, 9, 15].

Rather, evaluation of the choice between malleable-pre-curved and custom-made prostheses is important since, ever mindful of the superiority of titanium, the two types of implant do differ in cost, user-friendliness and in the long-term results. Within the literature there are several reports dealing with cranioplasty performed using custom-made prostheses, although relatively few articles discuss the use of malleable pre-curved meshes.

In this regard, we have reviewed our clinical experience which is based on the use of a small selection of malleable titanium mesh, titanium standard pre-curved and custom-made prostheses. Malleable titanium meshes are used just for reconstruction of small defects. For this reason, we compared two different titanium prostheses for reconstruction of skull defects following craniectomy: a standard pre-curved mesh and 3D-printed custom-made prosthesis. The second aim was to assess whether one of the two prostheses should be excluded, or whether both could be useful in different situations [21].

For this study we selected and included patients undergoing cranioplasty for large or near large skull defect. We reviewed the medical records, radiological data (pre- and postoperative CT scans) and operating reports; we reported the demographic data, age, surgical time, cause of skull bone defect, time elapsed between defect acquisition and reconstruction, any clinical systemic and local risk factors eventually related for cranioplasty failure, molding prosthesis time and any other kind of complications (early or late), objectively aesthetic results (comparison with pre-pathological photos). Finally, we created a specific questionnaire for patients (or their caregivers for patients with persistent neuro-cognitive deficits) covering subjectively-experienced satisfaction in terms of cosmetic result based on 100-mm-long VASs (VASC: visual analogue scale for cosmesis) [9]. Statistical analysis was performed using the t-test. A p value <0.05 was considered statistically significant.

Two types of prostheses were used: pre-curved (CranioCurve Preformed Mesh Zimmer Biomet) and 3D-printed custom-made (MT Ortho). During the study period the two types of prosthesis were not always available in our department, and the choice of which prosthesis to use was partly dependent on the financial readiness of our hospital to purchase one or the other prosthesis. From January 2014 to January 2019, 23 patients, 16 males and 7 females, underwent cranioplasty using titanium prostheses. Average age 47.6 years (minimum 16 years, maximum 71 years); average follow-up time 813 days (minimum 120 days, maximum 2105 days). 3 patients underwent tumour removal surgery with intradiploic extension (radical resection) and immediate reconstruction technique using pre-curved titanium mesh (single stage resection-reconstruction). The remaining 20 patients were submitted for delayed cranioplasty after decompressive craniectomy for severe head trauma (14 patients), intraparenchymal haemorrhage (2 patients), subarachnoid haemorrhage (2 patients), cerebral venous thrombosis (1 patient), subdural empyema (1 patient). The mean time interval between craniectomy and cranioplasty was 89 days (minimum 15 days, maximum 327 days). 20 patients had cranial defect in the fronto-temporo-parietal region, 1 fronto-temporal defect, 1 fronto-temporo-orbital defect and 1 bi-parietal defect at the vertex. Pre-curved titanium meshes were used in 13 patients (10 patients undergoing decompressive craniectomy and 3 undergoing single-step resection-reconstruction). Custom-made titanium prostheses were used in 10 patients. In 8 of the 13 pre-curved mesh patients the fitting of the mesh was inaccurate with persistence of slit irregular surface, especially on the edge of the prostheses, and a small area of the bone defect uncovered by the prosthesis (Fig. 10.3). In all these cases prosthesis defects were identified by palpation; in two cases the prosthesis defect was seen on visual inspection. In 10 custom-made prosthesis patients we observed a perfect fitting of the mesh confirmed by the revision of post-op CT scan (Fig. 10.4).

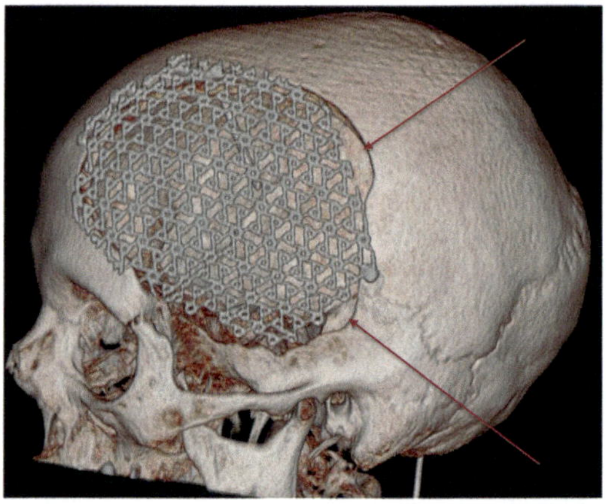

Fig. 10.3 Postoperative 3D CT reconstruction of a patient treated using pre-curved titanium mesh; the cranial defect is not completely covered (red and white arrow) with persistent small defect in the posterior and inferior portion of the defect

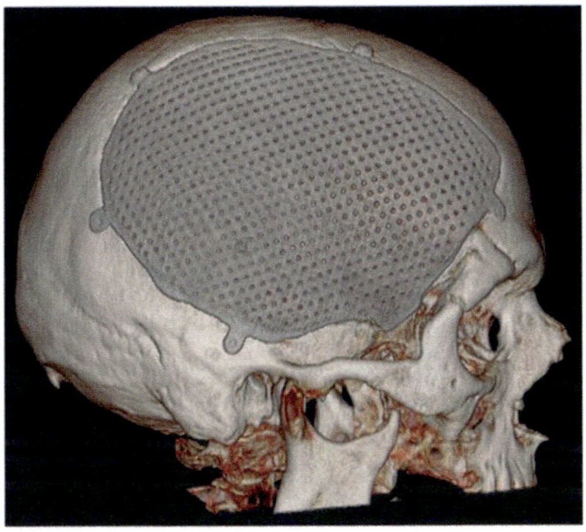

Fig. 10.4 Postoperative 3D CT reconstruction of a patient treated using custom-made titanium cranioplasty; the implant completely cover cranial defect and obtain adequate cosmetic result

Average surgical time in pre-curved mesh was 186 min (min 110–max 240), as against 141 min (minimum 115–maximum 200) for custom-made prostheses: an average difference of 45 min with a p value = 0.04. The three patients who underwent immediate reconstruction after tumour removal were not considered in this evaluation. In the pre-curved group 2 patients had early complications: 1 patient had a wound drainage incarceration needing surgical reoperation in local anaesthesia and 1 patient developed a subcutaneous serose liquid treated conservatively. In the custom-made group 2 early complications were seen: 1 acute epidural hematoma surgically evacuated; 1 subdural hygroma conservatively treated. Late complications involved 1 skin dehiscence with underlying pre-curved mesh exposure, in a patient with multiple cranial surgeries and radiotherapy. The skin atrophy occurred along the prosthesis border either a perfect fitting in the bone defect and no tilt or lump present. Reoperation for removing prosthesis was not performed because patient declined surgery. In the following months we observed a progressive worsening of dehiscence (Fig. 10.5). No other late complications occurred in this group of patients. Standard pre-curved patients show a VASC of 68 (40–100), compared to 94 (80–100) in the custom-made group (test t p = 0.002) [21].

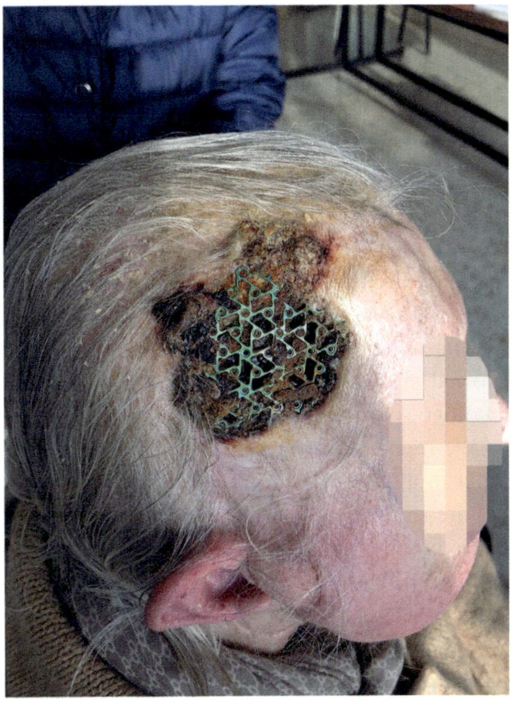

Fig. 10.5 Largeskin dehiscence with exposure of the underlying pre-curved titanium mesh

We evaluated the results in terms of incidence of complications, surgical times, cosmetics and failure of the cranioplasty. Failure here means the need to remove the prostheses (prematurely or later), of which the most common causes are infections, exposure of the prostheses to skin lesions, reabsorption of the graft or of the bone edges on which it is fixed with consequent mobility. We reported only one major complication for each type of prostheses: a failure (skin dehiscence with prostheses exposure) for the pre-curved, and an epidural haematoma surgically evacuated for the custom-made group. Actually, our data showed no infections in either group, confirming data from the literature reporting a very low infection rate in titanium prostheses compared to other materials [3, 5, 11]. In cranioplasty surgery, infection is the most serious complication because it can induce neurological impairment, and/or systemic clinical deterioration (local infection, sepsy), usually requiring immediate surgical removal of the prosthesis (failure of cranioplasty). Infection rates vary from 0.6% to 25% depending on the series considered [1, 4, 9–11].Van de Vijfeijken et al. reviewed the literature, including 228 articles, for a total of 10,346 cranioplasty procedures; infection was the most common complication (about 6% of the total). In their review, autologous bone and PMMA had the highest rate of infection (6.9% and 7.8% respectively) compared to hydroxyl-apatite (3.3%) and titanium (5.4%) [14]. Titanium's low infection rate is confirmed by Matsuno's work in which titanium prostheses showed significantly lower infection rates than autologous bone, PMMA and ceramic [11].

We reported only one early epidural haematoma in a custom-made prosthesis group which required emergent surgical evacuation. In our entire group of patients, we had 4.3% of post-op epidural hematoma, which is in line with the literature data (between 2 and 5%) [3–5, 12, 22]. In other reports the incidence of epidural hematoma is much higher, around 10% [13, 23, 24]. Generally, it represents the third cause of complication in cranioplasty surgery, after infection and bone resorption [4]. We think that this kind of complication is much more frequent in prostheses that do not allow easy absorption of the liquids produced by the inflammatory process of the tissue around the bone defect, including the accumulation of blood. We believe that this phenomenon can be reduced with widely fenestrated prostheses such as those in titanium. In fact, the communication of the epidural space with the sub-galeal space allows the galea and the skin tissues to absorb these collections even if only in part. This complication is more frequent in cases with important preoperative brain and skin depression over the skull defect. The large space created by the prosthesis over the depressed brain and dura mater facilitates fluid and blood accumulation and retention. In addition, scar tissue around the craniectomy is richly vascularized facilitating postoperative bleeding. The grid structure of both pre-curved and custom-made meshes reduces the risk of collection of liquid and blood extradurally thanks to the absorptive capacity of the galea and cutaneous tissues. Moreover, in titanium mesh, extradural and sub-galeal compartments are well interconnected, so a single sub-galeal suction tube can drain both compartments. This observation is also reported in a randomized clinical trial published by Lindner et al. in 2017, in which custom-made cranioplasty in titanium and hydroxyapatite are compared. They found a significantly higher number of epidural hematomas in the HA group compared to the titanium group [13]. Probably this is due mainly to the grid structure of the titanium prosthesis rather than the biophysical properties of the material used.

In our series we observed only one case with skin dehiscence (skin ischemia) with underlying pre-curved mesh exposure. Although the patient denied surgery for removal of the prosthesis, it must be counted as a failure because of the very high infection complication and progressive skin dehiscence. This patient had had multiple previous surgeries and radiotherapy for skull base metastatic tumour. In this case we believe that late cranioplasty failure is related to the patient's clinical history rather than a prosthesis-related event.

Our observation is supported by data on risk factors inducing poor outcome and failure in cranioplasty surgery: pre-cranioplasty irradiation, multiple previous operations, skull bone defect communicated with paranasal sinuses and mastoid cells, long delay between craniectomy and cranioplasty, previous local infection [5, 25]. Time to discharge appeared to be mainly dependent on the patient's clinical status rather than on the type of prosthesis.

The main differences between our groups of patients were surgical time, cosmetic result, cost and availability of prostheses. The surgical time was significantly shorter (45 min) in the custom-made group ($t < 0.05$). This difference is mainly related to the molding of standard pre-curved mesh to get better fitting on bone defect, as it is almost always necessary to adapt the mesh as best as possible by trimming excess parts and molding it to minimize the disparity between the mesh curvature and the skull surface. From a theoretical point of view, longer surgical time and prolonged manipulation of the prosthesis might be considered risk factors for cranioplasty failure. Infact, Matsuno et al. [11], performed an analysis on factors influencing local infection after delayed cranioplasty. They reviewed a total of 206 cases, 25 infected and 181 non-infected. They reported that mean surgical time for the infected group was longer (146.0 min) than the non-infected group (142.2 min). However, this difference was not statistically significant ($t > 0.05$).

The cosmetic result was assessed using a visual analogue scale for cosmesis (VASC scale). The score was assigned by the patient or family caregiver. In all cases the patient VASC score is in line with the clinicians' evaluations. 3D-printed custom-made cranioplasty obtained a higher score (94 vs. 68, $p = 0.002$) [21]. This result was easy predictable given the technical difficulties to reproduce the normal shape and conformation of the cranial vault. These aspects have been widely discussed in literature, where several authors have shown the superiority of 3D-printed custom-made prostheses concerning cosmetic result, both with prostheses in titanium [9, 15, 22] and biomaterials (HA, PMMA and PEEK) [24, 26–30], highlighting the advantage of 3D-printed custom-made cranioplasty. A good aesthetic result has, firstly, psychological and sociological implications for patients, family members and the community respectively; secondly, it furthers a good long-term clinical result, whereas prostheses with inadequate curvature or inexact shape can give rise to local chronic pain and / or skin decubitus resulting in treatment failure. For these reasons cosmetic results must be considered one of the most important aspects when selecting the prosthesis [4, 5, 9, 15, 22].

From an economical stance, 3D-printed custom-made meshes are notably much more expensive than standard pre-curved meshes, even if pre-curved meshes need a higher number of screws for fixing and molding. Nevertheless, costs of custom-made prostheses commonly depend on their size and construction material: for example, PMMA is less expensive than some other materials (titanium or PEEK) but we know it has an higher risk of local infection [4, 9, 22]. Gilardino et al. [31] carried out a cost-effectiveness study evaluating the clinical and economic aspects when comparing autologous bone versus custom computer-generated implant cranioplasty. Results of this study demonstrated no significant increase in overall treatment cost associated with the use of custom-made cranioplasty. In addition, the use of this technique was associated with a statistically significant decrease in surgical time and early clinical complications needing ICU recovery. Our data confirm these observations; if we consider the clinical outcome of cranioplasty made with 3D-printed custom-made prostheses, the cost-effectiveness of these products is much lower than other types of cranioplasty: less risk of failure, less clinical discomfort with subsequent improved psychological and social behaviour on the part of the patient.

In our current study, the last difference between different cranioplasty techniques considers the availability of the prosthesis in terms of the time it takes to become available for use. Comparison of the data is difficult because of the wide variation in products and their manufacture in the various economic and geographical areas. In almost any country, after hospital purchase, standard pre-curved meshes are always available for implant even in emergency surgery. On the other hand, in our geographical area the entire production period for 3D-printed custom-made prostheses to become available (from the pre-modelling CT scan to hospital delivery) is about 25 days (20–30 days). This time lapse is unimportant for patients who require delayed cranioplasty, for example after decompressive craniectomy. This category of patients (who represent the majority in almost all the series), usually requires a reasonable period of time before cranioplasty in order for clinical conditions to stabilize and to allow regression of cerebral swelling. In such cases, cranioplasty is usually planned in advance, so 3–4 weeks for prosthesis manufacture does not cause any clinical or organizational problems. However, manufacturing time might be a problem in those cases where it is advisable to shorten the interval until cranioplasty, as well as in patients eligible for single stage surgery (resection-reconstruction), with tumour and bone involvement, head trauma with large comminute fracture, local infectious diseases with bone involvement. For example,

Ehrlich et al. performed a single stage surgery cranioplasty (resection-reconstruction), with standard pre-curved titanium mesh, for treatment of 24 patients with post-craniotomy infection. In their series only two patients were early reoperated after reconstruction, but not for prosthesis infection, and all patients had a good clinical outcome. Patients who completed the aesthetic evaluation questionnaire (20/24), were highly satisfied [32]. As mentioned before, early skull defect reconstruction has many advantages: it avoids visible cosmetic deformity which can be sometimes difficult to restore, reduces the vulnerability of the unprotected brain, prevents additional patient distress for the reoperation, eliminates additional medical and surgical related risks and, finally, reduces the extra costs induced by longer hospital stay, surgical time, recovery and work inhability [32–34].

In conclusion, we have seen that, even if the two types of prosthesis showed overlapping rating of clinical complications in line with data in literature, 3D-printed custom-made cranioplasty gives much better aesthetic results, permits complete and precise coverage of the skull bone defect, requires forward planning to become available, allows shorter surgical times and uses an easier surgical technique. Standard malleable pre-curved cranioplasty is cheaper, gives satisfactory aesthetic results mainly in small defects, and is always available even for emergencies or single stage surgery (resection-reconstruction. So, despite the higher costs, we believe that a 3D-printed custom-made prosthesis should be considered the first choice, especially in young patients with large cranial defects [21].

10.6 Single Step Surgery (Resection–Reconstruction)

The use of custom-made prostheses produced with 3D printing technology, as already discussed in the previous paragraphs, is very useful in the treatment of cranial defects treated in delayed mode. However, in the case of cranial resections for neoplasms, trauma or infection it would be useful to be able to perform an immediate reconstruction of the cranial bone defect, especially if this is extensive. As previously stated, in such cases the reconstruction using standard malleable pre-curved mesh was mainly used, adapting the prosthesis to the patient's cranial conformation as best as possible. While this strategy guarantees an immediate reconstruction avoiding lengthy waiting times for any subsequent therapies (radiotherapy) and the potential complications of a second procedure, the aesthetic and functional result may be less satisfactory. Recently, however, technological evolution has made it possible, through the use of neuro-navigation, to prepare the construction of the prosthesis before surgery. In selected cases of neoplasms or post-traumatic craniofacial reconstructive surgery, the use planning procedures for bone removal in a preoperative phase can allow the production of 3D-printed custom-made prostheses to be used with a single step surgery. The planning of the prosthesis involves the creation of a cut-out mask of the skull that forms a bone defect complementary to the prosthesis itself. The cutting lines and consequently the size of the bone defect are planned in detail on the 3D reconstructions of the patient's skull taking into account the extent of infiltration of the skull cavity and the neoplastic mass to be removed. This allows immediate reconstruction with considerable benefits for the patient. Della Puppa A [35] and Broeckx CE [36] have shown, in line with our experience, how the preoperative design of the prosthesis is feasible by defining the cutting lines of the skull on the three-dimensional image of the patient's skull. Unlike our experience, the authors ~~have~~ identified and recorded the contours of the cranial prosthesis on the navigator and used this to perform the cutting lines. This strategy allows ~~to obtain~~ optimal cranial reconstructions in a single surgical step [35, 36].

10.7 Conclusions

Reconstructive surgery for cranial defects is a very common problem for neurosurgeons. Its purpose is to restore aesthetics and safe protection of brain structures. While seemingly a procedure that appears simple and risk-free, compared to other neurosurgical procedures it shows a rather high 10–20% complication rate, and the choice of surgical techniques and prosthetic materials to be used are still under discussion. For a long time, autologous bone reconstruction was considered the gold standard. However, growing clinical experience and scientific evidence has shown that allograft reconstructions guarantee better results both in the short and long term. In this context, many types of cranial prostheses have been proposed, differing both in construction techniques and in the materials used. The use of 3D printing technology for the construction of these has without doubt implemented the possibility and ease of obtaining complex-shaped reconstructive cranial prostheses. These prostheses are made to measure for the individual patient 's defect, ensuring perfect fitting of the prosthesis in the bone defect, making reconstructive surgery easy and quick. They reduce the need to manipulate the prosthesis intra-operatively with consequent reduction of the risk of contamination and consequently of infection of the surgical flap, offer a perfect aesthetic result and, in terms of cost-effectiveness, the data suggest that in the long run they can reduce economic costs by reducing the number of complications.

References

1. De Bonis P, Frassanito P, Mangiola A, Nucci CG, Anile C, Pompucci A. Cranial repair: how complicated is filling a "hole"? J Neurotrauma. 2012;29(6):1071–6. https://doi.org/10.1089/neu.2011.2116.
2. De Bonis P, Pompucci A, Mangiola A, D'Alessandris QG, Rigante L, Anile C. Decompressive craniectomy for the treatment of traumatic brain injury: does an age limit exist? J Neurosurg. 2010;112(5):1150–3. https://doi.org/10.3171/2009.7.JNS09505.
3. Honeybul S, Morrison DA, Ho KM, Lind CR, Geelhoed E. A randomized controlled trial comparing autologous cranioplasty with custom-made titanium cranioplasty. J Neurosurg. 2017;126(1):81–90. https://doi.org/10.3171/2015.12.JNS152004.
4. Van de Vijfeijken SECM, Münker TJAG, Spijker R, Karssemakers LHE, Vandertop WP, Becking AG, Ubbink DT, CranioSafe Group. Autologous bone is inferior to alloplastic cranioplasties: safety of autograft and allograft materials for cranioplasties, a systematic review. World Neurosurg. 2018;117:443–452.e8. https://doi.org/10.1016/j.wneu.2018.05.193.
5. Williams LR, Fan KF, Bentley RP. Custom-made titanium cranioplasty: early and late complications of 151 cranioplasties and review of the literature. Int J Oral Maxillofac Surg. 2015;44(5):599–608. https://doi.org/10.1016/j.ijom.2014.09.006.
6. Annan M, De Toffol B, Hommet C, Mondon K. Sinking skin flap syndrome (or syndrome of the trephined): a review. Br J Neurosurg. 2015;29(3):314–8. https://doi.org/10.3109/02688697.2015.1012047.
7. Kuo JR, Wang CC, Chio CC, Cheng TJ. Neurological improvement after cranioplasty—analysis by transcranial doppler ultrasonography. J Clin Neurosci. 2004;11(5):486–9.
8. Sakamoto S, Eguchi K, Kiura Y, Arita K, Kurisu K. CT perfusion imaging in the syndrome of the sinking skin flap before and after cranioplasty. Clin Neurol Neurosurg. 2006;108(6):583–5.
9. Cabraja M, Klein M, Lehmann TN. Long-term results following titanium cranioplasty of large skull defects. Neurosurg Focus. 2009 Jun;26(6):E10. https://doi.org/10.3171/2009.3.FOCUS091.
10. Corliss B, Gooldy T, Vaziri S, Kubilis P, Murad G, Fargen K. Complications after in vivo and ex vivo autologous bone flap storage for cranioplasty: a comparative analysis of the literature. World Neurosurg. 2016 Dec;96:510–5. https://doi.org/10.1016/j.wneu.2016.09.025.
11. Matsuno A, Tanaka H, Iwamuro H, Takanashi S, Miyawaki S, Nakashima M, Nakaguchi H, Nagashima T. Analyses of the factors influencing bone graft infection after delayed cranioplasty. Acta Neurochir. 2006;148(5):535–40; discussion 540.
12. Kim JK, Lee SB, Yang SY. Cranioplasty using autologous bone versus porous polyethylene versus custom-made titanium mesh: a retrospective review of 108 patients. J Korean Neurosurg Soc. 2018;61(6):737–46. https://doi.org/10.3340/jkns.2018.0047.
13. Lindner D, Schlothofer-Schumann K, Kern BC, Marx O, Müns A, Meixensberger J. Cranioplasty using custom-made hydroxyapatite versus titanium: a randomized clinical trial. J Neurosurg. 2017;126(1):175–83. https://doi.org/10.3171/2015.10.JNS151245.
14. Tellisi N, Ashammakhi NA, Billi F, Kaarela O. Three dimensional printed bone implants in the clinic. J Craniofac Surg. 2018;29(8):2363–7. https://doi.org/10.1097/SCS.0000000000004829.
15. Joffe J, Harris M, Kahugu F, Nicoll S, Linney A, Richards R. A prospective study of computer-aided design and manufacture of titanium plate for cranioplasty and its clinical outcome. Br J Neurosurg. 1999;13(6):576–80.
16. Baldo S, Tacconi L. Effectiveness and safety of subcutaneous abdominal preservation of autologous bone flap after decompressive craniectomy: a prospective pilot study. World Neurosurg. 2010;73(5):552–6. https://doi.org/10.1016/j.wneu.2010.02.018.
17. Fan MC, Wang QL, Sun P, et al. Cryopreservation of autologous cranial bone flaps for cranioplasty: a large sample retrospective study. World Neurosurg. 2018;109:e853–9. https://doi.org/10.1016/j.wneu.2017.10.112.

18. Sundseth J, Sundseth A, Berg-Johnsen J, Sorteberg W, Lindegaard KF. Cranioplasty with autologous cryopreserved bone after decompressive craniectomy: complications and risk factors for developing surgical site infection. Acta Neurochir. 2014;156(4):805–11. https://doi.org/10.1007/s00701-013-1992-6.
19. Chan DYC, Mok YT, Lam PK, et al. Cryostored autologous skull bone for cranioplasty? A study on cranial bone flaps' viability and microbial contamination after deep-frozen storage at −80°C. J Clin Neurosci. 2017;42:81–3. https://doi.org/10.1016/j.jocn.2017.04.016.
20. Khan NAJ, Ullah S, Alkilani W, Zeb H, Tahir H, Suri J. Sinking skin flap syndrome: phenomenon of neurological deterioration after decompressive craniectomy. Case Rep Med. 2018;2018:9805395. Published 2018 Oct 23. https://doi.org/10.1155/2018/9805395.
21. Policicchio D, Casu G, Dipellegrini G, Doda A, Muggianu G, Boccaletti R. Comparison of two different titanium cranioplasty methods: custom-made titanium prostheses versus precurved titanium mesh. Surg Neurol Int. 2020;11:148. https://doi.org/10.25259/SNI_35_2020.
22. Luo J, Liu B, Xie Z, Ding S, Zhuang Z, Lin L, Guo Y, Chen H, Yu X. Comparison of manually shaped and computer-shaped titanium mesh for repairing large frontotemporoparietal skull defects after traumatic brain injury. Neurosurg Focus. 2012;33(1):E13. https://doi.org/10.3171/2012.2.FOCUS129.
23. Jaberi J, Gambrell K, Tiwana P, Madden C, Finn R. Long-term clinical outcome analysis of polymethylmethacrylatecranioplasty for large skull defects. J Oral Maxillofac Surg. 2013;71(2):e81–8. https://doi.org/10.1016/j.joms.2012.09.023.
24. Jonkergouw J, van de Vijfeijken SE, Nout E, Theys T, Van de Casteele E, Folkersma H, Depauw PR, Becking AG. Outcome in patient-specific PEEK cranioplasty: a two-center cohort study of 40 implants. J Craniomaxillofac Surg. 2016;44(9):1266–72. https://doi.org/10.1016/j.jcms.2016.07.005.
25. Baumeister S, Peek A, Friedman A, Levin LS, Marcus JR. Management of postneurosurgical bone flap loss caused by infection. Plast Reconstr Surg. 2008;122:195e–208e. https://doi.org/10.1097/PRS.0b013e3181858eee.
26. Fiaschi P, Pavanello M, Imperato A, Dallolio V, Accogli A, Capra V, Consales A, Cama A, Piatelli G. Surgical results of cranioplasty with a polymethylmethacrylate customized cranial implant in pediatric patients: a single-center experience. J Neurosurg Pediatr. 2016;17(6):705–10. https://doi.org/10.3171/2015.10.PEDS15489.
27. Fricia M, Nicolosi F, Ganau M, Cebula H, Todeschi J, Santin MDN, Nannavecchia B, Morselli C, Chibbaro S. Cranioplasty with porous hydroxyapatite custom-made bone flap: results from a multicenter study enrolling 149 patients over 15 years. World Neurosurg. 2019;121:160–5. https://doi.org/10.1016/j.wneu.2018.09.199.
28. Kasprzak P, Tomaszewski G, Kotwica Z, Kwinta B, Zwoliński J. Reconstruction of cranial defects with individually formed cranial prostheses made of polypropylene polyester knitwear: an analysis of 48 consecutive patients. J Neurotrauma. 2012;29(6):1084–9. https://doi.org/10.1089/neu.2011.2247.
29. Kim BJ, Hong KS, Park KJ, Park DH, Chung YG, Kang SH. Custojmizedcranioplasty implants using three-dimensional printers and polymethyl-methacrylate casting. J Korean Neurosurg Soc. 2012;52(6):541–6. https://doi.org/10.3340/jkns.2012.52.6.541.
30. Stefini R, Esposito G, Zanotti B, Iaccarino C, Fontanella MM, Servadei F. Use of "custom made" porous hydroxyapatite implants for cranioplasty: postoperative analysis of complications in 1549 patients. Surg Neurol Int. 2013;4:12. https://doi.org/10.4103/2152-7806.106290.
31. Gilardino MS, Karunanayake M, Al-Humsi T, Izadpanah A, Al-Ajmi H, Marcoux J, Atkinson J, Farmer JP. A comparison and cost analysis of cranioplasty techniques: autologous bone versus custom computer generated implants. J Craniofac Surg. 2015;26(1):113–7. https://doi.org/10.1097/SCS.0000000000001305.
32. Ehrlich G, Kindling S, Wenz H, Hänggi D, Schulte DM, Schmiedek P, Seiz Rosenhagen M. Immediate titanium mesh implantation for patients with postcraniotomy neurosurgical site infections: safe and aesthetic alternative procedure? World Neurosurg. 2017;99:491–9. https://doi.org/10.1016/j.wneu.2016.12.011.
33. Kshettry VR, Hardy S, Weil RJ, Angelov L, Barnett GH. Immediate titanium cranioplasty after debridement and craniectomy for postcraniotomy surgical site infection. Neurosurgery. 2012;70(1 Suppl Operative):8–14; discussion 14-5. https://doi.org/10.1227/NEU.0b013e31822fef2c.
34. Wind JJ, Ohaegbulam C, Iwamoto FM, Black PM, Park JK. Immediate titanium mesh cranioplasty for treatment of postcraniotomy infections. World Neurosurg. 2013;79(1):207.e11–3. https://doi.org/10.1016/j.wneu.2011.02.013.
35. Della Puppa A, Mottaran R, Scienza R. Image-guided cranial osteoma resection and bioceramic porous hydroxyapatite custom-made reconstruction in a one-step surgical procedure. Technical notes and illustrative case. Acta Neurochir. 2010;152(1):155–9. https://doi.org/10.1007/s00701-009-0374-6.
36. Broeckx CE, Maal TJJ, Vreeken RD, Bos RRM, Ter Laan M. Single-step resection of an intraosseous meningioma and cranial reconstruction: technical note. World Neurosurg. 2017;108:225–9. https://doi.org/10.1016/j.wneu.2017.08.177.

11 3D Facial Prosthesis

Stefano Fusetti and Federico Apolloni

11.1 Introduction

Imaging and medical software advancements have determined a paradigm shift towards 3D technologies in diagnosis and virtual surgical planning in the field of maxillofacial surgery. 3D printing (3DP) is a computer-aided manufacturing (CAM) method based on computer-aided design (CAD) for the production of a 3D object; these customized devices are currently used to translate the virtual surgical planning (VSP) to the surgical field.

To date, there are two streams in CAM: additive manufacturing and subtractive manufacturing; the differences reside in the processing protocol, material used and their respective accuracy. The first CAM process was an additive manufacturing called "stereolithography" (STL), developed in the early 1980s by Charles W. Hull; later other additive processes like selective laser sintering (SLS), selective laser melting (SLM), and inject printing (IP) were set up. Subtractive manufacturing, on the other hand, is based on milling the workpiece from a larger blank by a computer numeric controlled (CNC) machine [1, 2].

S. Fusetti (✉) · F. Apolloni
Department of Neuroscience DNS, Maxillofacial Surgery Unit, University Hospital of Padova, Padova, Italy
e-mail: Stefano.fusetti@unipd.it

Several materials are used in additive and subtractive manufacturing: a detailed description of them and their technical properties is beyond the aim of this chapter. Briefly, the main material currently used for 3DP in maxillofacial surgery can be summarized in non-resorbable materials (such as titanium, polyethylene, polyether ether ketone (PEEK), and hydroxyapatite (HA)) and absorbable materials (such as poly-DL-lactic acid (PDLLA), polylactic-co-glycolic acid (PLGA), and calcium phosphate).

3DP is nowadays widely applied in maxillofacial surgery; compared to a "non-3DP guided surgery" several papers have reported the improvement in the esthetical and function outcome, the reduction in the operation time and postoperative complication, a greater accuracy and reliability resulting in predictive results. These improvements are enabled by a surgeon's more accurate preoperative diagnosis in the 3D environment, a more precise osteotomy design and more detailed reconstructive plan through CAD technologies; finally, by tailored devices or patient-specific implant (PSI) through CAM technologies [3].

The main superficial drawback related to 3DP is financial; cost analysis showed that customized devices are more expensive compared to the traditional procedure; however, in the authors opinion additional costs should be considered together with several parameters such as the reduction in surgery time and hospitalization period; further

C. Zoccali et al. (eds.), *3D Printing in Bone Surgery*, https://doi.org/10.1007/978-3-030-91900-9_11

investigations are needed to assess the real economic impact of these devices.

The 3DP technique in the cranio-maxillofacial area surgery includes contour models, guides, splints, and patient-specific implants (PSI).

- *3D model* are accurate replicas of patient-specific anatomy; these replicas can be utilized in several ways in trauma surgery (i.e., orbital mesh pre-bending), dysmorphic surgery (i.e., asymmetric osteotomy design), and oncological resection (i.e., segmental osteotomy planning). These models, better known as stereolithographic models or just STL, are produced from the preoperative CT dataset, potentially just with a CAM phase;
- *Guides* are patient-specific templates that guide precise cutting and/or drilling, as virtually planned. Guides are more sophisticated devices than STL: they are designed on the VSP, necessarily with a CAD phase; this implies both the use of dedicated software and precise informatic-surgical skill in the planner.
- *Splints* are similar devices compared to the guide; however, they are the replica of a patient structure in a virtual postoperative position; these devices are widely used in orthognathic surgery to guide the osteotomized bone repositioning according to the VSP.
- *PSI* are three-dimensionally printed objects that are directly implanted in the patients. PSI are frequently used with cutting/drilling guide, resulting in maximization of the surgical accuracy (i.e., oncological bone resection and primary free-flap reconstruction). Currently, the most used materials for PSI production in maxillofacial surgery are titanium and PEEK.

This chapter presents an overview of 3D printing technology for state-of-the-art application in craniofacial dysmorphic, oncologic, and reconstructive surgery. To simplify the discussion, the authors will consider the CAD/CAM application in the three main anatomic regions of the face: upper, middle, and lower third. Finally, the authors will consider the application of 3DP in orthognathic surgery.

11.2 Upper Third: Naso-Fronto-Orbital Region

Orbital and naso-ethmoidal defects are among the most frequent problem oral and maxillofacial surgeons have to deal with; these are frequently associated with primary or secondary trauma, occasionally with primary oncological resection or associated secondary reconstruction. The adequate repair of the orbital wall in challenging: in front of a high anatomical complexity the surgeon has to deal with a limited surgery field; moreover, an unsatisfactory reconstruction con result in a change of the orbital volume, resulting in diplopia, enophthalmos, and even vision loss [4].

Craniofacial reconstruction or remodeling surgery is complex and presents a multidisciplinary challenge. The indication for surgery is mainly to correct post-traumatic or congenital deformity, such as craniosynostosis. The challenge in this surgery is to symmetrically reconstruct/reshape the fronto-orbital bandeau [5].

The advent of 3D technologies has improved the surgical efficiency and effectiveness in such complex anatomical field; the authors will now consider the more common application of 3D models, guides, splints, and PSI in the upper third of the face.

3D Models 3DP models fabricated from patient's CT is currently used as a template to presurgically reshape a titanium mesh/plate to precisely fit the defects of the orbital wall/rim, thus creating patient-specific implants for orbital floor reconstruction. This pre-bent implant has been found to be more accurate than conventional, freehand bent mesh/plates for reconstruction of orbital fracture, particularly when the unaffected orbit is virtually mirrored, and 3D printed. Another advantage is the significant reduction in surgery time, estimated in 30–40 min by different authors; having that the material cost for one orbital 3DP models is relatively low compared to the surgical theater cost, a significant monetary saving can be expected in the use of pre-bent mesh/plates for orbital per periorbital defects [6–8].

Guides These devices are particularly attractive in the management of the deformities that need three-dimensional orbital repositioning, for example in orbital hypertelorism or post-traumatic telecanthus correction. These procedures entail osteotomies in a tortuous region followed by a combination of translational and rotational movements which are very difficult to control by using the traditional freehand method. Furthermore, currently, template and CAD/CAM based bone remodeling for craniosynostosis surgery is an emerging topic, with a few novel techniques described in the literature over the last few years [5, 9].

Splints The surgical molding of the bone is only one of the variables affecting the long-term cosmetic outcome in craniosynostosis; the degree of the cranial base deformity, which is not corrected through the fronto-orbital advancement, might have an impact on long-term outcome. However, surgical procedures for craniosynostosis lack methods simplifying and objectifying the cranial remodeling process. Several groups have recently described cranial vault remodeling with prefabricated templates using the preoperative CAD/CAM technique; they concluded that this method allows for more precise, accurate, efficient, and rapid surgery, without the need for subjective assessment of the desired calvaria shape. In addition, it accelerates the learning curve for young and less experienced surgeons and helps families gain a better understanding of the disease and the surgery [5].

PSI CAD/CAM fabricated PSI in orbito-frontal cranioplasty can be suitable option in several circumstances: comminuted fracture, residual skeletal defects following trauma, tumor removal, resorption of an original bone flap, unsatisfying shape of the artificial skull. Since their first description in cranio-maxillofacial surgery in 2007, these implants have rapidly become a standard in calvaria reconstructive surgery and are also progressively gaining popularity in maxillofacial rehabilitation. CAD/CAM techniques include the designing of a CAD model and computer-based processing to manufacture custom-made skull implants from alloplastic materials such as titanium, PEEK, and PMMA. Advantages have been shown in accumulating the literature to apply PSI implants for craniofacial skeletal reconstruction in terms of excellent cosmesis and few complications when compared to autogenous or alloplastic bone grafts. The great advantage is that CAD/CAM implants can be tailored to the individual's anatomy: this eliminates the need for tedious and long intraoperative manipulations for the adaptation of traditional non-custom-made implants so that they fit the defect as precisely as possible; the use of CAD tools that support the "mirroring" of the healthy side onto the affected side has led to create specular implants that reproduce the unaffected side profile, thus precisely restoring facial symmetry; moreover, other algorithms allows contour elevation or depression, with the aim to compensate soft tissue deficit (contour elevation) or subcranioplasty dead space (contour depression) [7, 10].

One other important application of PSI meshes (Fig. 11.1) is individualized orbital wall reconstruction (i.e., secondary to trauma or oncological resection) or orbital volume restoring (i.e., post-traumatic enophthalmos or in oncological secondary reconstruction). The CAD phase is based on "mirroring" a symmetrical and chiral image of the contralateral healthy orbital wall, having the restitution of the anatomical symmetry with decreasing of operating time and morbidity. Moreover, planning allows control of several measures (including length, thickness, angle, weight, volume) in addition to spatial position relative to other virtual object; for these reasons many authors consider PSI the first choice when dealing with late or secondary correction of the orbital floor [11, 12].

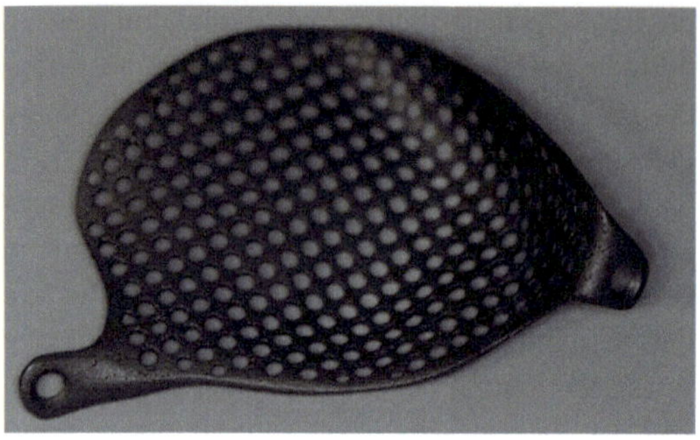

Fig. 11.1 Orbital floor PSI

11.3 Middle Third: Maxillary Region

Various prefabricated maxillofacial implants are used in the clinical routine for the surgical treatment of patients. In addition to these prefabricated implants, customized CAD/CAM implants become increasingly important for a more precise replacement of damaged anatomical structures. The clinical outcomes of reconstruction of complex 3D maxillary defect have always been very challenging. Recently, 3D-printed titanium mesh implants have been successfully used to reconstruct the maxilla after ablation surgery. 3D individualized maxillary model based on mirror images of the unaffected maxilla can be obtained to fabricate anatomically adapted titanium mesh using computer-assisted design and manufacture. The individual titanium mesh can be inserted into the maxillary complex defect after total maxillectomy. Using VSP, the orbital volume and protrusion degree of eye can be measured and planned for the reconstruction. Reconstruction of complex maxillary defect with 3D-printed titanium mesh can achieve successful clinical outcomes, which recovered orbital volume and protrusion degree of eye [13].

One other application of 3D printed maxillary implants is in the field of dental rehabilitation of the atrophic maxilla, with the use of subperiosteal jaw implant. A few authors have suggested the use of such devices as an alternative to large bone grafting technique followed by traditional dental implant rehabilitation. Architectural changes, topological optimization, and amendments to biofunctionalization of these implants are performed through the use of computer-aided design, finite element analysis, and VSP [14].

One other field of application of facial prostheses is in cases of complex 3D defect after resection of the entire nasal region or after orbital exenteration, in patients that are not candidate for surgical reconstruction. Traditionally a labor intensive process, the fabrication of craniofacial prostheses (epithesis), involves taking a plaster cast of the area to be treated, hand carving wax models of the restoration, and multiple meetings with the patient to alter this wax restoration before making a final prosthesis in silicone. Using the patient's pre-existing computed tomography (CT) images and 3D printing technology, a patient-specific silicone prosthesis can be created with improved efficiency and accuracy. The benefits of using this method include reduced manufacturing time, decreased outpatient appointments, improved personalized outcomes, and a repeatable process allowing multiple prostheses to be made [15].

11.4 Lower Third: Mandibular Region

Mandible acquired defects following oncological resection or traumatic events are challenging for the surgeon: comprehensive reconstruction strategies require the restoration of the 3D facial buttresses, the restoration of the internal/external envelope and last, but not least, dental rehabilitation. Mandible congenital defects are even more challenging for the surgeon given the complex variation from the normal anatomy and the small surgical field, especially when the correction of a pediatric malformation is required. For these reasons, mandible reconstruction has long been a daunting task for the reconstructive surgeons: ambitious and thoughtful undertakings have led to technical innovations that have ultimately been translated into improvement of patient outcome [16].

With the recent advances in medical imaging and 3DP, the reconstruction modalities have been widely implemented: the preoperative planning has moved from physical or stereolithographic model into ad almost completely virtual environment. The feasibility of these CAD/CAM based procedures has been widely demonstrated in several studies; these studies pointed out several advantages apported by 3DP in mandibular surgery: accuracy in oncological resection, appropriate functional and esthetic reconstruction based on mirroring tools, tailored osteotomies, quicken in free-flap harvesting, intraoperative time saving. Finally, with the aim of 3D technologies applied on mandibular oncological resection and corresponding free-flap harvesting, a paradigm shift from secondary to primary reconstruction has occurred [17, 18].

Many reconstruction modalities have been attempted and reported: they can briefly be resumed in reconstruction plates, non-vascularized bone graft, vascularized free flap, mandible distraction osteogenesis. The current use of 3DP in each of these categories had greatly improved the outcome of mandible surgery; the authors will briefly discuss the application of 3D technologies in this field.

3D Models Historically, mandible bone reconstruction relied on intraoperative subjective evaluation of the post-ablative defect. The introduction of the CT-based stereolithographic models allowed a 3DP model of the mandible, used for different purpose in preoperative planning depending on the reconstructive strategy selected. When reconstruction plate is indicated, the stereolithography of the mandible allows precise diagnosis and osteotomy line definition, precise reconstruction plate adaptation with considerably short operation time. When bone graft is indicated, the mandible stereolithography gives the exact amount of bone needed for harvesting; furthermore, for a precise evaluation of the graft shape, a 3DP of the harvesting site should be performed: this is particularly important to achieve an acceptable prosthodontic position of future dental implant rehabilitation.

Guides 3D models helped to save valuable intraoperative time, but the cumbersome bone model surgery resulted in a considerable preoperative time commitment and failed to simulate the shape of the reconstructed mandible. With the advent of VSP, the CAD phase allowed the surgeon to mirror the anatomy of the unaffected side, plan osteotomies, and manipulate bony segments; with the CAM technologies, these information was translated to the operation theater with cutting and drilling guides, either used for oncological or reconstructive purpose. Not surprisingly, the use of cutting-drilling guides improved the accuracy of mandible reconstruction with the aim of bone graft (either vascularized or non-vascularized) [19].

Splints Based on a CT scan and a digitized tooth setup, the prosthetically ideal implant positions can be planned virtually with the help of a guided surgery software allowing for three-dimensional visualization prior to implant surgery. Furthermore, the possibility to transfer the virtually planned implant position to the real clinical situation is provided by a stereolithographically fabricated surgical template. While only few guided implant placement systems were available at the time, today, multiple computer-assisted implantology software are available on the market [20].

PSI Although a reasonably high level of accuracy should be achieved with template-assisted mandibular reconstruction, it is technically challenging and time-consuming not only because of the microvascular anastomosis procedure, but also for the shaping of the graft to resemble the configuration of the mandible; moreover, in more complex scenario, pre-bent reconstruction plates should make the realization of the virtual plan rather insufficient [21]. Individualized or patient-specific reconstruction plates, shaped on a digital database and transformed in a numerically controlled 3D manufacturing process, offer a reliable improvement, yielding a precise fit to the neo-mandibular contours [18].

Reconstruction with customized plates is an alternative surgical option if microvascular reconstruction using bone free flap is not possible and the patient has poor general condition: in these cases, one of the main solutions is the creation of customized bridging mandibular prosthesis, based on patient's specific mandibular prototyping of the native mandible. Printing titanium CAD/CAM prosthesis gives the opportunity to have larger anchorage surface on the bone and larger bone contact, reducing the problem relative to plate fracture for inadequate biomechanical forces on the hardware surface. Furthermore, virtual planning is of crucial importance for the setting of the new screw holes in the right points of the bone, making this procedure surgically safer. The main drawback of this technique is the cost and the impossibility to obtain future dental rehabilitation (Figs. 11.2 and 11.3) [22].

In pediatric dysmorphic patient, recent advances in computer-aided design and manufacturing (CAD/CAM) technology allow for precise planning and production of customized mandibular distractors, ultimately leading to more reliable surgery, especially in such a complex field. The traditional approach for surgical planning of mandibular distraction osteogenesis was mostly based on surgeons' experience; modern CT-based 3D reconstructions and simulations which emerged in the last decade represent an efficient tool for an accurate preoperative qualitative and quantitative determination of mandible deformities for precise diagnosis, surgical planning, and follow-up. VSP allows the surgeon to design safer osteotomy line and screw holes with respect to teeth buds and the inferior alveolar nerve, and to plan the best position of the distraction device; CAD/CAM technologies allow the manufacture of customized cutting guides which are used in vivo with respect to the surgical plan and customized distractors with predetermined arcs of rotation and precise uniplanar or multi-planar movement vectors; all of these are critical factors for a successful outcome. In Fig. 11.4 is reported the CAM workflow used by the authors to treat a Treacher Collins infant, using mandible customized distractors and cutting-drilling guides [23].

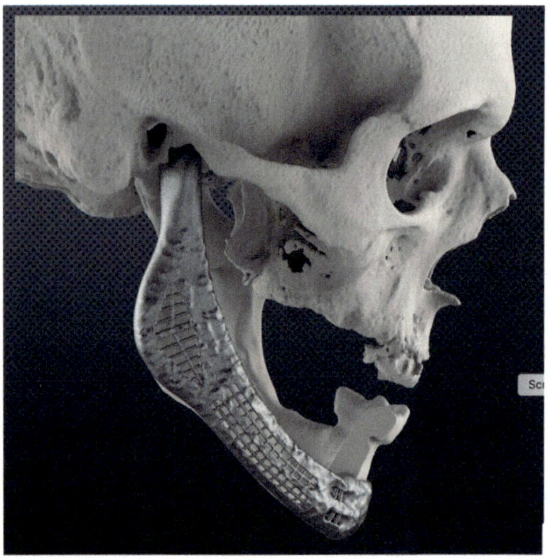

Fig. 11.2 Customized mandible plate that includes the condyle region; sagittal view

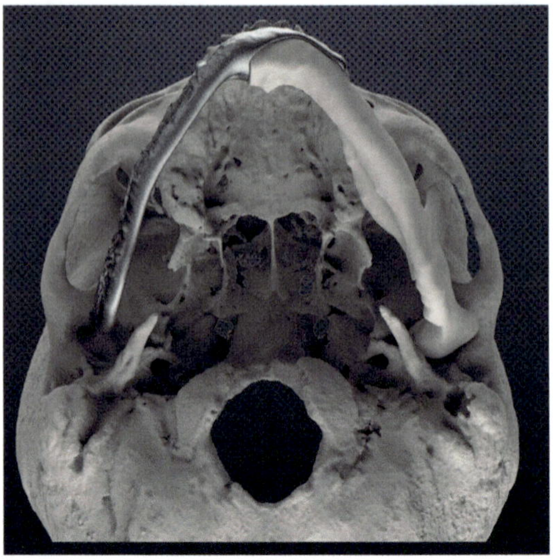

Fig. 11.3 Customized mandible plate that includes the condyle region; axial view

11.5 Maxillo-Mandibular Complex: Orthognathic Surgery

In orthognathic surgery, the "traditional surgical planning" (TSP) is based on two-dimensional (2D) latero-lateral (L-L) teleradiograph, 2D cephalometric analysis, model surgery, and fabrication of surgical acrylic splints as intraoperative guides. Although cheap and available, 2D teleradiographs have several problems, such as anatomical distortion and magnification; furthermore,

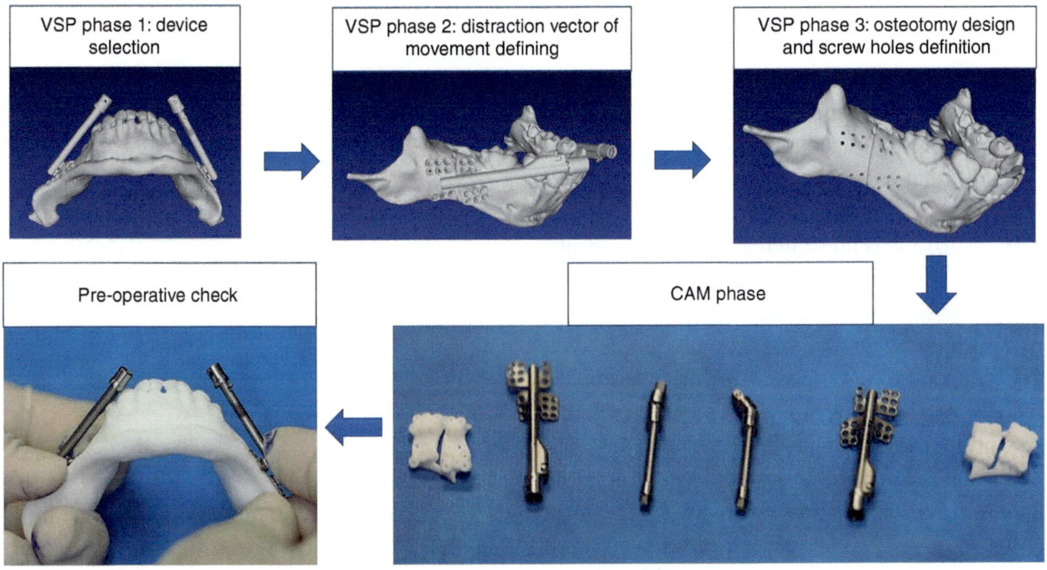

Fig. 11.4 CAM phase of mandible distractors (phase 1,2,3); consequent CAD phase

the traditional splints could create several errors related to the complex process of splint production. All these limitations are illustrated by poor accuracy in different case study analysis.

The benefit of computer-assisted planning in orthognathic surgery has been extensively documented over the last decade; with the use of "virtual surgical planning" (VSP) and the production of 3DP devices, orthognathic procedure can be improved, especially in the term of feasibility, accuracy, operating time, and clinical outcome [24].

3D Models The possibility to produce 3DP models using DICOM files from preoperative CT dataset has significantly improved preoperative assessment, orthognathic surgical planning, as well as intraoperative orientation. Furthermore, if the 3DP models derive from VSP, thus containing the surgical movement, the surgeon has the possibility to pre-bend the fixation plate.

Splints Over the past few years, after the introduction of three-dimensional (3D) cephalometric analysis based on computer tomography (CT) or cone beam computer tomography (CBCT), virtual surgical planning (VSP) has become the new paradigm in preoperative orthognathic planning; the application of computer-aided design and computer-aided manufacturing (CAD/CAM) techniques to the virtual planning allows the fabrication of CAD/CAM splint. With this technology, it was possible to skip all the manual steps of the traditional planning in order to reduce potential errors in the preoperative phase, resulting in more accurate repositioning of dental arches. Moreover, it was possible to reduce planning times, especially in patients with complex maxillofacial deformities. Nevertheless, occlusal guiding with splints maintained some sources of errors in the procedure, both in maxilla-first and in mandible-first sequences: these are related to a poor control in the maxillary vertical dimension and an intraoperative condylar position.

Guides In order to overcome these issues, new devices have been developed: these are based upon patient-customized devices to guide maxillary repositioning after Le Fort I down-fracture. Although no accuracy analysis has been carried out until now, the use of "orthognathic positioning system" (OPS) in maxilla-first sequence seems to solve the aforementioned couple of problems.

Cutting and predrilling guides are also used by several authors during guided bilateral sagittal split osteotomy; the intent is to control the buccal vertical osteotomy and positioning of the screw holes, taking into account the movements of the skeletal fragments [25].

PSI In 2013 was presented a new surgical protocol able to reproduce in operating room the maxillary repositioning and the Le Fort I osteotomy using a cutting guide; because no splints were used during the maxillary or the mandibular repositioning, this protocol was named "splint-less orthognathic surgery" [26]. Traditional titanium plates were used for osteosynthesis. Since then, several "splint-less protocols" have been described by different authors: differences could be found in the type of cutting guide (dental-borne or bone-borne), in the manufacturing material of the cutting guide (titanium or plastic), in the type of osteosynthesis (traditional or CAD/CAM), the number and shape of the titanium plates (Figs. 11.5 and 11.6).

The authors cost analysis showed that the splint-less technique is more expensive compared to the standard one (in which an additional cost estimated in 1000–1300€ have). Time needed from digital planning to hospital delivery was about 30 days, about twice the time needed for CAD/CAM splints: this can be explained by the higher complexity in the design and manufacturing of the devices. Moreover, in authors' experience, a reduction in the operative time of about 30 minutes (compared to splint surgery) has been observed; time reduction is due to the fact that there is no need for intermaxillary fixation during maxillary repositioning, no need for vertical assessment, no need for plate bending during osteosynthesis, and predefined screw locations by the cutting guide. We believe that additional costs related to splint-less surgery should be considered together with the reduction in operating time (especially in complex case such as asymmetry) and the reduction in the number of conventional plates and screws needed. Further studies are needed to assess the real cost of this splint-less protocol.

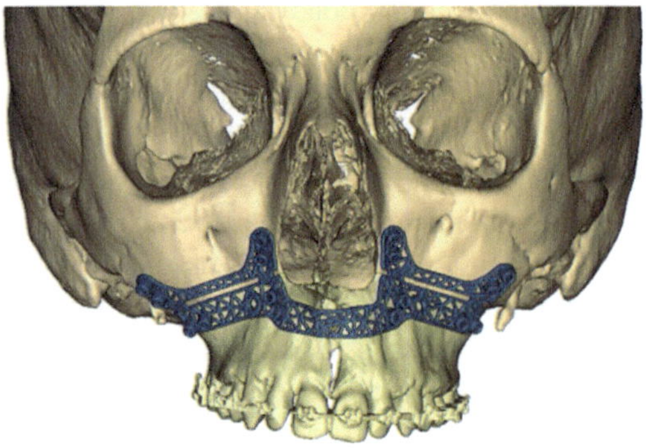

Fig. 11.5 Customized Lefort I osteotomy cutting guide

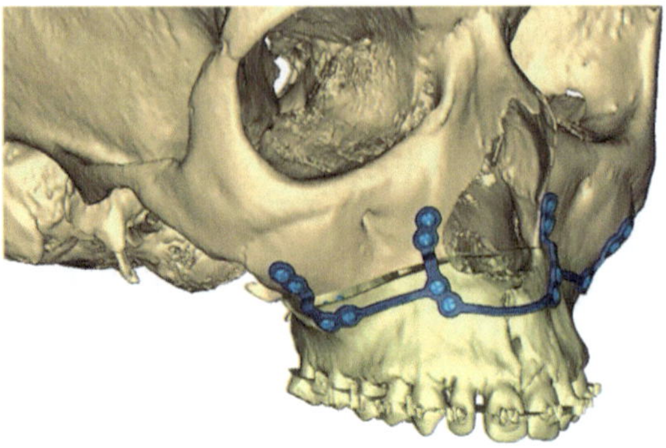

Fig. 11.6 Customized Lefort I osteotomy plate (Patient-specific implant)

As better accuracy in maxillary repositioning seems to be reached, mandibular proximal segment is still challenging for surgeons; its adequate intraoperative position and skeletal fixation appear to be the key for preventing relapse; moreover, adequate intraoperative positioning of proximal segments in bilateral sagittal split osteotomy (BSSO) can also be performed using drilling and cutting guide [27]; finally, in the last few years, several publications have described encouraging results with the mandible-first sequencing protocol [28].

Whereas there are several reports in scientific literature on the success of "splint-less protocol" for maxillary orthognathic surgery, mandibular repositioning by means of patient-specific implants is still limited, especially when mandible-first sequence is scheduled. The authors are performing a clinical study; the primary aim is to evaluate the first case-series of a bi-maxillary orthognathic surgery with mandible-first timing, in which mandibular repositioning is accomplished without surgical intermediate wafer; secondly, the accuracy of the technique is assessed to investigate its efficacy. In this case report mandibular repositioning of the distal segment is performed using CAD/CAM-produced surgical drilling and cutting guides, as well as patient-specific implants for rigid fixation. The accuracy of the technique is estimated via a surface analysis, superimposing the preoperative data set corresponding to the surgical planning and the one obtained from the postoperative computer tomography. The adequate fitting of both surgical osteotomy and drilling guides on the bony surface of the lateral mandible has made it possible to reposition and fix the distal mandibular segment in a splint-less way. The computation of surface-to-surface linear distances through the superimposition of preoperative and postoperative stereolithographic models has pointed out a low discrepancy between the planned and actual surgical results; the control on the rotational movements seems promising. This preliminary experience supports the use of the waferless repositioning of the mandible. Nonetheless, additional prospective studies with a larger sample size are essential in order to statistically confirm the efficacy of this customized repositioning system in mandibular orthognathic surgery, as well as its accuracy.

Conflict of Interest Statement None to declare.

References

1. Martelli N, Serrano C, Van Den Brink H, Pineau J, Prognon P, Borger I, el Batti S. Advanges and disadvantages of 3-dimensional printing in surgery: a systematic review. Surgery. 2016;159(6):1485–500. https://doi.org/10.1016/j.surg.2015.12.017.Epub.
2. Abduo J, Lyons K, Bennamoun M. Trends in computer-aided manufacturing in prosthodontics: a review of the available streams. International journal of dentistry volume. 2014;2014:783948, 15 pages. https://doi.org/10.1155/2014/783948.
3. Oh J. Recent advanced in the reconstruction of cranio-maxillofacial defects using computer-aided design/computer aided manufacturing. Maxillofac Plast Reconstruct Surg. 2018;40:2. https://doi.org/10.1186/s40902-018-0141-9.
4. Sigron G, Ruedi N, Chammartin F, Meyer S, Msallem B, Kunz C, Thieringer F. Three-dimensional analysis of isolated orbital floor fractures pre- and post-reconstruction with standard titanium meshes and “hybrid” patient-specific implants. J Clin Med. 2020;9(5):1579.
5. Soleman J, Thieringer F, Beinemann J, Kunz C, Guzman R. Computer-assisted virtual planning and surgical template fabrication for Fronto-orbital advancement. Neurosurg Focus. 2015;38(5):E5.
6. Kim YC, Jeong WS, Park TK, Choi JW, Koh KS, Oh TS. The accuracy of patient specific implant prebented with 3D-printed rapid prototype model for orbital wall reconstruction. J Cranio-Maxillofac Surg. 2017;45:928–36.
7. Kozakiewicz M, Elgalal M, Piotr L, Broniarczyk-Loba A, Stefanczyk L. Treatment with individual orbital wall implants in humans-1-year ophthalmologic evaluation. J Craniomaxillofac Surg. 2011;39:30–6.
8. Strong EB, Fuller SC, Wiley DF, Zumbansen J, Wilson MD, Metzger MC. Preformed vs intra-operative bending of titanium mesh for orbital reconstruction. Otolaryngol Head Neck Surg. 2013 Jul;149(1):60–6. https://doi.org/10.1177/019459981.
9. Scolozzi P. Application of 3D orbital computer assited surgery (CAS). J Stomatol Oral Maxillofacial Surg. 2017;118(4):217–23.
10. Kung W, Tzwng I, Lin M. Three-dimensional CAD in skull reconstruction: a narrative review with focus on Cranioplasty and its potential relevance to brain sciences. Appl Sci. 1847;2020:10. https://doi.org/10.3390/app10051847.
11. Bachelet JT, Cordier G, Porcheray M, Bourlet J, Gleiza A, Foletti JM. Orbital reconstruction by patient specific implant printed in porous titanium: a retrospective case series of 12 patient. J Oral Axillofac Suger. 2018;76:2161–7.
12. Tarsitano A, Badiali G, Pizzigallo A, Marchett C. Orbital reconstruction: patient specific orbital floor reconstruction using a mirroring techniques and a customized titanium mesh. J Craniofac Surg. 1822;2016(27):1825.
13. Liu BY, Cao G, Dong Z, Chen W, Xu JK, Guo TJ. The application of 3D-printed titanium mesh in maxillary tumor patients undergoing total maxillectomy. Mater Sci Mater Med. 2019;30(11):125. https://doi.org/10.1007/s10856-019-6326-7. PMID: 31728639
14. Mommaerts MY. Evolutionary steps in the design and biofunctionalization of the additively manufactured sub-periosteal jaw implant ‘AMSJI’ for the maxilla. Int J Oral Maxillofac Surg. 2019 Jan;48(1):108–14. https://doi.org/10.1016/j.ijom.2018.08.001.
15. Sherwood RG, Murphy N, Kearns G, Barry C. The use of 3D printing technology in the creation of patient-specific facial prostheses. Ir J Med Sci. 2020 Nov;189(4):1215–21. https://doi.org/10.1007/s11845-020-02248-w.
16. Bp K, Venkatesh V, Kumar KAJ, Yadav BY, Mohan SR. Mandibular reconstruction: overwiew. J Maxillofac Oral Surg. 2016;15(4):425–41.

17. Maurer P, Ecjer AW, Kriwalsky MS, Schubert j. Scope and limitations of methods of mandibular reconstruction: a long term follow-up. Br J Oral Maxillofac Surg. 2010;48:100–4.
18. Cornelius CP, Smolka W, Giessler GA, Wilde F, Probst FA. Patient specific reconstruction plates are the missing link in computer assisted mandibular reconstruction: a showcase for technical description. J Cranio-Maxillofac Surg. 2015;43(5):624–9.
19. Foley B, Thayer WP, Honeybrook A, McKenna S, Press S. Mandibular reconstruction using computer-aided design and computer-aided manufacturing: an analysis of surgical results. J Oral Maxillofac Surg. 2013;71:e111–9.
20. Spielau T, Uli H, Katsoulis J. Computer assited, template-guided immediate implant placement and loading in the mandible: a case report. BMC Oral Healt. 2019;19:55.
21. Roser SM, Ramachandra S, Blair H, Grist W, Carlson GW, Christensen AM, et al. The accuracy of virtual surgical planning in free fibula mandibular reconstruction: comparison of planned and final results. J Oral Maxillofac Surg. 2010;68:2824–32.
22. Tarsitano A, Battaglia S, Sandi A, Marchetti C. Design of a customized bridging mandibular prosthesis for complex reconstruction: a pilot study. Acta Otorhinolaryngol Ital. 2017;37:195–200. https://doi.org/10.14639/0392-100X-1250.
23. Apolloni F, De Leonardis L, Sagron M, Tore C, Crivellaro G, Baietto F. Mandible customized distraction osteogenesis in a Treacher-Collins patient: literature review, report of a case and post-distraction 3D analysis. Interdiscip Neurosurg. 2020;21:100761. https://doi.org/10.1016/j.inat.2020.100761.
24. Heuefelder M, Wilde F, Pietzka S, Mascha F, Winter K, Schramm A, Rana M. Clinical accuracy of waferless maxillary position using customized surgical guides and patient specific osteosynthesis in bimaxillary orthognatic surgery. J Craniomaxillofac Surg. 2017;45(9):1578–85.
25. Philippe B. Accuracy of positioning of cutting and drilling guides for sagittal split guided surgery: a proof of concept study. Br J Oral Maxillofac Surg. 2020;58:940–6.
26. Li B, Zhang L, Sun H, Yuan J, Shen SG, Wang X. A novel method of computer aided orthognathic surgery using individual CAD/CAM templates: a combination of osteotomy and repositioning guides. Br J Oral Maxillofac Surg. 2013;51(8):e239–44.
27. Suojanen J, et al. The use of patient-specific implants in ortho- gnathic surgery: a series of 30 mandible sagittal split osteotomy patients. J Craniomaxillofac Surg. 2017;45(6):990–4.
28. Brunso J, et al. Custom-machined Miniplates and bone- supported guides for orthognathic surgery: a new surgical procedure. J Oral Maxillofac Surg. 2016;74(5):1061.e1–1061.e12.

3D Carpal (Hand) Prosthesis

12

Alessia Pagnotta and Iakov Molayem

12.1 Introduction

The hand is a complex of multiple structures that form an elegant and sophisticated motor-sensitive organ. Although it is a perfect mechanism when intact, its lesion inevitably causes dysfunction of the hand and thus the entire upper extremity.

Reconstruction of losses of substance has always been a challenge for hand surgeons; in orthopedics, autograft, allograft, and prosthesis have been largely used for treatment of bone defects, but hand anatomy and biomechanics limit the use of allografts and prosthesis.

3D printing is an emerging technology that permits simpler and faster design and manufacture of customized prosthesis than standard procedures. Although it may provide interesting solutions in reconstructive orthopedics, the applications in hand surgery are still controversial.

12.2 Indications

The possible indications for 3D printed prosthesis in hand surgery are severe bone defects secondary to:

- Tumors, if total or subtotal bone excision is needed.
- Fractures or their sequelae, when repair or reconstruction is not possible.
- Bone necrosis, if revascularization is not feasible.

12.3 Review of Literature

The customized 3D printed titanium prosthesis was proved to be effective in bone defect reconstructions [1]. However, few studies focus on its application in hand surgery.

Punyaratabandhu et al. [2] report a case of first metacarpal giant-cell tumor of bone (GCTb) treated with metacarpal and trapezium excision, cement spacer and subsequent metacarpal prosthesis replacement. Although the range of motion and strength was diminished at the follow-up, the patient was satisfied with the cosmetic and functional outcome. The authors conclude that customized prosthesis is a valid alternative for entire first metacarpal bone loss treatment, and it has the benefit of sparing autograft for any revision surgery.

Beltrami [3] reports a case of GCTb recurrence in fourth ray proximal phalanx treated with phalanx excision and its prosthesis replacement. At the follow-up the patient had returned to his daily and leisure activities, despite the proximal interphalangeal joint ankylosis. The author

A. Pagnotta (✉) · I. Molayem
Hand Surgery and Reconstructive Microsurgery Unit, Jewish Hospital, Rome, Italy

C. Zoccali et al. (eds.), *3D Printing in Bone Surgery*, https://doi.org/10.1007/978-3-030-91900-9_12

believes the surgical option was effective in this case, considered the previous oncological failure of a more conventional treatment.

Xie et al. [4] report a case of stage IIIc Kienbock disease treated with lunate excision and its prosthesis replacement. They consider the 3D printing technology a new solution to fabricate an anatomically matched lunate, thus improving the inherent implant stability.

Finally, Rossello [5] reports a case of scaphoid non-union with necrosis of both bone fragments and no sign of secondary arthritis treated with scaphoid excision and its prosthesis replacement. He concludes that implant should be considered in selected patients; moreover, in case of failure, alternative procedures are still possible.

Although their experience is limited to single cases, authors agree that 3D printed implants may be an interesting option but a longer follow-up is needed to evaluate the results.

Summary of literature is reported in Table 12.1.

12.4 Discussion

Treatment of severe bone loss is still a challenge for hand surgeons. In the past decades, various methods including vascularized and non-vascularized autograft, allograft, and prosthesis have been used for reconstructions. Each has its own advantages and limits.

Autograft, especially if vascularized, has superior healing capability due to excellent osteogenic, osteoconductive, and osteoinductive properties, but it requires invasive collection and supply is limited. Unlike non-vascularized bone graft, vascularized bone graft remains alive and dynamic in its recipient site; consequently, viable bone does not undergo creeping substitution, the process of gradual vascular ingrowth, resorption, and replacement of necrotic bone that permits the incorporation of "conventional" bone graft. The result is an improved healing, especially in difficult circumstances, and also superior material properties and stress responsiveness [6].

Vascularized bone (or osteochondral) graft may be applied in septic or aseptic non-union, traumatic or tumor loss of substance and traumatic or idiopathic avascular necrosis; most common indications are scaphoid non-union with avascular necrosis and idiopathic lunate necrosis (Kienbock disease), but are also described applications in metacarpal, phalanx and joint pathology [7].

Allografts withdrawal in fingers or wrists can be critical for ethical reasons. Allografts has only osteoconductive property, but avoids donor-site morbidity.In hand surgery, allografts have mostly been used in isolated cases. Adani et al. [8, 9] report 12 patients treated with metacarpal, phalanx, metacarpophalangeal (MCP) and proximal interphalangeal (PIP) joint allograft replacement in bone loss secondary to recurrent neoplasm or trauma. Complications have been skin necrosis, requiring treatment with local flap, and plate failure. Authors conclude that allograft main limits are the need of a stable and durable osteosynthesis, the joint stiffness and also its uncertain future (resorption?).

Prosthesis can provide an "immediate support" of bone defect, but it is also associated with important complications such as implant dislocation, fracture, and infection.

The traditional prosthesis is custom-made, but may cause some delay in treatment for its complex productive process; the most modern implant is manufactured by machining a solid titanium block, which is followed by applying different surface and geometry treatments in multiple steps. In recent years, the modular prosthesis has been developed and extensively used because of being readily available. Although it meets requirements in most surgeries, customized prosthesis is still needed in some anatomic sites and in complex cases [10].

The rapid prototyping is a process that directly generates physical objects on the basis of virtual mode data. It includes different techniques among which the electron beam melting (EBM), a 3D printing technology, can be used to fabricate complex metallic components, therefore it may be a feasible solution to design a customized

Table 12.1 Summary of literature

Author	Age, Sex	Pathology	Site, Side	Treatment	Stabilizer reconstruction	Immobilization	Functional outcome	Follow up	3D printing technique, material	Alternative procedures proposed
Punyaratabandhu et al. [2]	37yy, F	GCTb	1st MC, L	MC and trapezium excision + cement spacer; 6 mm later, MC prosthesis replacement	MCP Collateral ligaments + dorsal capsule reconstruction with PL tendon graft TMC Deep anterior oblique and dorsal radial capsular ligaments reconstruction with FCR emi-tendon + posterior ligament reconstruction with EPB tendon + interposition arthroplasty with FCR emi-tendon and EPB tendon	4 + 2ww	No pain MCP, stable ROM F30/E0 TMC, stable ROM F5/ E25/Abd45 Grip strength 9 kg Key-pinch strength 2 kg Kapandji thumb opposition score 4 Thumb shortening 5 mm	2yy	EBM, mirror image from contralateral hand, titanium	Autograft
Beltrami [3]	64yy, M	GCTb recurrence	4th ray P1, R	P excision + prosthesis replacement	MCP and PIP Ligament reattachment and reconstruction (not specified)	–	No pain MCP, stable ROM maintained (not specified) PIP F80 ankylosis	2yy	EBM, mirror image from contralateral hand, titanium	Amputation, arthrodesis, allograft, allograft prosthesis composite, autograft prosthesis composite

(continued)

Table 12.1 (continued)

Author	Age, Sex	Pathology	Site, Side	Treatment	Stabilizer reconstruction	Immobilization	Functional outcome	Follow up	3D printing technique, material	Alternative procedures proposed
Xie et al. [4]	41yy,–	Kienbock disease	Lunate, –	Lunate excision + prosthesis replacement	None (only dorsal capsule repair)	4ww	VAS score 2 Wrist ROM E54.2/F50.5/ UD23.8/ RD16.4 Grasp force 36.2 kg Cooney score 91	1yy	3D printing (not specified), mirror image from contralateral hand, titanium	None
Rossello [5]	34yy, M	Non-union	Scaphoid,–	Scaphoid excision + prosthesis replacement	IC, distally STT arthrodesis-like with prosthetic stem IC, proximally SL reconstruction with labral tape	4ww	VAS score At rest 0 Under load 1 Wrist ROM E70/F70/ UD35/RD30 Grip strength 30 kg Pinch strength 9 kg DASH score General 13.3 Work 12.5 Sport/music 12.5 PRWE 11	1yy	EBM, mirror image from contralateral hand, titanium	Proximal row carpectomy, scaphoidectomy +3 or 4 corner fusion, wrist denervation

ww weeks, *yy* years, *M* male, *F* female, *R* right, *L* left, *GCTb* giant-cell tumor of bone, *MC* metacarpal, *P* phalanx, *MCP* metacarpophalangeal, *TMC* trapeziometacarpal, *PIP* proximal interphalangeal, *IC* intercarpal, *STT* scaphotrapeziotrapezoid, *PL* palmaris longus, *FCR* flexor carpi radialis, *EPB* extensor pollicis brevis, *SL* scapholunate, *VAS* visual analog scale, *ROM* range of movement, *F* flexion, *E* extension, *Abd* abduction, *UD* ulnar deviation, *RD* radial deviation, *EBM* electron beam melting, – not reported

prosthesis and manufacture it simply and in reduced time [11].

Hand function needs a perfect balance between stability and movement that depends not only on bone and ligament interaction, but also on tendons, muscles, capsule, and nerves. For this reason, a functional replacement of its bones is a hard challenge.

Examples of "critical structures" in hand reconstructions:

- *Scapholunate (SL) and lunotriquetral (LT) ligaments* are C-shaped structures that span the dorsal, proximal, and palmar margins of their respective joint spaces; the thickest and strongest region of SL ligament is located dorsally, while that of LT ligament is located palmary. This structure supports the "balanced lunate" concept, meaning that the lunate is under the influence of two opposite moments (scaphoid flexion and triquetral extension) which counteract each other [12].

  SL and LT ligaments are essentials for maintenance of a normal carpal kinematic. Particularly, the SL ligament lesion causes wrist instability and, as a consequence, a predictable pattern of osteoarthritis called "scapholunate advanced collapse" (SLAC). Actually, reconstruction of SL ligament and prevention of its sequelae remain problematic, representing the main limits to scaphoid replacement.
- *MCP and PIP joints* have little bone intrinsic stability and depend on a complex arrangement of capsular, ligamentous, and musculotendinous structures. Proper collateral ligament supports the joint laterally being the primary restraint to varo-valgus deviation. It arises dorsally from the lateral condyle of the metacarpal or proximal phalanx and inserts on the volar third of the proximal or middle phalanx, respectively; collateral ligament has also an accessory component situated more palmary. Volar plate forms the floor of the joint preventing hyperextension. Its distal portion is thick and fibrocartilaginous, whereas the proximal one is thin and membranous; moreover, volar plate forms proximally a pair of checkrein ligaments, especially in the PIP joint, and is suspended laterally by collateral ligaments.

  This configuration produces a three-dimensional structure called "three-sided ligament box," that is resistant to displacement while permitting movement [13]; an inadequate bone and soft-tissue restoration of this fine balance is at the base of most MCP and PIP joint replacement failures.

Hand complexity, and our inability to completely reproduce it, is probably the main impediment for the long-term success of bone prosthesis. In hand surgery non-prosthetic reconstructive procedures such as autograft, selective arthrodesis, and functional amputations have had more predictable results until now. Current investigations are exploring biological enhancers, new graft substitutes, and more biocompatible materials.

Acknowledgments We want to thank Mrs. Susanna Fusco for the English revision of the chapter.

References

1. Li J, Li P, Lu H, Shen L, Tian W, Long J, Tang W. Digital design and individually fabricated titanium implants for the reconstruction of traumatic zygomatico-orbital defects. J Craniofac Surg. 2013;24:363–8. https://doi.org/10.1097/SCS.0b013e3182701243.
2. Punyaratabandhu T, Lohwongwatana B, Puncreobutr C, Kosiyatrakul A, Veerapan P, Luenam S. A patient-matched entire first metacarpal prosthesis in treatment of Giant cell tumor of bone. Case Rep Orthop. 2017; https://doi.org/10.1155/2017/4101346.
3. Beltrami G. Custom 3D-printed finger proximal phalanx as salvage of limb function after aggressive recurrence of giant cell tumour. BMJ Case Rep. 2018; https://doi.org/10.1136/bcr-2018-226007.
4. Xie MM, Tang KL, Yuan CS. 3D printing lunate prosthesis for stage IIIc Kienböck's disease: a case report. Arch Orthop Trauma Surg. 2018;138:447–51. https://doi.org/10.1007/s00402-017-2854-0.
5. Rossello MI. A case of total scaphoid titanium custom-made 3D-printed prostheses with one-year follow-up. Case Rep Plast Surg Hand Surg. 2020;7:7–12. https://doi.org/10.1080/23320885.2019.1708203.
6. Bishop AT, Shin AY. Vascularized bone grafting. In: Wolfe SW, Hotchkiss RN, Pederson WC, Kozin SH,

Cohen MS, editors. Green's operative hand surgery. 7th ed. Philadelphia: Elsevier; 2017. p. 1612–42.
7. Malizos KN, Dailiana ZH, Innocenti M, Mathoulin CL, Mattar R Jr, Sau-erbier M. Vascularized bone grafts for upper limb reconstruction: defects at the distal radius, wrist, and hand. J Hand Surg Am. 2010;35:1710–8. https://doi.org/10.1016/j.jhsa.2010.08.006.
8. Adani R, Tarallo L, Innocenti M, Delcroix L, Rollo G, Bassi A. The use of allograft in reconstructive surgery of the hand. G I O T. 2006;32:205–14.
9. Innocenti M, Adani R, Boyer MI. Nonvascularized osteoarticular allograft replacement of the proximal interphalangeal joint after extensive loss of bone, joint, and extensor tendon. Tech Hand Up Extrem Surg. 2007;11:149–55. https://doi.org/10.1097/bth.0b013e318033c824.
10. Fan H, Fu J, Li X, Pei Y, Li X, Pei G, Guo Z. Implantation of customized 3-D printed titanium prosthesis in limb salvage surgery: a case series and review of the literature. World J Surg Oncol. 2015; https://doi.org/10.1186/s12957-015-0723-2.
11. Rengier F, Mehndiratta A, von Tengg-Kobligk H, Zechmann CM, Un-terhinninghofen R, Kauczor HU, Giesel FL. 3D printing based on imaging data: review of medical applications. Int J Comput Assist Radiol Surg. 2010;5:335–41. https://doi.org/10.1007/s11548-010-0476-x.
12. Apergis E. Wrist anatomy. In: Apergis E, editor. Fracture-dislocations of the wrist. Milan: Springer-Verlag Italia; 2013. p. 7–41.
13. Merrell G, Hastings H. Dislocations and ligament injuries of the digits. In: Wolfe SW, Hotchkiss RN, Pederson WC, Kozin SH, Cohen MS, editors. Green's operative hand surgery. 7th ed. Philadelphia: Elsevier; 2017. p. 278–317.

13 3D Tarsal (Foot) Prosthesis

Francesco Malerba, Giovanni Romeo, and Nicolò Martinelli

13.1 Introduction

Management of large bone defects, advanced osteoarthritis (OA) of the ankle and midtarsal joints particularly when in association, talus or navicular severe avascular necrosis (AVN), and malignant tumors around the foot and ankle represent a major challenge for the orthopedic surgeons with limited treatment options [1–7]. Current techniques include bone grafting procedures sometimes carried out with bone transport, extensive arthrodesis and amputations are associated with high costs, failures, and relevant complications rates. Furthermore, revision surgery is burdened with critical bone loss, poor bone quality, deformities, and disrupted soft tissues [8–10].

Since the early 2000s custom-made implants were made following the subtractive manufacturing technique of 3D CT scan reconstruction and favorable results were reported at long-term follow-up. The emerging and increasingly popular field of 3D printed custom-made implants (additive manufacturing process) and special implants (e.g., cages) have been proposed as an option to achieve better anatomical replica in very complicated cases of bone loss requiring limb-salvage surgery. The efficacy of this technique at medium\long term is unreported, no surgeons have enough cases to contribute significantly to the literature, only anectodical reports are available. New technologies lead to innovative options which are mandatory in the evolving practice of medicine. We should in any case consider that the surgeons' community has often hindered innovations as surgery relies on tradition and innovators are respected but inconsistently supported [11].

3D printings expand rapidly and are expected to revolutionize health care in creation of customized prosthetics, implants, and anatomical models. Although there are several examples of tissue engineering using the 3D printing technology, in foot and ankle surgery the more frequently used custom-made implants included: cages to fill bone defects, total talar or calcaneal implants to replace missing or severely deteriorated bones [12–15].

An ideal 3D printing implant would possess trabecular titanium surfaces capable of mimicking the structure of the cancellous bone and which are able to promote osseointegration where an arthrodesis is expected or specially prepared for motion where the surface of the implant is a part of a joint [16].

F. Malerba · N. Martinelli (✉)
IRCCS Istituto Ortopedico Galeazzi, Milan, Italy
e-mail: N.Martinelli@unicampus.it

G. Romeo
Istituto Clinico Città Studi, Milan, Italy

C. Zoccali et al. (eds.), *3D Printing in Bone Surgery*, https://doi.org/10.1007/978-3-030-91900-9_13

13.2 Indications and Contraindications

As previously reported, the indications in foot and ankle pathology include massive bone loss with or without joint involvement, total lack of one bone, i.e., talus, navicular or calcaneus, in general due to the outcome of high energy trauma, severe avascular necrosis, severe osteomyelitis, failure of total ankle replacement, failure of ankle or subtalar arthrodesis, and un-recoverable bone tumors [1, 17, 18].

Everyone knows treating these cases the difficulties of massive bone graft rehabilitation, the functional problems connected to a pantalar arthrodesis, and the complexity in case of missing bones (especially the calcaneus).

3D printing may quickly produce prosthetics, implants, and anatomical models with a great capability of osseous integration and could solve the abovementioned problems.

The ethical approach to 3D custom-made implants should include a severe selection of the eligible patients (pathology and personality), a specific consent, a well-designed revision surgical plan, an accurate oversight of the outcomes, and the consensus of the scientific board of the operative structure.

From a technical point of view, the customized implant should perfectly fit the defect and stay immediately stable, we should also consider and control pathological forces and restore the anatomical alignment and achieve a plantigrade foot, which is mandatory for osseointegration of the implant.

Contraindications to the procedure include active infection, significant peripheral arterial disease, poor glycemic control, poor nutritional status, and tobacco abuse [19], acute Charcot disease, skin necrosis and severe comorbidities such as cardiac and renal disease [20].

This chapter provides a brief overview and our experience in recent developments and application of 3D printing technology to treat foot and ankle pathologies, its controversies as well as the future.

13.3 3D Printed Custom Cages

Large osseous defects in specific sites after resection of bone tumors or difficult revision surgery remains a difficult challenge for foot and ankle surgeons. Current application of 3D printing technology could be used as alternative to massive bone allografts or in other sites where modular prosthesis is not available [20].

Two case reports on the same patient reported short- to long-term outcomes of a patient-specific 3D printed titanium implant used to treat traumatic distal tibia bone loss [1, 17]. It is interesting that the authors used a truss cage to reconstruct an intra-articular distal tibia segmental bone defect with concomitant comminuted talus fracture and multiple additional foot fractures that would have possibly gone on to amputation. The final design was made of 3D printed porous titanium; the implant was cannulated to accept an intramedullary nail and packed with morselized bone allograft that was able to promote osseointegration. Outcomes showed that patient returned gradually to routine activities of daily living and unlimited walking for exercise and pain-free status at 12 months after surgery. The five-year follow-up demonstrated successful bone incorporation of the talus, calcaneus, and tibia with a rating of "nearly normal" regarding her current level of function.

More recently, Dekker et al. reported the largest known follow-up study of patient-specific 3D titanium implants for a variety of tibia, ankle, and hindfoot defects [14]. They presented a cohort of 15 consecutive patients treated with custom-designed 3D printed implant cages for severe bone loss, deformity correction, and/or arthrodesis procedures with a mean follow-up of 22 months. All patients who went on to fusion were satisfied with their surgery with an overall clinical success rate of 87%. Despite good clinical results and satisfaction, there were two failures, one infection and one nonunion.

Currently, total ankle replacement (TAR) has shown promising results for the treatment of end stage ankle osteoarthritis. TAR could preserve ankle motion and preserve joint function, with little or no pain, although revision surgery for prosthetic loosening may be problematic [10]. Tibiotalar arthrodesis and tibiotalocalcaneal arthrodesis have proven to be acceptable surgical treatment options for salvage of failed TAR [21–23]. In case of severe bone loss after the prosthesis removal bone allografts, autografts, or replacement materials (porous metals such as Trabecular Metal™) can be used to bridge the defect [18].

13.4 Total Talar Prosthesis

The ability of the foot to accommodate uneven surfaces and maintain stability is accomplished as long as the motion of the peritalar joints (ankle, subtalar, and midtarsal joints) is maintained. Talus integrity is the key factor in ankle and foot biomechanics which can be greatly impaired in case of severe damages requiring extensive arthrodesis.

Arthrodesis of the peritalar joints, in particular tibiotalar and talo-navicular joints results in a very limited function with overloading of the adjacent joints and subsequent risk of degenerative arthritis [24].

Different studies reported the experience with custom-made talar implants, produced from a stereolithographic model through subtractive manufacturing technique, with favorable results. In 1997, Harnroongroj et al. reported 16 cases of AVN of the talus treated with a stainless-steel prosthesis designed to replace the body of the talus (first implant in 1974), and in 2014, the same authors published a report with longer follow-up and satisfactory ankle and foot function [25, 26]. In 2012, Taniguchi et al. reported variable outcomes in patients with aseptic necrosis of the talus treated with partial talar body or total talar prostheses. The partial alumina ceramic prostheses showed fair results and their use was not recommended [27]. Taniguchi et al., in 2015, reported about 55 alumina ceramics total talar prosthesis for AVN of the talus with mid-term follow-up and concluded that total talar replacement is a useful procedure maintaining an acceptable foot function [28].

Magnan et al. reported a complete extrusion of the talus treated with the implant of a custom-made talus in association with a total ankle prosthesis (Scandinavian total ankle replacement) [29].

Kurokawa et al. combined a custom-made total talus to a standard total ankle replacement (TAR) in patients with poor bone stock of the talus (12 ankles) and compared the functional and clinical outcomes of the "combined" TAR with a standard TAR. Patients with the "combined" TAR resulted in better clinical results [30].

Based on literature review, we conclude that total talar anatomic custom-made implants, produced from stereolithographic models through the subtractive manufacturing technique, demonstrated favorable results at long-term follow-up.

3D printing technology represents an important step forward for a near perfect match of the customized implants and potentially stands as the best option for accuracy, complete congruency, capability to fabricate parts with complex designs and excellent material properties, almost no porosity if not required, reduced productive costs with short waiting time and multiple providers. In addition, 3D technology permits to manufacture modular talar implants even combining different materials [31]. Scott et al. presented in 2019, early outcomes in 15 patients (AVN of the talus) and concluded that total talar replacement with 3D printed implants (cobalt-chrome alloy) showed significant clinical scores improvement and represents an exciting treatment option [32]. Tracey et al. in the same group of patients observed that the accuracy of 3D implants allowed to restore and maintain an absolute normal radiographic alignment of the ankle and subtalar joint [33].

As previously reported, the most frequent indications in literature for 3D printed total talar implants are AVN of the talus, failed TAR, tumors, severe post-traumatic talar damages and missing talus (Table 13.1).

Implants may be manufactured with different materials (alumina, cobalt-chrome alloy, titanium); however, the lack of guidelines makes difficult the material choice.

Table 13.1 3D printed total talar prostheses in literature

Study	Indication	Prosthesis type	Material	Surgery approach	Clinical outcomes
Tracey [33]	AVN (N = 14)	Total talus	Nickel-cobalt	Anterior	None
Scott [32]	AVN (N = 15)	Total talus	Cobalt-chrome	Anterior	Average F/U follow-up of 12.8 months – Mean pre/postop VAS: 7 to 3.6 – FAOS improved in all subscales
Patel [34]	Talar subsidence after TAR (N = 1)	Talar component with truss cage implant	Titanium	Anterior	F/U of 11 months: Pain free with no activity restrictions
Papagelopoulos [35], 2019	Ewing's sarcoma (N = 1)	Total talus	Titanium		
Fang [36]	Mesenchymal sarcoma (N = 1)	Total talus	UHMWPE and titanium	Anterior	6 months of F/U – AOFAS score = 91/100 – DF = 10°, PF =30°
Belvedere [37]	AVN (N = 1)	Total talus and navicular	Cobalt-chrome	Antero-medial	30 months of F/U – AOFAS score = 81/100 – DF/PF range = 20°

In case of an anatomic talar implant with a quite normal anatomy of the contiguous bones and cartilage, the implant should be manufactured with cobalt-chrome alloy or alumina ceramic which have an optimal surface roughness with a theoretical residual articulation and demonstrated, at medium-term follow-up, good tolerance by cartilage and subchondral bone (mild sclerosis in 50% of the cases defined as irrelevant in previous paper) [28]. An implant manufactured with cobalt-chrome alloy or alumina ceramic is also recommended in case of TAR coupled with total talar implant: the dome should be designed to accommodate the talar and tibial component of standard TAR.

Fang et al. implanted one total talar replacement with a 3D printed modular prosthesis for a malignant tumor: the lower modular component was made of titanium alloy to facilitate subtalar arthrodesis and the upper modular component was made of ultrahigh molecular weight polyethylene for articulation with the tibia and facilitate the revision [36].

Bacterial adhesion is an issue of great concern in the choice of implant's materials. Kazmier investigated the bacterial adhesion to alumina ceramic or cobalt-chrome femoral heads and found that a significantly greater number of microbes adhered to cobalt-chrome surfaces than to alumina ceramic [38]. Yoshinaga in an experimental study reported that alumina ceramic wear less than 316 L stainless steel and considered it an ideal material for an artificial talus [39]. 3D printing alumina ceramic implants are more complex to manufacture and there are few manufacturers available on the market. Therefore, materials should be chosen mainly in relation to the availability.

In case of subtalar arthrodesis, the lower part of the implants should be made with osteoinductive material with appropriate mechanical properties, substantial corrosion resistance, and full biocompatibility (i.e., open-cellular titanium alloy). In case of ankle osteoarthritis with very poor talar bone stock, a 3D printed total talus should be designed to accept the components of a standard TAR. Any combination (titanium/cobalt-chrome, titanium/alumina ceramic, UHMWPE/titanium) is available, but fixation of the different modular components should be firmly impacted or fixed (e.g., cement).

Post-traumatic cases required meticulous surgical planning.

We implanted three 3D printed total talus implants (1 idiopathic AVN and 2 severe post-traumatic talus damage). In all patients, there was

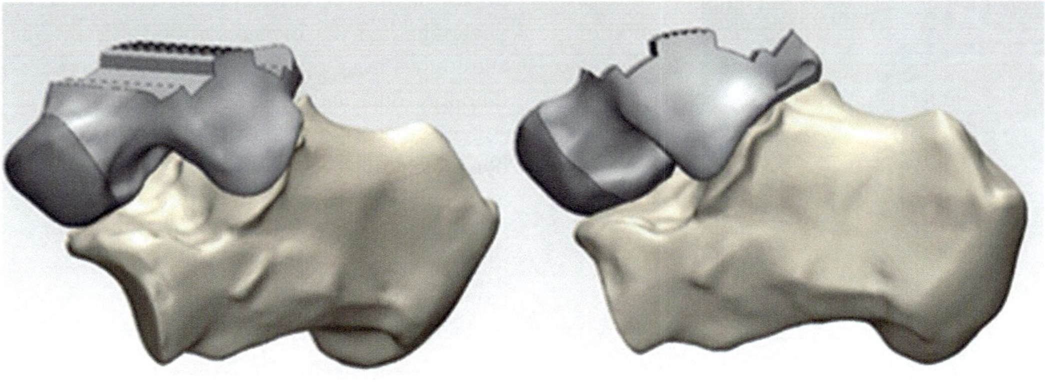

Fig. 13.1 3D model of the implanted total talar prostheses

a severe involvement of the subtalar and tibiotalar joint requiring a subtalar arthrodesis associated to a TAR. A modular 3D printed total talar implant was designed (Fig.13.1) with the following characteristics:

- the body with the lower surface manufactured in trabecular porous coating titanium with holes for screws fixation to achieve an immediate stability, essential for bone ingrowth,
- the head of the talus manufactured with cobalt-chrome alloy, polished and fixed to the talar body with a conical sleeve system,
- the dome of the implant designed to accept the talar component of the Zimmer Trabecular Metal Total Ankle™ (Fig. 13.2).

The talar component of the prosthesis was fixed to the total talar implant with bone cement (polymethyl methacrylate).

The prostheses were implanted through a lateral trans-fibular approach: the removal of the existing talus and the positioning of each part of the implant was easier, with anterior and medial ligamentous structures spared (Fig. 13.3).

All the cases were treated by the senior author and the total talus implant was provided by the same manufacture (Figs. 13.4, and 13.5).

3D-printing technology has many advantages when treating AVN of the talus; however, total talar replacement is not without limitations. Here we present the case of total talar prosthesis failure in a patient with idiopathic AVN of the talus.

A 41-year-old male was admitted to our outpatient clinic with a 12-month history of progressive swelling of the right ankle and severe pain during walking. The patient, with no history of trauma or previous fractures, was diagnosed with idiopathic AVN of the talus. We decided to proceed with limb salvage using a custom 3D printed total talar prosthesis and a tibial component. For the production of the implant, the relevant dimensions were measured on CT scans of the contralateral normal talus. To account for the initial ankle osteoarthritis, the dome shape was further adjusted to customize the fit to receive the talar component of the Zimmer Trabecular Metal Total Ankle™ and the corresponding component was used for the tibial surface. The implant had two holes to place screws and perform subtalar joint arthrodesis in order to increase implant's stability. The surgery was performed via a lateral approach to the ankle joint with a fibular osteotomy, following the manufacturer's guidelines with the original Zimmer Total ankle instrumentation (Fig. 13.6).

During the radiographic follow-up, subsidence of the tibial component was detected 6 months after surgery (Fig. 13.7).

The patient underwent tibial component repositioning with cement fixation (12 months after surgery) and calcaneal Z-osteotomy to correct a hindfoot varus (Fig. 13.8).

Two months after the revision of tibial component, the patient developed a draining sinus tract and implant's loosening was radiographically

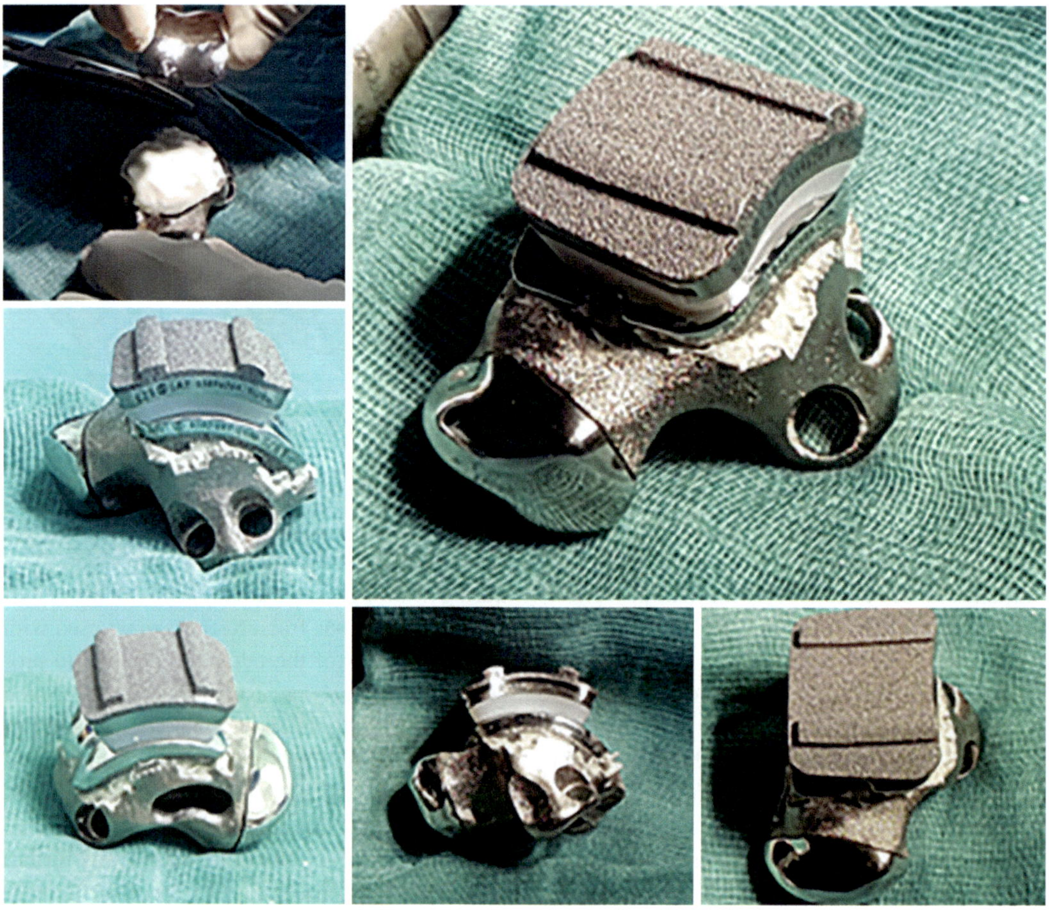

Fig. 13.2 3D printed total talus implant coupled with Zimmer TAR

detected. Surgery was considered as failed, and a two-stage procedure (debridement/implant removal/antibiotic-loaded cement spacer and ankle arthrodesis/tibia lengthening) was conducted to control the infection and maintain tibial length (Figs. 13.9, and 13.10).

At the time of writing this chapter, the patient is waiting for definitive bone consolidation of the ankle arthrodesis and at the level of proximal tibial, he walks with two crutches and partial weight-bearing.

13.5 Total Calcaneus Prosthesis

The calcaneus has a unique design and structure, acting as a short lever for the calf muscles. The heel provides the insertion site for the Achilles tendon and functions well as a shock absorbing structure, with tightly packed plantar fat pad engulfing the calcaneus on its posterior and plantar surfaces. The surgical method in case of malignant tumors or large bone defect is represented by calcanectomy or amputation [40, 41]. In recent years, thanks also to the advances in surgical techniques and biomedical engineering, 3D printed titanium implant offers a new paradigm of limb-salvage surgery. This procedure is safe and effective for the management of large bone defects where modular prosthesis is not available, and where providing durable stability and function is difficult with autogenous or allogenous bone grafts.

The first surgery implanting a 3D printed titanium calcaneal implant was performed in 2014 on a 71-year-old male patient who has chondrosarcoma in the heel [15]. The printed heel prosthesis was designed based on his specific defect. First, a total calcanectomy was performed, and the defect was fitted with a patient matched 3D printed titanium calcaneal prosthesis. Next, ligaments including the Achilles tendon, and plantar fascia were reattached without bone fixation. The postoperative course was uneventful, and at the 5-month clinical follow-up, the patient was fully weight-bearing, with a mobile ankle without pain.

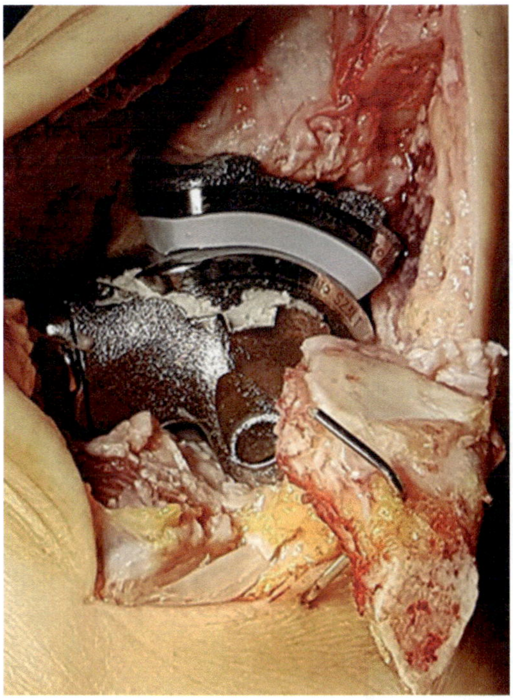

Fig. 13.3 Definitive implantation of total talar implant and TAR (Zimmer) through a trans-fibular approach

Park et al. reported their experience in a young man who underwent reconstructive surgery for a calcaneal desmoplastic fibroma with use of a 3D printed personalized implant [42]. The designed prosthesis matched and fixed simultaneously with multiple free suture holes for attaching soft tissues with proper tension. The clinical and functional outcomes of the surgery were acceptable.

The authors' personal experience is that bone fixation is necessary. Here, we report a five-month follow-up with imaging and patient-reported outcomes. The patient was a 56-year-old man who was involved in a rollover motor vehicle collision and sustained a right open calcaneal fracture with substantial bone loss at the scene of the injury. The wound was laterally based and severely contaminated. Additional injuries included a bimalleolar fracture and navicular dorsal avulsion fracture. The first surgical treatment was percutaneous fixation of calcaneal fracture, but the infection was early in the postoperative period, and there was nonviable bone. Then, he underwent a total calcanectomy (Fig. 13.11).

The patient self-referred to our Orthopedic Foot and Ankle Service 8 months after calcanectomy. Amputation and multiple limb salvage options were discussed with the patient via the shared decision-making process. The patient

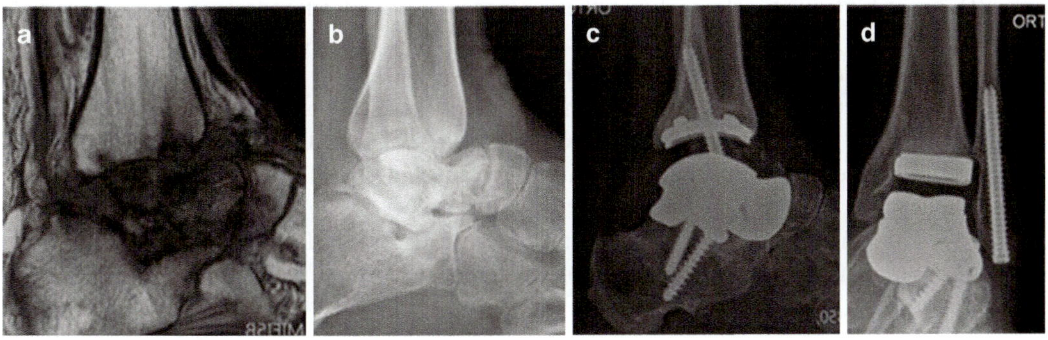

Fig. 13.4 43-year-old female patient with post-traumatic damage of the talus (**a**, **b**). Follow-up radiographs 16 months after total talar implant+ TAR and lateralizing calcaneal osteotomy (**c**, **d**) showed a well-positioned implant

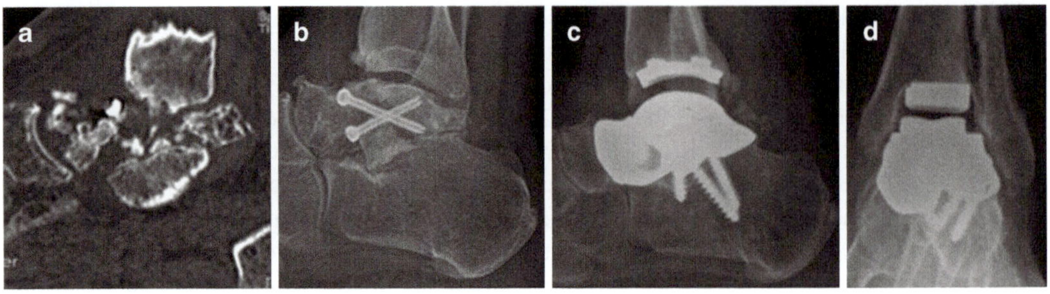

Fig. 13.5 37-year-old male patient with post-traumatic damage of the talus (**a, b**). Follow-up radiographs 12 months after surgery (**c, d**) showed a well-positioned implant with no radiographic abnormalities. Lateral fibular plate was removed 6 months after the index procedure for superficial infection

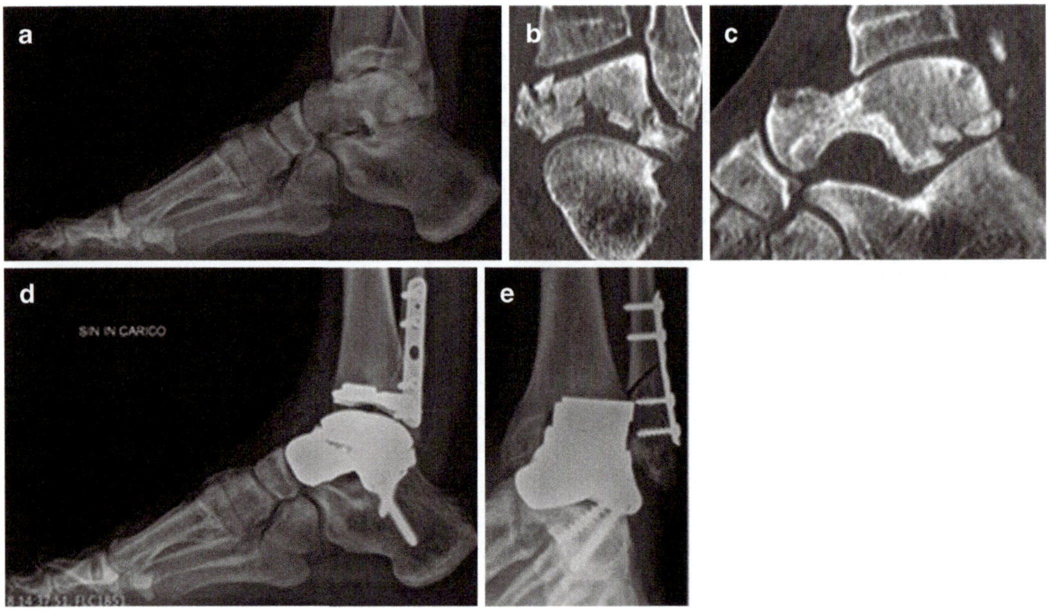

Fig. 13.6 Custom-made talus implant in a patient with idiopathic AVN of the talus (**a, b, c, d, e**)

opted to proceed with limb salvage using a custom 3D printed titanium calcaneal prosthesis (Fig. 13.12).

To prevent wound complications and skin irritation, we designed the implant to be smaller than the original bone so that there would be sufficient soft-tissue coverage. We considered the long-term complications, including painful subtalar or calcaneocuboid joint osteoarthritis because of the young age of the patient. The implant had 3 holes to place screws and perform subtalar and calcaneocuboid joint arthrodesis in order to provide soft-tissue stiffness around the heel bone (Fig. 13.13).

The designed prosthesis matched and fixed simultaneously with multiple free suture holes for attaching Achilles tendon and plantar fascia with proper tension. No adverse postoperative events occurred. Intravenous antibiotics were administered for 1 week. An oral antibiotic was

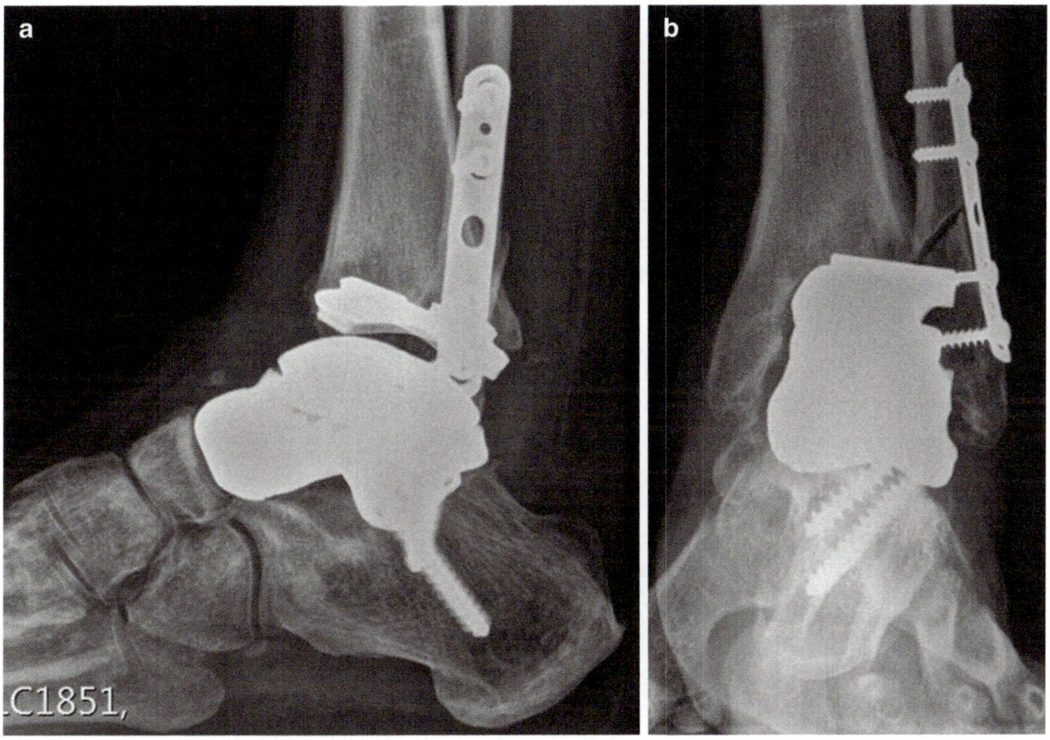

Fig. 13.7 Radiographic loosening of the tibial component 6 months after surgery (**a, b**)

used for another 2 weeks. For the first 6 weeks, a short-leg splint with ankle plantar flexion was applied.

After suture removal without wound complications at 2 weeks postoperatively, a short-leg splint with a neutral ankle position was applied. Primary complication of surgery was wound healing problem after 3 weeks postoperatively. Dehiscence rates are higher when tension is increased; non-weight-bearing crutch ambulation was allowed for the first 8 weeks, and partial weight-bearing was started after complete wound healing. At 12 weeks postoperatively, fullweight-bearing walking was permitted. At the last follow-up at 5 months postoperatively, potential complications, such as implant dislocation or painful peri-implant osteoarthritis, had not occurred. Mild discomfort on the plantar side of the heel was sensed when the patient started to walk, but diminished after the initial steps. He was able to walk without limping and required no support.

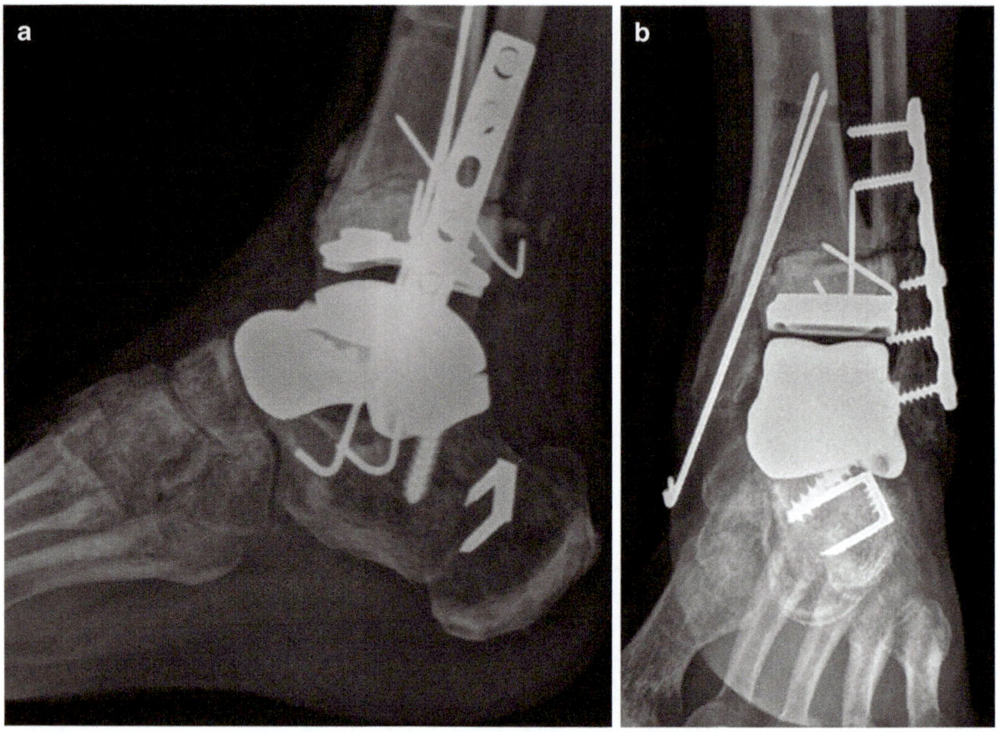

Fig. 13.8 Tibial component repositioning with cement fixation and calcaneal Z-osteotomy, 12 months after the index surgery (**a, b**)

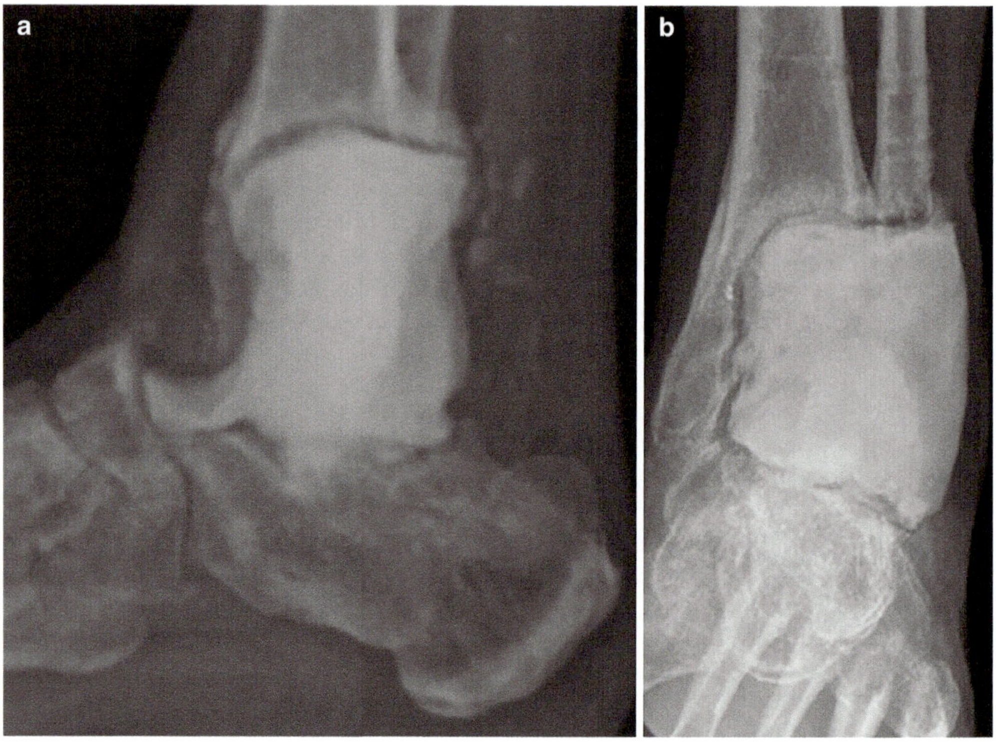

Fig. 13.9 Antibiotic-loaded cement spacer (**a, b**)

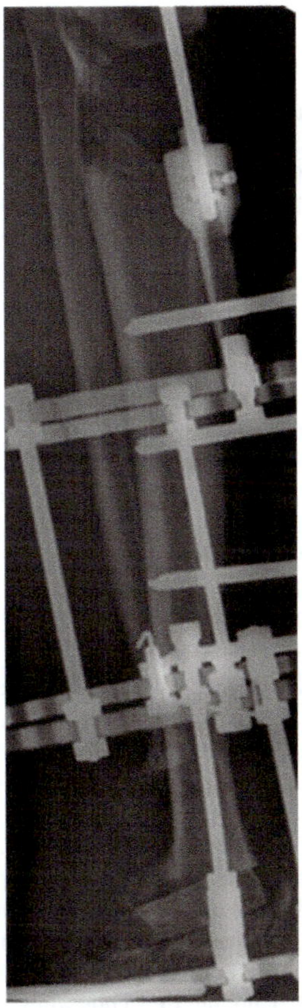

Fig. 13.10 Ankle arthrodesis with homologous bone graft and tibial lengthening with bone transport technique

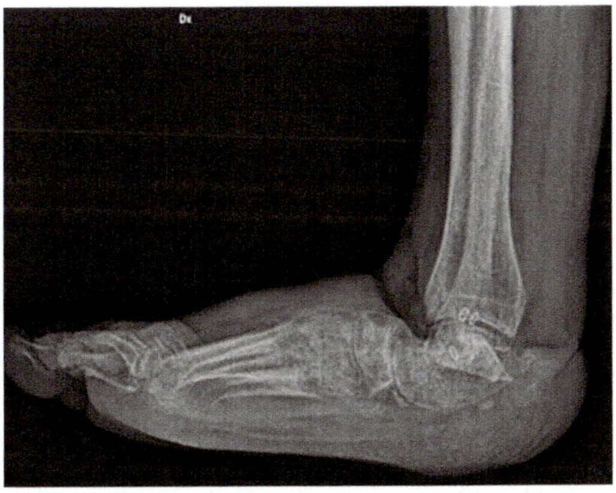

Fig. 13.11 Preoperative lateral x-ray 1 year after calcanectomy

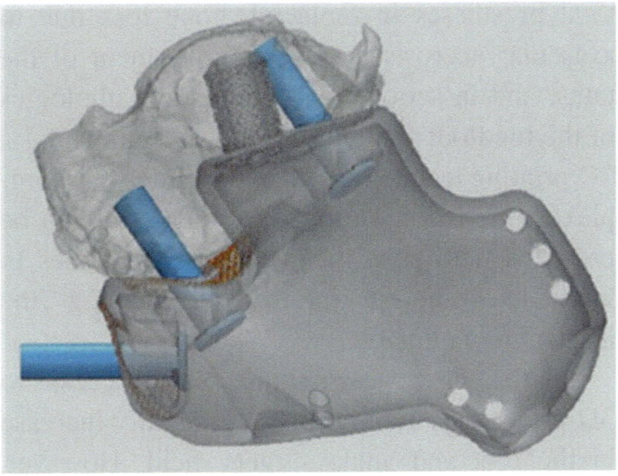

Fig. 13.12 The prosthesis design. Talar fixation was obtained using a titanium porous press-fit stem. Three pre-drilled holes for screws can be seen. Articular facet for cuboid bone and subtalar surface have a porous surface for potential bone ingrowth. Anchor points were used to attach ligaments (Achilles tendon and plantar fascia) to the prosthesis

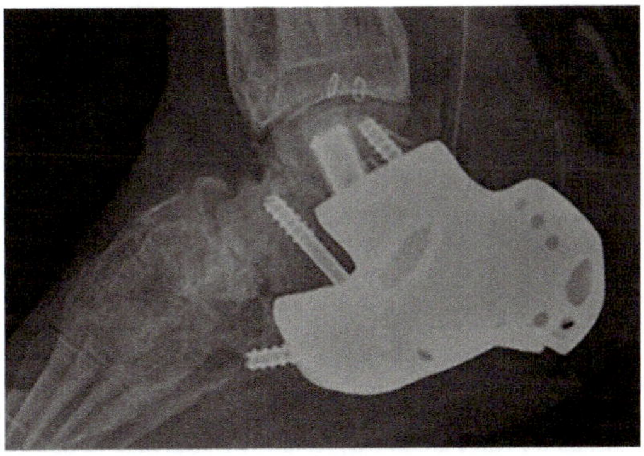

Fig. 13.13 Postoperative lateral x-ray after 3D printed calcaneal prosthesis. The implant and the screws are in good position

13.6 Conclusions

In recent years, 3D printing technologies for foot and ankle surgery have received increased attention as shown by the numerous papers published on this topic. Applications of these technologies evolved from models used for preoperative planning and education to construction of a custom

total prostheses in replacing bone loss due to avascular necrosis or severe impairment of the talus, and in serious post-traumatic pathologies of the hindfoot and midfoot including bone loss. 3D printing technologies can generate very complex forms tailored to an individual and can be provided with porosities and reticular zones to facilitate osteo-integration and making the implant more flexible.

In the next near future, easy access to 3D-printing technologies will gradually increase in the foot and ankle surgery field. However, orthopedic surgeons look forward to seeing larger prospective clinical studies, since worldwide and national guidelines are still lacking. Different evaluation standards should be also assessed in depth and progressively formed. Furthermore, given the individual nature of these "custom-made" implants, studies and arguments will be required for ethical issues related to the safety and rationality of such implants, as well as the registration and supervision of custom-made medical devices produced in different countries.

Acknowledgments We would like to thank Dr. Farnetti, for providing the photographs of 3D printed calcaneal prosthesis.

References

1. Hamid KS, Parekh SG, Adams SB. Salvage of severe foot and ankle trauma with a 3D printed scaffold. Foot Ankle Int. 2016;37:433–9.
2. Hsu AR, Ellington JK. Patient-specific 3-dimensional printed titanium truss cage with tibiotalocalcaneal arthrodesis for salvage of persistent distal tibia nonunion. Foot Ankle Spec. 2015;8:483–9.
3. Thomason K, Eyresl K. A technique of fusion for failed total replacement of the ankle: tibio-allograft-calcaneal fusion with a locked retrograde nail. J Bone Joint Surg Br. 2008;90:885–8.
4. Tenenbaum S, Stockton KG, Bariteau JT, Brodsky JW. Salvage of avascular necrosis of the talus by combined ankle and hindfoot arthrodesis without structural bone graft. Foot Ankle Int. 2015;36:282–7.
5. Hsu AR, Szatkowski JP. Early tibiotalocalcaneal arthrodesis intramedullary nail for treatment of a complex tibial pilon fracture (AO/OTA 43-C). Foot Ankle Spec. 2015;8:220–5.
6. Bussewitz B, DeVries JG, et al. Retrograde intramedullary nail with femoral head allograft for large deficit tibiotalocalcaneal arthrodesis. Foot Ankle Int. 2014;35:706–11.
7. Thomas JL, Jaffe KA. Use of polymethylmethacrylate in large osseous defects in the foot and ankle following tumor excision. J Foot Ankle Surg. 1999;38:208–13.
8. Overley BD Jr, Rementer MR. Surgical complications of ankle joint arthrodesis and ankle arthroplasty procedures. Clin Podiatr Med Surg. 2017;34:565–74.
9. Kunutsor SK, Barrett MC, et al. Clinical effectiveness of treatment strategies for prosthetic joint infection following Total ankle replacement: a systematic review and meta-analysis. J Foot Ankle Surg. 2020;59:367–72.
10. Maffulli N, Longo UG, Locher J, Romeo G, et al. Outcome of ankle arthrodesis and ankle prosthesis: a review of the current status. Br Med Bull. 2017;124:91–112.
11. Riskin DJ, Longaker M, Gertner M, Krummel T. Innovation in surgery, a historical perspective. Ann Surg. 2006;244:686–93.
12. Cohen MM, Kazak M. Tibiocalcaneal arthrodesis with a porous tantalum spacer and locked intramedullary nail for post-traumatic global avascular necrosis of the talus. J Foot Ankle Surg. 2015;54:1172–7.
13. Shnol H, La Porta GA. 3D printed Total Talar replacement. Clin Podiatr Med Surg. 2018;35:403–22.
14. Dekker TJ, Steele JR, et al. Use of patient-specific 3D-printed titanium implants for complex foot and ankle limb salvage, deformity correction, and arthrodesis procedures. Foot Ankle Int. 2018;39:916–21.
15. Imanishi J, Choong PF. Three-dimensional printed calcaneal prosthesis following total calcanectomy. Int J Surg Case Rep. 2015;10:83–7.
16. Ventola CL. Medical applications for 3D printing: current and projected uses. P T. 2014;39:704–11.
17. Nwankwo EC, Chen F, Nettles DL, Adams SB. Five-year follow-up of distal tibia bone and foot and ankle trauma treated with a 3D-printed titanium cage. Case Rep Orthop. 2019;3:1–6.
18. Mulhern JL, Protzman NM, et al. Salvage of failed total ankle replacement using a custom titanium truss. J Foot Ankle Surg. 2016;55:868–73.
19. Angthong C. Anatomic total talar prosthesis replacement surgery and ankle arthroplasty: an early case series in Thailand. Orthop Rev (Pavia). 2014;6:5486.
20. Angelini A, Kotrych D, Trovarelli G, Szafrański A, Bohatyrewicz A, Ruggieri P. Analysis of principles inspiring design of three-dimensional-printed custom-made prostheses in two referral centres. Int Orthop. 2020;44:829–37.
21. McCollum G, Myerson MS. Failure of the agility total ankle replacement system and the salvage options. Clin Podiatr Med Surg. 2013;30:207–23.
22. Donnenwerth MP, Roukis TS. Tibio-talo-calcaneal arthrodesis with retrograde compression intramedullary nail fixation for salvage of failed total ankle replacement: a systematic review. Clin Podiatr Med Surg. 2013;30:199–206.

23. Kitaoka HB, Romness DW. Arthrodesis for failed ankle arthroplasty. J Arthroplast. 1992;7:277–84.
24. Ling JS, Smyth NA, Fraser EJ, et al. Investigating the relationship between ankle arthrodesis and adjacent-joint arthritis in the hindfoot: a systematic review. J Bone Joint Surg Am. 2015;97:513–20.
25. Harnroongroj T, Vanadurongwan VJ. The talar body prosthesis. Bone Joint Surg Am. 1997;79:1313–22.
26. Harnroongroj T, Harnroongroj T. The Talar body prosthesis: results at ten to thirty-six years of follow-up. J Bone Joint Surg Am. 2014;96:1211–8.
27. Taniguchi A, Takakura Y, Sugimoto K, et al. The use of a ceramic talar body prosthesis in patients with aseptic necrosis of the talus. J Bone Joint Surg Br. 2012;94:1529–33.
28. Taniguchi A, Takakura Y, Tanaka Y, Kurokawa H, Tomiwa K, Matsuda. An alumina ceramic total talar prosthesis ceramic for osteonecrosis of the talus. J Bone Joint Surg Am. 2015;97:1348–53.
29. Magnan B, Facci E, Bartolozzi P. Traumatic loss of the talus treated with a talar body prosthesis and total ankle arthroplasty. A case report. J Bone Joint Surg Am. 2004;86:1778–82.
30. Kurokawa H, Taniguchi A, Morita S, Takakura Y, Tanaka Y. Total ankle arthroplasty incorporating a total talar prosthesis: a comparative study against the standard total ankle arthroplasty. Bone Joint J. 2019;101-B:443–6.
31. Sing SL, An J, Yeong WY, Wiria FE. Laser and electron-beam powder-bed additive manufacturing of metallic implants: a review on processes, materials and designs. J Orth Res. 2015;34:369–85.
32. Scott D, Steel J, Fletcher A, Parekh G. Early outcomes of 3D printed total talus arthroplasty. Foot Ankle Spec. 2019; https://doi.org/10.1177/1938640019873536.
33. Tracey J, Arora D, Gross CE, Parekh SG. Custom 3D-printed Total Talar prostheses restore Normal joint anatomy throughout the Hindfoot. Foot Ankle Spec. 2019;12:39–48.
34. Patel H, Kinmon K. Revision of failed Total ankle replacement with a custom 3-dimensional printed Talar component with a titanium truss cage: a case presentation. J Foot Ankle Surg. 2019;58:1006–9.
35. Papagelopoulos PJ, Sarlikiotis T, Vottis CT, Agrogiannis G, Kontogeorgakos VA, Savvidou OD. Total Talectomy and reconstruction using a 3-dimensional printed talus prosthesis for Ewing's sarcoma: a 3.5-year follow-up. Orthopedics. 2019;42:e405–9.
36. Fang X, Liu H, Xiong Y, et al. Total talar replacement with a novel 3D printed modular prosthesis for tumors. Ther Clin Risk Manag. 2018;14:1897–905.
37. Belvedere C, Cadossi M, Mazzotti A, Giannini S, Leardini A. Fluoroscopic and gait analyses for the functional performance of a custom-made Total Talonavicular replacement. J Foot Ankle Surg. 2017;56:836–44.
38. Kazmier P, Gornowicz BA, Crow B, Christensen GD, Bal S. Bacterial adhesion to alumina ceramic versus cobalt-chrome femoral heads. In: 49th Annual Meeting of the Orthopaedic Research Society, Denver Post.
39. Yoshinaga K. Replacement of femoral head using endoprosthesis (alumina ceramics vs metal)-an experimental study of canine articular cartilage. Nihon Seikeigeka Gakkai Zasshi. 1987;61:521–30.
40. Geertzen JH, Jutte P, Rompen C, Salvans M. Calcanectomy, an alternative amputation? Two case reports. Prosthet Orthot Int. 2009;33:78–81.
41. Choong PF, Qureshi AA, Sim FH, Unni KK. Osteosarcoma of the foot: a review of 52 patients at the Mayo clinic. Acta Orthop Scand. 1999;70:361–4.
42. Park JW, Kang HG, Lim KM, Kim JH, Kim HS. Three dimensionally printed personalized implant design and reconstructive surgery for a bone tumor of the calcaneus: a case report. JBJS Case Connect. 2018;8(2):e25.

The Composite Custom-Made Prosthesis

14

Carmine Zoccali, Nicola Salducca, Fabio Erba, and Giovanni Zoccali

14.1 Introduction

3D-Printed Titanium Custom-Made Prostheses (3DPTCMP) are currently a reality in reconstruction after complex resections; in cases in which standard modular prostheses are not able to restore the anatomy, a custom-made construct is considered a valid solution [1].

Indeed, Custom-Made Prosthesis (CMP) plays a role moreover in the pelvis where modular prostheses are not so efficient in guaranteeing stability and function [2].

In some cases, the use of composite massive allografts is still the best solution, because allograft osseointegration can guarantee a greater stability and a longer result, increasing also the bone stock even if the bone quality is low [3].

CMPs were already used in the early 1970s at the beginning of the limb savage surgery epoch, before the development of modular prostheses; nevertheless, they did not allow to fix tendon and muscles and they were characterized by an intrinsic instability. Moreover, they were characterized by a high complication rate, infections in the first place [4]. Also, prosthesis survival was limited and the patient could undergo several revisions during his lifetime.

Allograft Composite Prostheses (ACPs) were introduced to try to reduce the instability related to CMP.

An ACP consists in a revision prosthesis inserted in a massive allograft which maintains its tendons' insertions so that they can be sutured with the patient's residual tendons and muscles. Reattaching tendons should increase the joint stability, assuring a better function and increase the patient's bone stock [5].

Obviously, ACPs also present several complications as periprosthetic bone resorption, non-union at the graft-host bone interface, fractures, and infections [6].

Infection is considered the most important complication; the frequency can vary and depends on several factors as the infection site; indeed, the pelvis is considered at high risk. An ACP is actually a huge foreign body and acts as an optimal environment and culture medium for bacteria growth [7].

C. Zoccali (✉)
Department of Anatomical, Histological, Forensic Medicine and Orthopaedic Science, Sapienza University of Rome, Rome, Italy

Oncological Orthopedics, IFO - Regina Elena National Cancer Institute, Rome, Italy

N. Salducca
Oncological Orthopedic Department, IRCCS – Regina Elena National Cancer Institute, Rome, Italy
e-mail: nicola.salducca@ifo.gov.it

F. Erba
Regione Lazio Muscular-Skeletal Tissue Bank, Regina Elena National Cancer Institute, Rome, Italy
e-mail: fabio.erba@ifo.gov.it

G. Zoccali
Plastic Surgery - Queen Victoria Hospital NHS foundation trust, East Grinstead, West Sussex, UK

C. Zoccali et al. (eds.), *3D Printing in Bone Surgery*, https://doi.org/10.1007/978-3-030-91900-9_14

Another important factor which has to be taken in consideration is that these patients often have to undergo postoperative chemotherapy and radiotherapy which can decrease the fusion process, increase the infection risk and the incidence of allograft fractures [6].

Thus, while the use of the 3DPTCMP can be considered a new solution at a first glance, it actually is a return to the first reconstruction techniques. Obviously, the availability of new materials and new techniques can bring better results than in the past.

3DPTCMP should assure a more efficient reconstruction with better functional results, decreasing the high infection risk associated to ACP. Indeed, ACP prolongs surgery duration and therefore the related infection risk, while the possibility to fill the gap with a ready-made system decreases surgery time and maybe the infection risk. Moreover, the surface of 3DPTCMPs can be treated with several techniques to reduce bacteria surface adhesion and biofilm formation. Obviously, these factors must be considered hypothetic; more data are necessary to verify these intuitions.

One of the most important criticism associated to 3DPTCMP is the risk of mobilization, mostly at long-term follow-up, and the non-restoration of the bone stock. Indeed, the loss of bone stock associated to an important resection could make a successive revision after 3DPTCMP reconstruction very complex, with a high risk of infection and poor functional results.

A possible solution could be a Composite Custom-Made Prosthesis (CCMP) which could combine the primary stability and the fast assembly of a 3DPTCMP with a better integration derived from the graft component.

It comes from the union of a bone graft (human or animal), which can be processed, cut, and composed to adapt to and restore the anatomy of the gap after tumor removal, added to a custom-made structure which must give primary stability and reinforce the graft.

14.2 The Composite Custom-Made Prosthesis

The Composite CCMP is therefore composed by a biological component and a 3D-printed custom-made component.

The biological component should have the characteristics of the ideal bone graft, which means it has to encourage osteoinduction, osteoconduction, and osteogenesis.

Osteoinduction is the ability to stimulate primitive, undifferentiated pluripotent cells to differentiate into a bone-forming cell lineage [8]; osteoconduction is the ability of a structure to facilitate bone growth on its surface [8]. Osteogenic activity is the ability of cells already present in the tissue to produce bone [9].

Another important characteristic is osteointegration; this term strictly refers to a non-osseous structure as a prosthesis and the ability of bone to adhere and have a strong link with it [10]; this concept can also be applied to a graft.

The biological component can be of different origin:

- massive autograft (Fig. 14.1): it presents no osteogenic activity, low osteoconductiveness, and good osteoinductive activity; osseointegration is limited to the contact area for a few centimeters; the limits are similar to those of massive autografts in composite prostheses and are related to the low osseointegration which can cause failure at long-term follow-up. It is not easy to find a massive allograft with a shape that is perfectly compatible with the patient; a possible solution could be the manipulation and the specific cutting in white room (Class A) and the production of specific cutting guides to reproduce the programmed resection.
- engineered bone (Fig. 14.2): The characteristics depend on the specific type; nevertheless, they usually present low osteogenic and osteoconductive activity and good osteoinductive properties; osseointegration can also be subtotal.

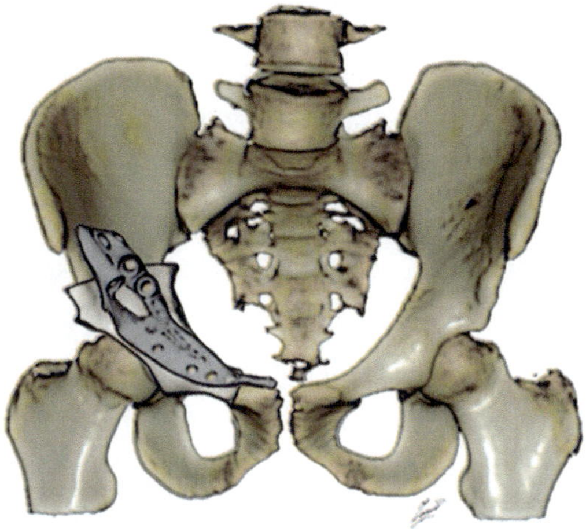

Fig. 14.1 Picture showing a composite allograft where the biological component is constituted by a standard massive allograft; the shape of the allograft can obviously be different from the resected part. Nevertheless, it can be precut in white room by a computer-guided system to better adapt to the patient's pelvic anatomy. A custom-made structure is then used to better stabilize the allograft

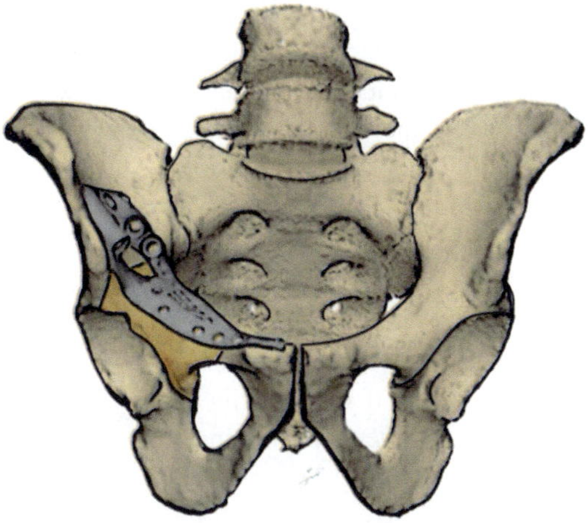

Fig. 14.2 A composite custom-made prosthesis where the biological component is represented by an engineered custom-made graft; in this case, the shape of the bone is identical to the resected part, but it could be modified to increase the bone stock in anticipation of a future revision surgery

– vascularized autograft (Fig. 14.3): It evidently presents the best biological properties: high osteogenicity, osteoinduction and osteoconduction activity; the possible donor areas are obviously limited, as the size of the graft.

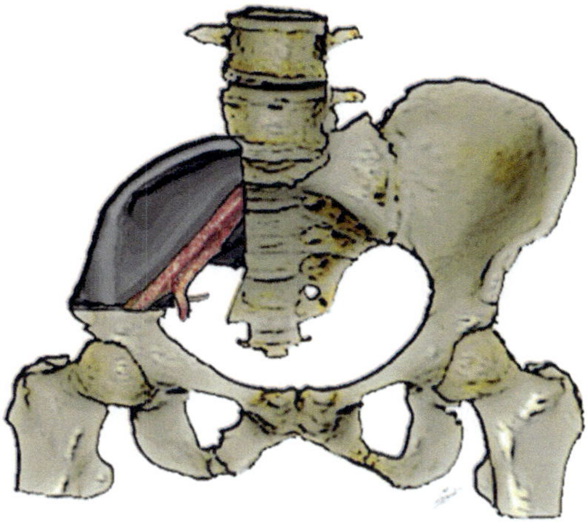

Fig. 14.3 A vascularized composite custom-made prosthesis; the 3D-printed titanium custom-made prosthesis provides primary stability and the vascularized fibular flap gives a long-term stability after consolidation, reducing the risk of mobilization

This technique could play a role in reconstruction after resection of the sacro-iliac joint. The CMP can present a slot where the vascularized autograft can be inserted assuring long-term stability and protecting the CMP from overload.

The 3D-printed custom-made components should guarantee stability to the system, moreover during the first time of osseointegration.

14.3 Exemplificative Case

Male patient, 63 years old, presented to our observation after discovering an osteolysis in his right acetabular roof. He complained a pain localized in his right hip onset about 3 months earlier. Considering that the symptoms did not improve with pain killers, his general practitioner proscribed an X-ray which showed the tumor and addressed the patient to a specialized tumor center (Fig. 14.4a). The patient underwent an MRI that displayed a cartilaginous-like nature, and a CT scan which evidenced an osteolytic mass with the presence of rare calcifications, suggestive of chondrosarcoma (CS) (Fig. 14.4b, c). The successive CT-guided biopsy confirmed the clinical suspect of CS-G1.

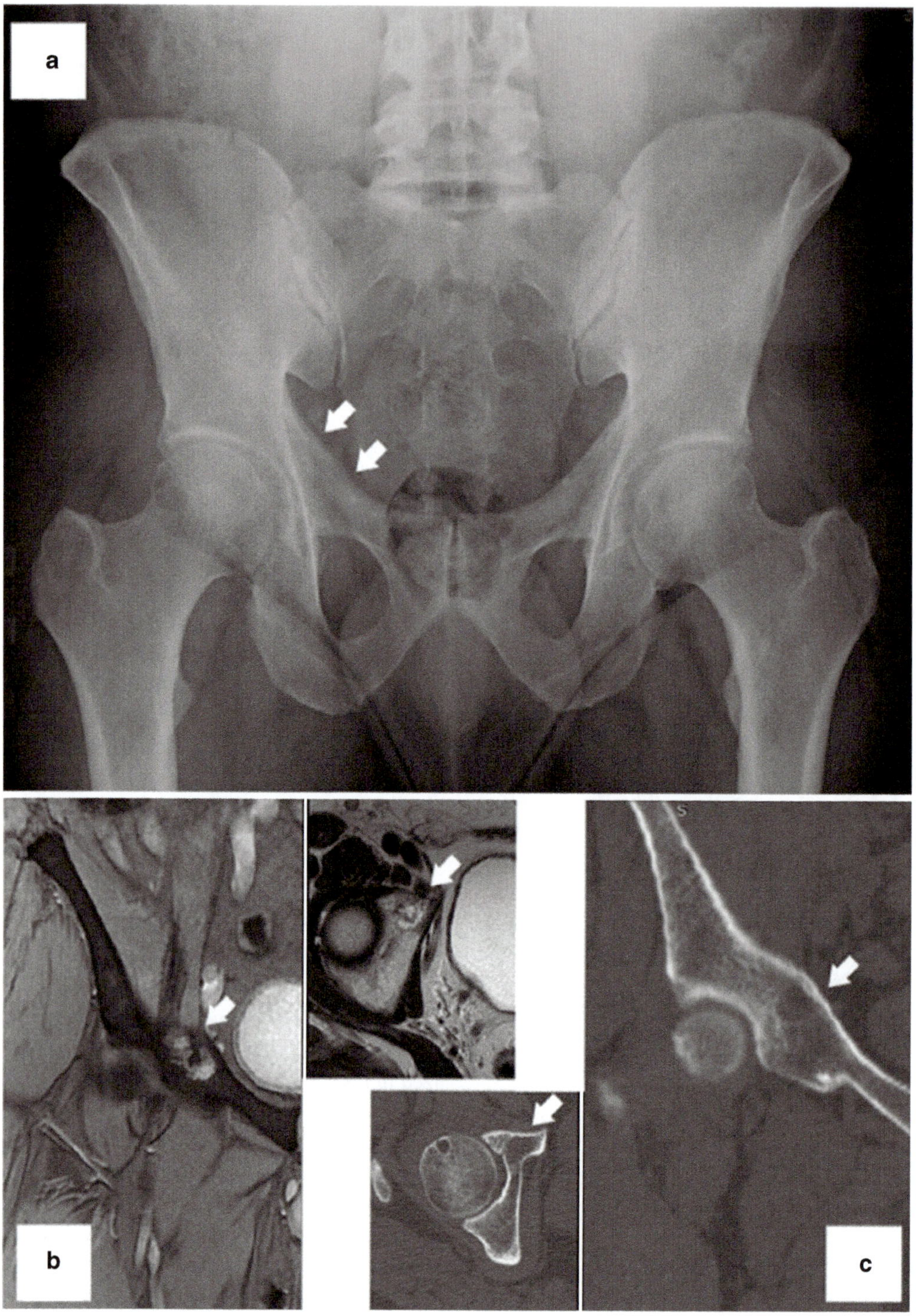

Fig. 14.4 (**a**) X-ray showing the partial osteolytic lesion in the right ileo-pubic ramus; the upper margin appears blown with a thin periosteal reaction; (**b**) Coronal and axial MRI scans evidencing cartilaginous-like tissue suggestive of chondroid tumor; (**c**) Axial and coronal CT scan showing the osteolytic lesion; some little calcification is present but not evident

The case was then discussed in a multidisciplinary team and the following possibilities were evaluated:

1. Standard resection and reconstruction with a composite allograft prosthesis: This technique can be considered the gold-standard treatment; after resection, a corresponding acetabular roof from a muscular-skeletal tissue bank is used to fill the gap and a standard Total Hip Arthroplasty (THA) is used to restore the joint.
2. Resection guided by cutting guides and reconstruction with 3D-printed titanium custom-made prosthesis and a standard THA. In this case the cutting guides should assure a safer and more accurate resection and the custom-made prosthesis should guarantee a more effective reconstruction.
3. Resection guided by cutting guides and reconstruction with a custom construct made of bone and a 3D-printed custom-made system that, like a plate, should give primary stability to the biological part.

Considering the low grade of aggressiveness and the possibility to perform a biological reconstruction, the third hypothesis was chosen.

The biological component was composed by several bone segments cut from larger bovine bones and shaped to reproduce the patient's specific anatomy (Fig. 14.5).

This bone is engineered to maintain osteoconductive and osteoinductive characteristics and allows a complete integration after a variable time period, depending on the dimensions of the graft.

The 3D-printed custom-made component is designed to adapt to the custom-made bone segments and stabilize them during the time necessary to obtain a first osseointegration.

Surgery was performed in supine position with an ileo-inguinal incision; the neurovascular bundle was isolated and dislocated medially and a cutting guide was applied on the anterior part of the iliac crest (Fig. 14.6a) to perform an accurate osteotomy, paying attention to not damaging the femoral head; then, the ileo-pubic rami was cut as medial as possible using a Gigli saw, as projected in preoperative planning (Fig. 14.6b) and the tumor was extirpated with an apparent wide margin (Fig. 14.6c).

The CCM was then composed starting from the different bone segments (Fig. 14.7a) which had to be assembled and stabilized with the 3DPTCM component (Fig. 14.7b).

The CCM was applied to fill the gap and was stabilized to the iliac wing and to the remaining symphysis using screws (Fig. 14.7c); a homoplastic fascia lata was placed between the bone graft and the femoral head to induce fibrosis and decrease its abrasion.

The immediate postoperative time elapsed without complications. The patient was allowed

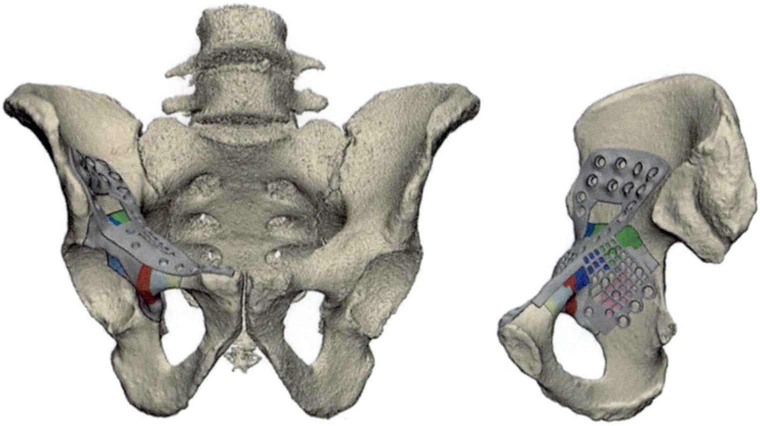

Fig. 14.5 The computerized rendering of the project; the 3DPTCMP was designed to give primary stability and to contain the xeno-segments (shown in different colors) cut to reproduce the anatomy

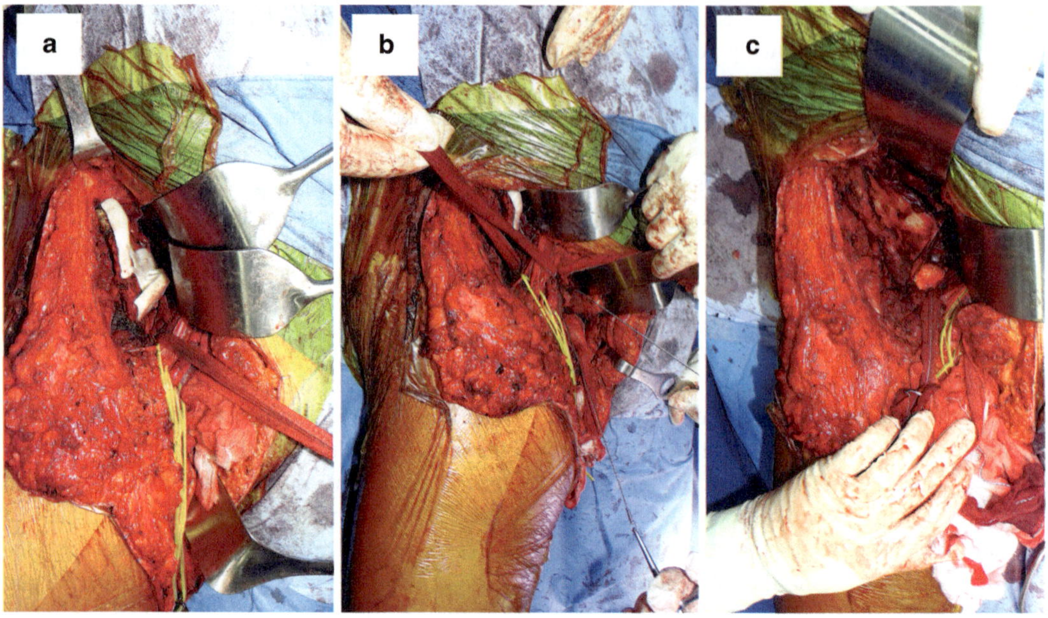

Fig. 14.6 (**a**): Intraoperative picture showing the isolated and medially dislocated neurovascular bundle and a cutting guide applied on the iliac crest to perform the lateral osteotomy; (**b**): successively, the neurovascular bundle was dislocated laterally and the ileo-pubic ramus osteotomy was performed with a Gigli saw, as medially as possible; (**c**): the surgical field after tumor resection, the femoral head is visible on the bottom

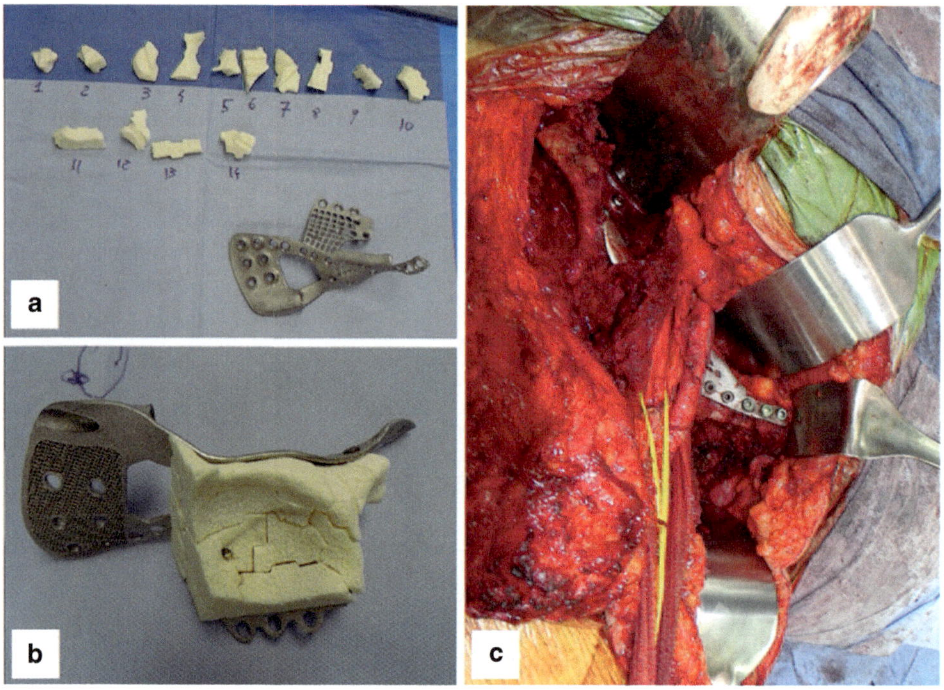

Fig. 14.7 The segments produced cutting bovine bone (**a**) were assembled and stabilized on a 3D-printed titanium custom-made construct (**b**) which was used to fill the gap that remained after tumor removal (**c**)

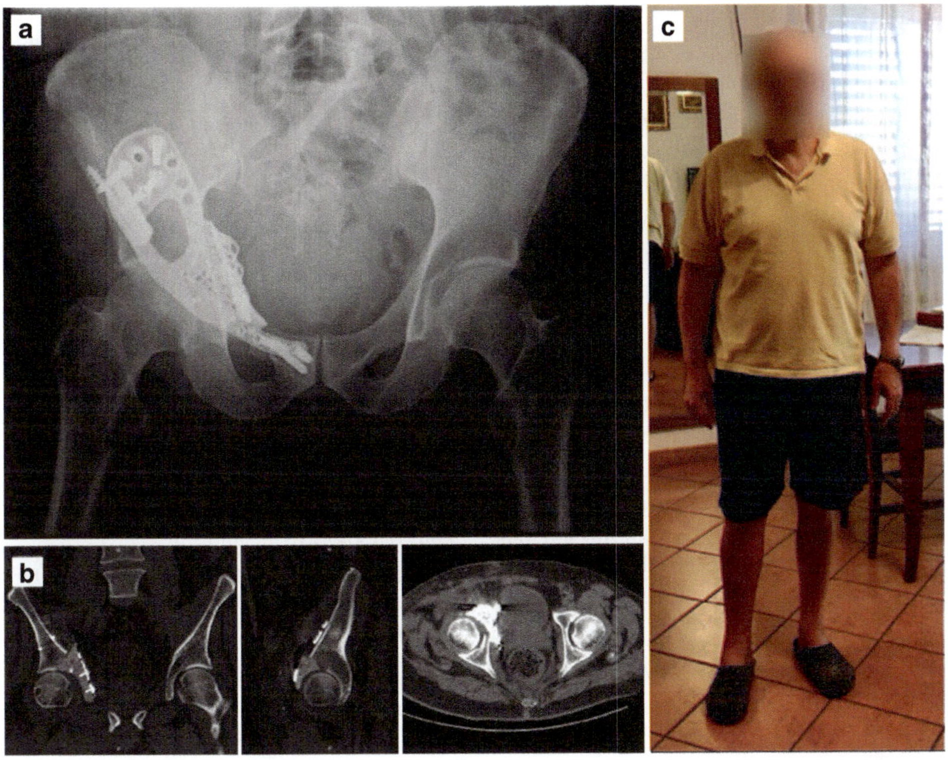

Fig. 14.8 X-ray (**a**) and CT scan (**b**) performed at 6 months of follow-up, showing the partially osseointegrated composite structure; (**c**) the patient weight bearing

to walk with two crutches without weight bearing after 3 weeks of bed rest. Progressive weight bearing was allowed after 3 months, reaching total bearing after 6 months from surgery.

The X-ray and CT scan performed at 6 months of follow-up showed a satisfying reconstruction (Fig. 14.8).

At 1 year of follow-up, the patient is able to walk with a crutch without significant pain.

14.4 Discussion

The duality between prosthesis and biological reconstruction is well known in literature. The first reconstruction techniques were based on custom-made prostheses; then allografts were matched to modular prostheses in composite constructs to overcome instability and try to improve functional outcomes. At present, CMPs and 3DPTCMPs are wide-spreading because they assure better and more accurate reconstructions and decrease the infection rate as well. The CCMP is a new attempt to add a biological value to the CMP, assuring better and longer results.

The periodic introduction of new techniques and new materials pushes the equilibrium from one side to the other and this could continue for the next decades since new technologies as bio-printing will allow to produce patient-specific replacement segments totally biocompatible with the originals.

The biological component added to CMPs should increase the bone stock with the intent to allow possible solutions in case of future revisions; moreover, when the biological component is constituted by a vascularized autograft, the intent is to give long-term stability, reducing the risk of mobilization.

In the proposed exemplificative case, our intent was to assure sufficient bone tissue to allow the use of a standard prosthesis when secondary arthritis will onset. Unfortunately, at present, we do not know the biomechanical and biological characteristics of the artificial bone and if it will be able to support a standard cup in case of a total hip arthroplasty.

More experience and randomized prospective studies are necessary to value the effectiveness of the technique and to understand if this could be considered a new step in limb-salvage surgery.

References

1. Liang H, Ji T, Zhang Y, Wang Y, Guo W. Reconstruction with 3D-printed pelvic endoprostheses after resection of a pelvic tumour. Bone Joint J. 2017 Feb;99-B(2):267–75.
2. Guo W, Li D, Tang X, Yang Y, Ji T. Reconstruction with modular hemipelvic prostheses for periacetabular tumor. Clin Orthop Relat Res. 2007 Aug;461:180–8. https://doi.org/10.1097/BLO.0b013e31806165d5.
3. Delloye C, Banse X, Brichard B, Docquier PL, Cornu O. Pelvic reconstruction with a structural pelvic allograft after resection of a malignant bone tumor. J Bone Joint Surg Am. 2007;89(3):579–87. https://doi.org/10.2106/JBJS.E.00943.
4. Kotz R, Ritschl P, Trachtenbrodt J. A modular femur-tibia reconstruction system. Orthopedics. 1986;9(12):1639–52.
5. Lee SH, Ahn YJ, Chung SJ, Kim BK, Hwang JH. The use of allograft prosthesis composite for extensive proximal femoral bone deficiencies: a 2- to 9.8-year follow-up study. J Arthroplast. 2009;24(8):1241–12481.
6. Mayle RE Jr, Paprosky WG. Massive bone loss: allograft-Prosthetic Composites and beyond. J Bone Joint Surg Br. 2012;94(11 Suppl A):61–4.
7. Deijkers RL, Bloem RM, Petit PL, Brand R, Vehmeyer SB, Veen MR. Contamination of bone allografts: analysis of incidence and predisposing factors. J Bone Joint Surg Br. 1997;79(1):161–6.
8. Wilson-Hench J. Osteoinduc- tion. In: Williams DF, editor. Progress in biomedical engineering, vol. 4. Amsterdam: Definitions in biomaterials, Elsevier; 1987. p. 29.
9. Baldwin P, Li DJ, Auston DA, Mir HS, Yoon RS, Koval KJ. Autograft, allograft, and bone graft substitutes: clinical evidence and indications for use in the setting of orthopaedic trauma surgery. J Orthop Trauma. 2019 Apr;33(4):203–13.
10. Zarb G, Albrektsson T. Osseointegration – a requiem for the periodontal ligament? – an editorial. Int J Periodont Rest Dentistry. 1991;11:88–91.

3D-Printed Custom-Made Instruments

15

Jacopo Baldi, Alessandro Grò, Umberto Orsini, and Leonardo Favale

15.1 3D-Printed Custom-Made Instrumentations

In traditional orthopedic procedures, surgeons mentally integrate all preoperative two-dimensional (2D) images and formulate a 3D surgical plan. This preoperative planning is particularly difficult in areas with complex anatomy and severe deformity, or in cases of bone tumor surgery. 2D axial images can be processed into other reformatted views (sagittal and coronal), and 3D virtual models with patient-specific anatomy can be created. Then, with improved visualization, surgeons can analyze this processed information to make a more detailed diagnosis, planning, and surgical intervention on a patient-specific basis [1].

3D printed models are useful for transferring information to the surgeon; moreover, they allow to test the procedure on patient-specific (PS) anatomy through the use of printing materials, able to resemble the mechanical properties of bone [2].

Actually, applying 3D printing technology for the development of dedicated tools that help the conduct of surgical procedures represents a chance for success rather than a real indication. Radermacher et al., for the first time in the 1990s, introduced the concept of Patient-Specific Instrument (PSI), a 3D printed intraoperative instrument [3]; PSI exists for total knee arthroplasty [4–7], hip resurfacing [8], pedicle screw insertion [9, 10], pelvic osteotomies [11], and long-bones corrective osteotomy.

In the treatment of axial or appendicular skeletal deformities the 3D printing technology allows the creation of instruments that facilitate the surgical procedure, making it safe and quick to perform. The execution of corrective osteotomies normally depends on the experience of the orthopedic surgeon who uses standard surgical instruments; osteotomy not only allows for angular correction in three different planes (varus/valgus, extension/flexion, and internal/external rotation) but also for displacement correction in three directions (lengthening/shortening, medial/lateral, dorsal/ventral). This 3D complexity means that these procedures benefit greatly from 3D planning. The suggested applications for PSI range from lower limb osteotomies [12–14] and upper limb osteotomies [15–17] to osteotomies to improve joint functions [18–21]. The availability of 3D printed instruments can also be a fundamental aid in the placement of screws such as pedicle screw placement in case of severe congenital scoliosis intending to design patient-specific instrumentations [9, 10].

Another example of PSI use can be the treatment of osteochondral autologous transplanta-

J. Baldi (✉) · A. Grò · U. Orsini · L. Favale
Oncological Orthopaedics Department, IRCCS - Regina Elena National Cancer Institute, Rome, Italy
e-mail: alessandro.gro@ifo.gov.it; leonardo.favale@ifo.gov.it

C. Zoccali et al. (eds.), *3D Printing in Bone Surgery*, https://doi.org/10.1007/978-3-030-91900-9_15

tions (OAT) [22] procedures as a treatment option for osteochondral cartilage defects. In the surgical plan, a set of customized guides could be designed and 3D-printed for each osteochondral graft as follows: a positioning template, a harvest guide cylinder, and a delivery guide cylinder. This means to obtain the desired grafts technically in the best way and to position them in the damage site respecting the preoperative planning as much as possible in order to restore the desired anatomy and function recovery [23, 24].

In traumatology, the possibility of creating 3D models reproducing the fracture pattern helps the surgeon to think about the reduction and the correct positioning of the synthesis instruments. The customized production of surgical instruments dedicated to trauma is difficult to speculate. The surgical timing required in this field of orthopedic surgery often incompatible with the once required for the production of PSI. In the polytraumatized patient, the need to treat, first of all, associated lesions of the splanchnic organs in order to obtain hemodynamic stability, can lead to a delayed treatment of the associated fractures. Especially in pelvic fractures, complex both for anatomical and three-dimensional reasons, the bone synthesis performed in emergency condition doesn't lead to satisfactory results; due to this a definitive surgical treatment is often required. In these cases, are treated the outcomes of the fracture rather than the fracture itself. Manufacturing of ad-hoc tools could be a great surgical opportunity. To achieve a stable anatomical synthesis, it is possible to create resection jigs and customized osteotomes for calloclasia, or corrective osteotomies; moreover, the use of guides for the introduction of free screws between the fracture fragments and the design of levers for the reduction maneuvers of the main fracture fragments guarantee the success of planned treatment.

Aimed to achieve surgical radicality, oncological orthopedics probably represents the branch in which 3D printing aimed at customizing surgical instruments finds its greatest use both for anatomically complex sites than for districts, easily accessible, where the disease has made the success of the surgery particularly difficult.

By using MRI and CT scan, it is possible to study exactly the tumor extension planning the resection levels in advance [25]; once these cutting levels are defined, thanks to 3D printing technology, it is possible to create real PSI. The surrounding structures, such as the soft tissues (e.g., ligaments, residual muscle tissue), can be considered, and, if needed, they can be the base for the creation of 3D study models. Once the margins, the resection planes, the type of reconstruction, and the fixation devices are defined, different types of patient-specific guides can be designed to transfer the preoperative plan to the surgery.

Basic guide, as reference guide once applied on the bone, serves as a registration tool between the 3D planning and the intraoperative situation. For accurate matching of the preoperative plan to the intraoperative setup, the guide needs to be placed exactly on the pre-planned position. The undersurface of the guide must be shaped as a negative of the bone surface in regions with distinct bone features ensuring that way the guide precisely apposed on the planned position. This use is allowed in regions where the tumor does not reach the surface of the bone; this means that in every case it is necessary to plan the part of the basic guide that matches the bone surface in safe distance to the affected bone area. When the right position for the guide is found, the placement of reference surgical pins must be performed. For this reason, it must have pre-planned drill sleeves attached. Every further step relies on these pins, including every additional placement of other guides.

Since tumor resection produces a bone defect, allograft size needs to be considered. For the reconstruction phase, the use of an equivalent bone (same bone in the same dimensions), when possible, must be kept in mind. An allograft construct has to perfectly fit in the bone defect. Starting from the allograft CT scan, 3D models are created similarly to what described for tumor resection jigs. Another option is to create a guide in which the allograft could be inserted, like a casket. Additional drill sleeves and cutting slits need to be added onto this guide in such a manner that the allograft could be prepared as needed, so that the drill bit or saw blade is constrained to the planned osteotomy planes, and proper customizing of the allograft will be achieved [26].

One of the most frequent application sites of PSI is the oncological pelvic surgery. Because of the complex geometry of the pelvis, tumor resection requires good cutting accuracy; the recurrence rates within the pelvis can be high, ranging from 28 to 35% [27]. To reduce this poor accuracy computer-assisted technologies have been developed for pelvic bone tumor surgeries. PSI technology was introduced alternatively to navigation systems. PSI is an intraoperative technology that allows the surgeon to replicate the preoperative resection strategy with relevant accuracy; this is consistent with the findings of Wong et al. [28] who assessed a millimetric resection accuracy during an extremity bone tumor surgery. Bellanova et al. [29] applied 3D printed technology to design PSIs to guide tumor resection cuts and allograft, shaping cuts for four pediatric patients undergoing tibial bone sarcoma resection, and bone-bank allograft reconstruction. Consequently, all resection margins were tumor-free. Postoperative imaging revealed satisfactory host-graft contact and no evidence of recurrent disease.

PSI guides and instruments are a relatively newly developed computer-assisted technology, and their application for orthopedic surgical interventions is in the beginning phase.

FDA has already cleared some 3D printed devices and issued more generalized draft guidance; the responsibility for appropriate long-term clinical evaluation rests with the individual surgeons and their institutions.

The results reported in the literature, regarding the quality of surgical operations performed with PSI rather than with conventional surgical instruments, especially in the field of conventional prosthetics and correction of skeletal deformities, and in some areas of oncological orthopedics, are encouraging. A series of technical and logistical limits remain to be reported.

The technical limitations of PSI usage include the need for adequate bone exposure intraoperatively to ensure a satisfactory fit. This could be challenging during the operation due to surrounding soft tissue and muscle. Also, the lack of real-time feedback when using PSIs, as compared to navigation systems, could potentially result in incorrect placement. Inexact placement of PSI could result in the subsequent inaccurate guided procedure and may result in deviation from the preoperative plan.

For what about logistics the use of PSI requires accurate preoperative planning and a timeframe of manufacturing of 4–5 days at least. This could be not acceptable in oncological orthopedics because it could result in tumor growth during the manufacturing period with a consequent mismatch of PSI with patient anatomy and an inaccurate or even an intralesional excision.

The customized surgical instruments provide a new method of planning the surgical intervention and effectively transfer the operative planning to the practice, making it easy to use.

According to the literature data, the customized cutting masks allow a reduction in surgical times [30]; intraoperative complications and blood loss can also be significantly reduced making the surgical procedure safer. The higher accuracy of the cuts makes safe resection margins and better surgical results possible to achieve.

Unlike freehand resection techniques and those that use navigation systems, which require great surgical experience, the use of cutting masks simplifies the technical execution of the intervention by reducing the operator's learning curve to the planning phase, for which it is essential to develop three-dimensional thinking. There might be a learning curve for researchers and technicians in the design of the guides too.

The future of PSI is not limited only to the creation of cutting jigs; 3D printing represents the opportunity to create with readymade, low-cost, easily re-use materials entire surgical sets, intended for conventional orthopedic surgery in economically disadvantaged places in the world or conflict situations.

David Armstrong, Professor of Surgery and Director of the Southern Arizona Limb Salvage Alliance (SALSA) at the University of Arizona, interested in 3D printing, about the realization of low-cost surgical instruments says: "It seems like there is a possibility there for low-resource settings or inaccessible areas" [31].

15.2 Clinical Applications

One of the first clinical cases we decided to use customized tools is that of a 37-year-old patient diagnosed with low-grade osteosarcoma (Fig. 15.1).

The lesion was classically located at the distal metaphyseal region of the femur, lateral surface. In order to achieve an adequate result both surgically and oncologically, we decided, starting from the preoperative thin-layer CT scan, to produce customized cutting jigs. One jig, applied in situ, made the *en-bloc* resection of the lesion possible achieving wide margins. The other cutting mask, applied to the distal femur provided by tissue bank, allowed us to obtain the massive graft to be placed in the bone defect we produced. Although the graft stability was absolute, we preferred to fix it with a compression screw. The postoperative radiographic control highlights the perfect congruence between the graft and the treated skeletal segment.

The custom instrumentation is quite versatile and blends well with common computed navigation systems.

An example of this is the case of a 27-year-old patient diagnosed with low-grade chondrosarcoma of the medial femoral condyle plus intercondylar region (Fig. 15.2).

To achieve an oncologically correct result and to remove both the lesions with wide margins, the surgical procedure was divided into two phases. During the first phase, by a medial access to distal femur, the use of the computed navigator system made the removal of the condylar lesion possible. Given the anatomical site of the second lesion, it was decided to overcome the possible technical difficulties by combining the information obtained from the navigation system with the use of a custom-made titanium burr; this allows us to control the exact direction of the burr moment by moment, achieving the adequate removal of the intercondylar lesion.

Using another customized burr, starting from the proximal epiphysis provided by tissue bank, we obtained a bone cylinder of equal size and volume than the one resected in order to fill the *minus* created and to achieve the anatomical

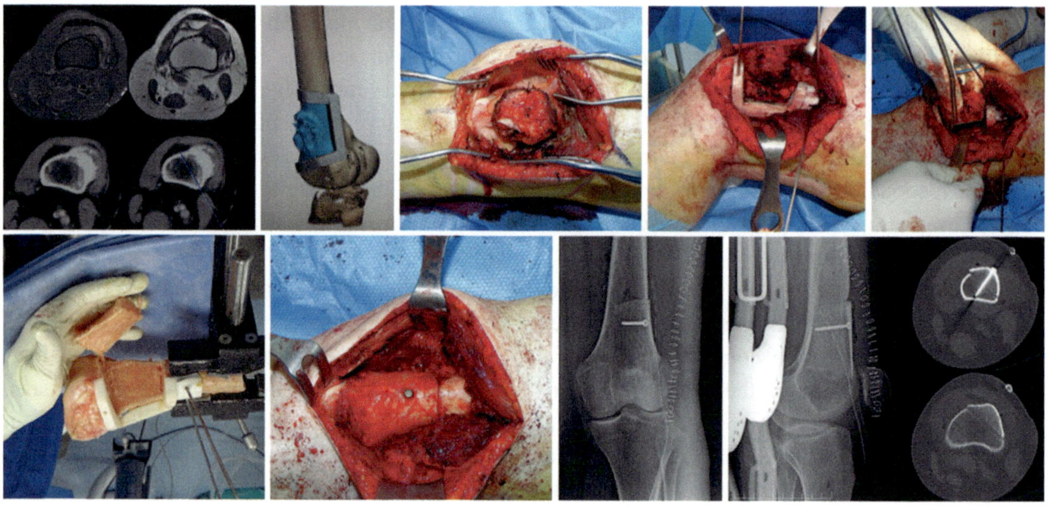

Fig. 15.1 37-year-old patient with low-grade osteosarcoma of the lateral part of the femoral metaphysis. The lesion was resected with a wide margin, using a 3D printed cutting jig manufactured on the basis of surgeon's needs and preoperative CT scan. The reconstruction was performed using a bone graft obtained from a distal femur provided by tissue bank, with a cutting mask similar to that used for resection

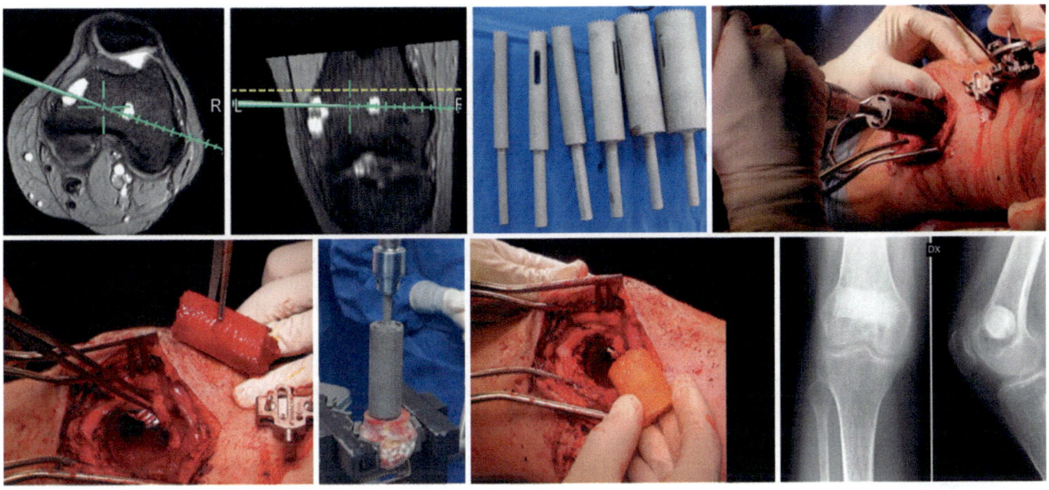

Fig. 15.2 27-year-old patient with histologically diagnosed low-grade chondrosarcoma of the medial epicondyle of the femur; there is the presence of further intercondylar neoformation. The two lesions were removed with a wide margin by using a titanium burr, manufactured on the basis of surgeon's indications and of the specific case with a 3D printer. The bone cylinder obtained, containing the two lesions, was removed with this burr and replaced by another bone cylinder obtained, using another similar custom-burr, from a femoral head provided by tissue bank. The procedure was totally guided by computerized navigation

reconstruction of the intercondylar region. Postoperative images and subsequent radiological controls documented the complete fusion of the graft to the host bone.

References

1. Zheng YX, Yu DF, Zhao JG, et al. 3D Print out models vs. 3D-rendered images: which is better for preoperative planning? J Surg Educ. 2016;73:518–23.
2. Bizzotto N, Sandri A, Regis D, et al. Three-dimensional print- ing of bone fractures: a new tangible realistic way for preoperative planning and education. Surg Innov. 2015;22:548–51.
3. Radermacher K, et al. Computer-assisted orthopedic surgery with image-based individual templates. Clin Orthop Relat Res. 1998;354:28e38.
4. Hafez MA, Chelule KL, Seedhom BB, Sherman KP. Computer-assisted total knee arthroplasty using patient-specific templating. Clin Orthop Relat Res. 2006;444:184–92.
5. Ng VY, DeClaire JH, Berend KR, Gulick BC, Lombardi AV Jr. Improved accuracy of alignment with patient-specific positioning guides compared with manual instrumentation in TKA. Clin Orthop Relat Res. 2012;470(1):99–107.
6. Nunley RM, Ellison BS, Zhu J, Ruh EL, Howell SM, Barrack RL. Do patient-specific guides improve coronal alignment in total knee arthroplasty? Clin Orthop Relat Res. 2012;470(3):895–902.
7. White D, Chelule KL, Seedhom BB. Accuracy of MRI vs CT imaging with particular reference to patient specific templates for total knee replacement surgery. Int J Med Robot. 2008;4(3):224–31.
8. Kunz M, Rudan JF, Wood GC, Ellis RE. Registration stability of physical templates in hip surgery. Stud Health Technol Inform. 2011;163:283–9.
9. Schkommodau E, Decker N, Klapper U, Birnbaum K, Staudte HW, Radermacher K. Pedicle screw implantation using the DISOS template system. In: Stiehl JB, Konermann WH, Haaker RG, editors. Navigation and robotics in Total joint and spine surgery. Berlin: Springer-Verlag; 2003. p. 501–5.
10. Thayaparan GK, Owbridge MG, Thompson RG, D'Urso PS. Designing patient-specific solutions using biomodelling and 3D-printing for revision lumbar spine surgery. Eur Spine J. 2018;28:18–24.
11. Staudte HW, Schkommodau E, Portheine F, Radermacher K. Pelvic osteotomy with template navigation. In: Stiehl JB, Konermann WH, Haaker RG, editors. Navigation and robotics in total joint and spine surgery. Berlin: Springer-Verlag; 2003. p. 455–63.
12. Munier M, Donnez M, Ollivier M, Flecher X, Chabrand P, Argenson JN, Parratte S. Can three-dimensional patient-specific cutting guides be used to achieve optimal correction for high tibial osteotomy? Pilot study. Orthop Traumatol Surg Res. 2017;103(2):245–50.

13. Hoekstra H, Rosseels W, Sermon A, Nijs S. Corrective limb osteotomy using patient specific 3D-printed guides: a technical note. Injury. 2016;47(10):2375–80.
14. Arnal-Burro J, Perez-Mananes R, Gallo-Del-Valle E, Igualada-Blazquez C, Cuervas-Mons M, Vaquero-Martin J. Three dimensional-printed patient-specific cutting guides for femoral varization osteotomy: do it yourself. Knee. 2017;24(6):1359–68.
15. Ranalletta M, Bertona A, Rios JM, Rossi LA, Tanoira I, Maignon GD, Sancineto CF. Corrective osteotomy for malunion of proximal humerus using a custom-made surgical guide based on three-dimensional computer planning: case report. J Shoulder Elb Surg. 2017;26(11):e357–63.
16. Bauer AS, Storelli DAR, Sibbel SE, McCarroll HR, Lattanza LL. Preoperative computer simulation and patient-specific guides are safe and effective to correct forearm deformity in children. J Pediatr Orthop. 2017;37(7):504–10.
17. Vlachopoulos L, Schweizer A, Graf M, Nagy L, Furnstahl P. Three-dimensional post- operative accuracy of extra-articular forearm osteotomies using CT-scan based patient-specific surgical guides. BMC Musculoskelet Disord. 2015;16:336.
18. Hirsiger S, Schweizer A, Miyake J, Nagy L, Furnstahl P. Corrective osteotomies of phalangeal and metacarpal Malunions using patient-specific guides: CT-based evaluation of the reduction accuracy. Hand. 2017;1(15 58944717726135):1558944717726135.
19. Weigelt L, Furnstahl P, Hirsiger S, Vlachopoulos L, Espinosa N, Wirth SH. Three-dimensional correction of complex ankle deformities with computer-assisted planning and patient-specific surgical guides. J Foot Ankle Surg. 2017;56(6):1158–64.
20. Schweizer A, Mauler F, Vlachopoulos L, Nagy L, Furnstahl P. Computer-assisted 3- dimensional reconstructions of scaphoid fractures and nonunions with and without the use of patient-specific guides: early clinical outcomes and postoperative assessments of reconstruction accuracy. J Hand Surg Am. 2016;41(1):59–69.
21. Schweizer A, Furnstahl P, Nagy L. Three-dimensional correction of distal radius intra-articular malunions using patient-specific drill guides. J Hand Surg Am. 2013;38(12):2339–47.
22. Sherman SL, Thyssen E, Nuelle CW. Osteochondral autologous transplantation. Clin Sports Med. 2017;36(3):489–500.
23. Sebastyan S, Kunz M, Stewart AJ, Bardana DD. Image-guided techniques improve accuracy of mosaic arthroplasty. Int J Comput Assist Radiol Surg. 2016;11(2):261–9.
24. Koh JL, Wirsing K, Lautenschlager E, Zhang LO. The effect of graft height mismatch on contact pressure following osteochondral grafting: a biomechanical study. Am J Sports Med. 2004;32(2):317–20.
25. Aisen AM, Martel W, Braunstein EM, McMillin KI, Phillips WA, Kling TF. MRI and CT evaluation of primary bone and soft-tissue tumors. Am J Roentgenol. 1986;146:749–56.
26. Luckas J, Daniel AM, Philipp F, Sandro FF, Lazaros V. Joint-preserving tumour resection around the knee with allograft reconstruction using three-dimensional preoperative planning and patient-specific instruments. Knee. 2019;26(3):787–93.
27. Dobbe JG, Pré KJ, Kloen P, Blankevoort L, Streekstra GJ. Computer-assisted and patient-specific 3-D planning and evaluation of a single-cut rotational osteotomy for complex long-bone deformities. Med Biol Eng Comput. 2011;49(12):1363–70.
28. Wong KC, Kumta SM, Sze KY, Wong CM. Use of patient-specific CAD/CAM surgical jig in extremity bone tumor resection and custom prosthetic reconstruction. Comput Aided Surg. 2012;17:1–10.
29. Bellanova L, Paul L, Docquier PL. Surgical guides (patient-specific instruments) for pediatric tibial bone sarcoma resection and allograft reconstruction. Sarcoma. 2013;2013:1e7.
30. Cartiaux O, Aurent P, Francq BG, Banse X, Docquier PL. Improved Accuracy with 3D Planning and Patient-Specific Instruments During Simulated Pelvic Bone Tumor Surgery. Annals of Biomedical Engineering. 2014;42(1):205–13.
31. Lee N. The lancet *technology: 3D printing for instruments, models, and organs?* Lancet. 2016;388:1368.

16 Future Developments of 3D Printing in Bone Surgery

Roberto Biagini, Alessandra Scotto di Uccio, Dario Attala, and Barbara Rossi

Today as never before, healthcare and surgery applications of 3D printing (3DP) represent a meeting point between dream and reality, present and future. This is especially true in the fields of cranial, maxillofacial, spinal, and orthopedic surgery, in case of cancer, trauma, or infection. 3DP aids all the stages of complex surgical reconstruction: imaging processing, planning, modeling, manufacturing, and operative implantation [1]. New generation splints, functional prosthetic hands, and even face masks for the pandemic COVID-19 outbreak are only a few examples of the new era of producing models, implants, and scaffolds [2, 3]. 3DP has tremendously grown in the fabrication of tailored prosthetics, medical implants, novel drug formulations, and bioprinting of bone and cartilaginous tissues in the past 10 years [2, 4]. The combination of 3DP technology with computer-assisted imaging and advanced anatomical models is a well-known, concrete possibility to use the novel additive manufacturing technique in clinical settings, educational presentations, surgical designs and to aid doctor–patient communication. The feasibility and effectiveness of 3DP are currently recognized to facilitate surgery: custom-made osteotomy guides and instruments decrease operative time and complications and problems related to donor site or bone flaps are avoided using patient-specific prostheses to replace joints, entire bones like scapulae and calcanei and parts of the spine, skull and pelvis [5–10]. As the personalization wave hits the healthcare industry and virtual software and technology meet biomaterial science and translational research, focusing on such a new born, rapidly growing 3D landscape is challenging, as perspectives have to face the limitations of actual viability, the small number of cases despite the numerous publications, the inhomogeneity of financial resources, the lack of standardized frameworks, and a yet too short learning (and training) curve. However, the analysis of recent literature on future directions of 3DP brings to an objective reflection on what will really be achievable in the next few years in the musculoskeletal surgery scenario (Fig. 16.1).

Since the Fused Deposition Modeling (FDM) patent expired in 2009, problems related to time and costs of manufacturing are likely to be overcome and 3DP technology will probably advance accordingly in clinical practice. The greatest expectations regard the possibility of creating printed human tissues and organs that

R. Biagini · B. Rossi (✉)
Oncological Orthopedics Unit, IFO - Regina Elena National Cancer Institute, Rome, Italy
e-mail: roberto.biagini@ifo.gov.it

A. Scotto di Uccio
Hepato-Biliary and Organ Transplant Unit, School of General Surgery, Sapienza University, Rome, Italy

D. Attala
Musculoskeletal Tissue Bank of the Lazio region, IFO - Regina Elena National Cancer Institute, Rome, Italy
e-mail: dario.attala@ifo.gov.it

C. Zoccali et al. (eds.), *3D Printing in Bone Surgery*, https://doi.org/10.1007/978-3-030-91900-9_16

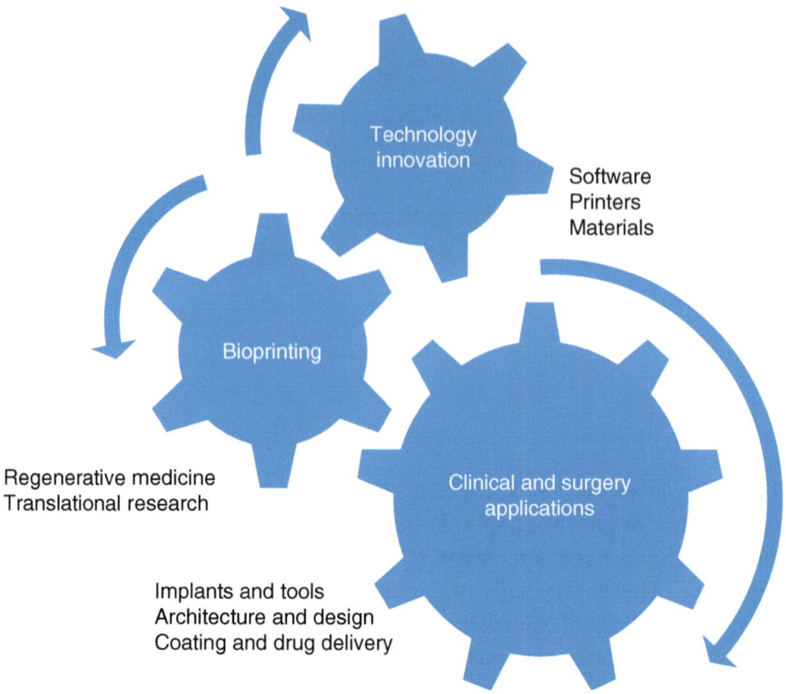

Fig. 16.1 Schematic integration of potential developments in 3D printing for bone surgery

can be transplanted like current grafts from donors [11, 12].

The aim of this study is a narrative overview on what is new in the use of 3DP in bone surgery and to investigate potential further developments. The authors' approach summarizes future perspectives in four main directions: technical innovations; clinical setting; bioprinting and 4D printing; 3DP banking.

16.1 Technical Innovations: New 3D Printers and Materials

The term "3D printing" refers to various technologies available for rapid prototyping (RP) through additive manufacturing, differently classified according to technique or basic material used (liquid, solid, or powder) [12, 13]. The 3DP systems most often used in biomedical applications are shown in Table 16.1.

Direct Metal Laser-based printing is mainly used for metal printing and implant manufacturing; with Selective Laser Sintering (SLS), a laser heats up the powdered material just below its melting point, whereas in Selective Laser Melting (SLM) the powder is heated just above its melting point. The final products differ in the porosity and fineness of the raw material: SLM requires a purer substance, while alloys with different porosity may be used in SLS.

The most promising new kind of 3DP technique is Electron Beam Melting (EBM). Metal powders can be consolidated into a solid mass using a computer-controlled electron beam as the heat source. Similar to SLM, parts are manufactured by melting metal powder, layer by layer, and the process takes place under vacuum, which makes it suited to manufacture parts made of reactive materials with a high affinity for oxygen, e.g., titanium. It allows to fabricate metallic components with complex shapes and porous structures or customized prostheses that replace irregular bones of unique dimensions. Furthermore, these devices and implants withstand autoclaving [13–15]. EBM greatly simplifies the processing steps and considerably reduced fabrication time. Besides producing customized implants, several companies have used EBM to manufacture special parts of standard prostheses. For example, the lattice structure of acetabular cups in hip replacement are fabricated

Table 16.1 Main features of different 3DP technologies used in the biomedical field

Types of techniques		Principle of working	Based-material state	Final manufacture type	Main use
Inkjet		The print head moves across a bed of powder, selectively depositing a liquid binding material	Liquid and powder	Plastic, ceramic, metal, hydrogel, gelatine (multicolored)	Modeling, bioprinting
Extrusion (nozzle)	FDM	Deposition of heat-softened thermoplastic materials	Solid	Thermoplastic, metal wires	
Laser heating	SLA	Polymerization of light-curable resin in layers or on mobile platforms	Liquid	Plastic	Implantation
	SLS	Molecular fusion of powder particles in upcoming layers in an adjustable bed of the desired shape	Powder	Plastic, metal alloys, ceramic	
	SLM	Similar to SLS but material powder is heated just above the melting point		Pure metal powder	
EBM		Material is melted layer by layer placed under a vacuum and different powders are fused together from heating by an electron beam	Solid or powder	Metal powder alloys or wire	

FDM Fused deposition modeling, *SLA* Stereolithography, *SLS* Selective laser sintering, *SLM* Selective laser melting, *EBM* Electron beam melting

by EBM [16]. Additive processes allow the structure of stems to be optimized to match the stiffness or flexibility of the host bone, reducing stress shielding [17]. Fan et al. were the first to describe in 2015 the use of prostheses manufactured by EBM to repair defects in unusual sites like clavicle, scapula, and ilium after malignant tumor resection [15]. Ti-6Al-4 V (TAV) alloy scaffolds manufactured by EBM have shown complete osteointegration within 60 days in an animal study [18].

Thus, metal RP processes like EBM and SLS can directly manufacture patient-specific medical TAV implants and devices at present. What we expect in the future is the possibility to integrate different 3DP modalities starting from the same computerized model in order to obtain complex multi-structured struts with different biomechanical features. Multi-tool printing with additional print heads or extruders will facilitate multi-material deposition in order to mimic the hierarchical complexity and heterogeneity of musculoskeletal tissues. A better performance in printer technology is the prerequisite for advances in 3DP engineering. In a recent study, vascularized bone was realized using polylactic acid (PLA) and gelatin methacryloyl (GelMA) enriched with BMP and VEGF, wherein PLA was deposited with FDM, while GelMA was printed using SLA [19].

Drawbacks include the inability to reproduce extremely small or thin structures because the printed products are excessively weak, and the necessity to improve the resolution of current cross-sectional scanners for CT or MRI which are responsible for the final accuracy of the 3D model.

While plastic materials are usually 3D-printed to be used as anatomic models and guiding instruments, metal powders, such as titanium or cobalt-chrome, are used to fabricate custom 3D-printed implants. Both SLM and DMLS can print a variety of metals and their alloys including stainless steel, aluminum and its alloys, titanium and alloy, cobalt-chrome and nickel alloys. Even precious metals like gold, silver, platinum, and palladium can be printed [12]. Biomimetic materials should be biocompatible and sterilizable for intraoperative use, with mechanical properties similar to those of native bone, which might help restore bony anatomical structures and biomechanical function. Polyether Ether Ketone (PEEK) offers exceptional strength along with superior heat and chemical resistance, and has excellent cell biocompatibility and a modulus of elasticity closer to that of cortical bone, which might help minimize stress-shielding effects in orthopedic implants [20]. PEEK has been used in trauma surgery as plates and in cervical spine surgery as reconstructive cages; carbon-fiber reinforced PEEK implants have recently been proposed for intramedullary nailing in patients affected by musculoskeletal tumors due to their positive biomechanical and structural properties, but above all for their advantages in performing radiotherapy and lesion monitoring during follow-up [21, 22]. This high-performance thermoplastic can now be 3D printed to make durable, lightweight and geometrically complex objects. The fabrication of 3D printed PEEK using FDM results in patient-specific implants with a smooth finish and no irregularities, of almost any complex geometry and which cannot be manufactured using other technologies [23]. Addition of bioactive materials such as calcium phosphates or bioglass and incorporation of porosity into PEEK improves bone-implant interfaces and osteointegration of PEEK-based devices. An innovative production technique based on the extrusion free-forming method realizes a bioactive PEEK/hydroxyapatite (PEEK/HA) composite with a unique configuration in which the HA bioactive phase distribution is accurately computer-controlled within a PEEK matrix [24]. The PEEK/HA biocomposites have exhibited a good biocompatibility and cell attachment, but the incorporation of HA into PEEK could result in modulation and reduction of mechanical strength which is also typical of carbon implants. It is yet to be demonstrated if 3D-printed PEEK artificial bones or implants are beneficial in patient-specific orthopedics [25].

16.2 Surgical Applications: Optimization of Constructs

Orthopedic applications include anatomic models that reproduce the patient's individual anatomy and pathology for surgical planning, education and training, patient-specific instruments for surgical procedures and fabrication of complex custom-made metal implants [25]. 3D Graphy is useful in acetabular and periarticular fractures, spinal and pediatric deformities, osteotomy planning, and reconstruction of bone defects [12]. 3DP technology can be used in surgery to manufacture prostheses and implants, used to reconstruct both soft tissues (arteries, muscles, tendons) and bone tissue [3]. Printing life-size anatomic models to aid tumor resection planning and trauma injury treatment is already a concrete opportunity in orthopedic surgery; the future developments should include the creation of models for preoperative distraction osteogenesis device selection, printing customized external fixators in fractures and mimicking expandable nailing or prostheses in limb salvage in children. The entire 3DP reproduction of a certain anatomical region can be shared by physicians of different specialties to improve the understanding of a complex procedure or the management of a challenging case, as in retroperitoneal or pelvic sarcomas. 3DP is emerging as the ideal reconstructive solution especially in musculoskeletal oncology since these implants can be customized to match the various shapes of bone defects after tumor resection [26, 27]. These bone defects do not simply need reconstruction to restore skeletal stability and function, but should adapt to skeletal growth in younger patients and ensure a valid anchoring to the surrounding soft tissues. Theoretical features of an optimal 3D printed implant should be: biocompatibility, appropriate mechanical properties, low risk of infections and loosening, predictable reabsorption and osteointegration; highly precise conformance to human anatomy; fast delivery to cancer and trauma patients. Theoretically, patient-specific implants in limb salvage surgery should be truly innovative "biological prostheses" that enclose all the advantages of grafts, such as osteointegration and to be anchors for reattaching ligaments and muscles and, on the other hand, are effective in mechanical restoration and anatomic reconstruction of joints and entire flat bones [15]. The combination of titanium implants with autogenous bone graft as well as PEEK and titanium for the reconstruction of load-bearing segments could lead to the creation of extremely performant biomimetic composites. The nature of additive layer manufacturing in 3DP allows the fabrication of custom implants with any complex shape or geometric feature. In addition to perfect anatomical conformation, modern 3D printing techniques could generate complex free-form surfaces such as scaffold lattice in a metal monoblock. This interconnected pore surface could facilitate osteointegration and reduce stiffness mismatch at bone–implant junctions [25]. Flanges can be added to the design of artificial acetabular defect reconstruction for optimum screw fixation to the remaining pelvic bone [28]. The problem of stress shielding may be further minimized by adapting porosity, pore sizes and therefore the elastic modulus of porous titanium to patient-specific loading conditions studied prior to implant fabrication [17, 29]. Other potential implementation of constructs could involve the architecture of 3D-printed prostheses, allowing to modulate the implant body (full rather than trabecular or trellis-made) and the shape of the primary fixation systems (cylindrical, triangular, conical stems or taps) or create conical funnels to allocate multidirectional screws in iliac and acetabular 3D-printed prostheses, as necessary. Another trick to improve the geometry of struts for pelvic reconstruction could be the creation of a metallic loop at the border of flat implants in order to gain a durable lumbosacral fixation. Cutting edge 3DP technology can help solve the expensive and devastating challenge of two-stage revision in septic or aseptic periprosthetic loosening by producing antibiotic-coated patient-specific spacers that perfectly fill the bone defect [3]. Amelioration of 3D-guided orthopedic surgery also deals with advances in personalized guiding templates, drilling and cutting guides, jigs and tools that result in shorter operation time, lower radiation exposure, less blood loss, and smaller incision size [13, 30]. The border between computer-assisted designed models, 3D-printed anatomical models, intraoperative navigation, and robotic surgery has not been completely explored yet and a potential integration still clashes with scarce financial resources and a poor learning curve for such a highly demanding technology. The concomitant availability of these technologies may become valued for the most difficult reconstructions in cervical spine surgery, as in neuro- or maxillofacial surgery. However, 3DP templates can nowadays guide the surgeon intraoperatively in case of difficult orientation and this should be even more easily accessible in robotic surgery, in which the operator sits far from the surgical field. In other words, with its wide applicability, high accuracy, and cost-effectiveness, the development of clinical applications of 3DP in surgery aims to achieve the best restoration of function with minimal invasiveness and complication rate.

16.3 Bioprinting: 3DP in Regenerative Medicine and Drug Delivery Systems

The future of 3DP finds its greatest expression in the field of bone and osteochondral repair and artificial generation. The development of prototypes for tissue engineering is addressed in 40% of scientific articles published in the last 5 years on the use of RP in bioengineering [3]. Bioprinting will be the ultimate solution to complications of alloplastic implants and poor availability of grafts. In bone tissue engineering, 3DP biomimicry can offer the desired spatial orientation to create a biological tissue through the combination of cells, extracellular matrix, controlled gradient of growth factors and supporting scaffold material with controlled chemistry, shape, and interconnected porosity [12, 13, 31, 32]. Different 3DP methods (SLA, SLS, FDM, bioinks) can be used to create different bioceramic scaffolds, with different compositions and hierarchical structures (macropores, micropores, nanostructured particles, nanolayers, and nanochannels) and specific features in terms of mechanical, degradation, permeability, and biological properties [2, 30]. 3D-printed scaffolds provide different potential applications in bone tissue engineering (Fig. 16.2) achieving satisfactory interconnectivity and porosity, pre-ordered macrostructure, and excellent mechanical strength when compared to traditional fabricated scaffolds.

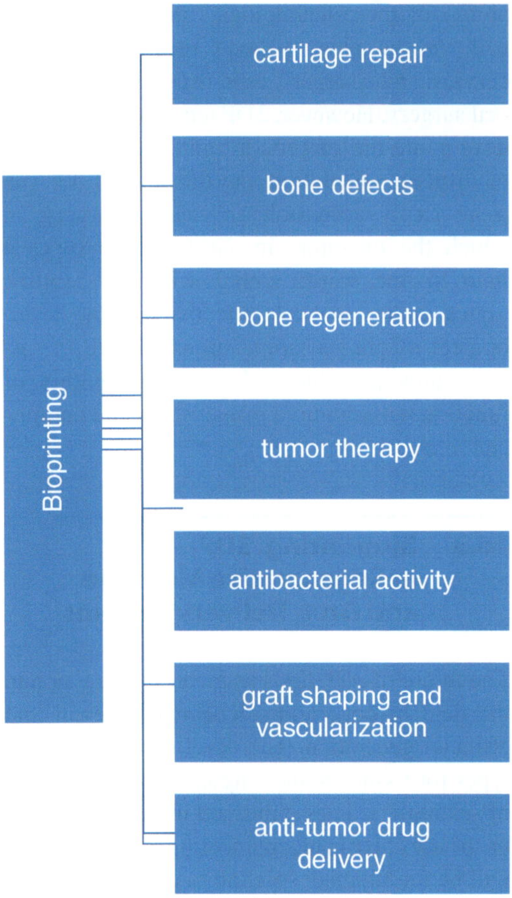

Fig. 16.2 Main applications of 3D bioprinting in bone tissue engineering

Bioceramic scaffolds play a crucial role in providing a predefined 3D architecture to create an environment for the adhesion, proliferation, and differentiation of mesenchymal stem cells (MSCs). Osteogenesis and osteoinduction are both promoted by the inclusion of bioactive composites/ceramic particles (from nano- to microsize range) in bioinks as osteo-promotive elements (silicate, borate, calcium, phosphate) that act either as nucleation centers which facilitate HA deposition on constructs or by releasing ions that induced MSCs differentiation [30, 33]. The hierarchic structure of 3D-printed bioceramic scaffolds can mimic the natural structure, as their osteogenic activity and bioactivity ensure anchoring sites for cell spreading throughout biomaterials. Since printable soft hydrogels for supporting biological factors have weaker mechanical properties than native bone, hybrid-tissue engineered constructs are realized combining them with rigid, porous additives that mimic structural strength of hard tissues [33]. For example, a 3D printed hypertrophic cartilage made from alginate bioink mechanically reinforced with PCL fibers was developed reproducing the architecture of the vertebral body: in vitro, the biocomposite successfully transitioned into vascularized bone via endochondral bone formation, similar to the physiological process of bone differentiation [34]. For osteochondral defects, human-derived induced pluripotent cell lines are increasingly being investigated for their potential use in cartilage 3DP, using nanofibrillated cellulose compositions with either alginate or hyaluronic acid hydrogels as supporting material conducive for miming a physiological environment [35]. In the field of meniscal lesions, 3D printed porous polycarbonate-urethane and ultra-high molecular weight polyethylene blends for the artificial meniscus are promising [36]. For bone defect repair in complex trauma, non-unions, tumors, and congenital anomalies, 3D-printed HA and tricalcium phosphate-based scaffolds and mesoporous bioactive glass composites showed a synergic capability in providing mechanical strength, osteogenesis, and angiogenesis in vitro and in vivo [30, 37].

Biodegradable, resorbable and biocompatible bioplastics as PLA and polycaprolactone (PCL) beads, discs, and filaments can be loaded with antibiotics or chemotherapy drugs for a more focused drug delivery system [38, 39]. The 3DP technique could generate devices, implants, and catheters specifically designed to reduce infections, treat osteomyelitis, tuberculosis, and cancer and help to prevent the spread of disease while controlling drugs release [2, 39, 40]. In addition to application in bone tissue regeneration, novel bifunctional bioceramic scaffolds with excellent photothermal or magnetothermal effects have proved to possess the ability to simultaneously treat tumors and regenerate bone. Local high temperature conductivity induced by functional scaffolds (graphene oxide (GO)-modified bioceramic scaffold, MoS2 nanosheets- or CuFeSe2 nanocrystals-covered ceramic scaffold) remarkably suppresses the proliferation of residual tumor cells and promotes tumor cell apoptosis while improving the osteogenic differentiation of rabbit bone MSCs [30, 33]. Sandwich-layered 3DP scaffolds, as GO-Fe3O4-GO or Silver/GO, represent a further optimization of these bioactive fillers, leading to the creation of superparamagnetic scaffolds with an oscillating magnetic field that locally kills the residual tumor cells or of scaffolds gifted with antibacterial activity, respectively [41, 42]. If 3DP tissue-engineered scaffolds are well able to support living cells, the novel frontier of biological 3DP is printing cells with the final aim of directly building living tissues. Through the combination of cellular assembly and biomimetic environments, bioprinting is intended to create new vital bone substitutes which are ink-printed in the required form and equipped with bone conduction and blood vessels, therefore capable to replace currently used grafts and allogenic bone marrow transplantation [3, 34]. It is now possible to realize the 3D micro-environmental niche for spatial tissue-specific differentiation by creating a gradient of VEGF within the 3D printed GelMA ink wherein the concentration of VEGF increases from the intramedullary cavity towards the cortex in order to ensure infiltration of blood vessels within the outer region of the bone tissue [43]. As concerning macroscopic creation of artificial functional tissue constructs of human-scale dimensions, development and availability of specialized 3D tissue-organ bioprinters are required. Some are already capable to reproduce mandible, calvarial bone, cartilage, and skeletal muscle of predefined geometry [33]. However, a probably not long but insidious way to actualization is due to the complexity of multiple cell types deployed during the bioprinting process, the risk of cellular damage during manufacturing and the intricate vasculature, nutrient and oxygen exchanges that are required to maintain long-term viability of tissue [3, 13, 30].

16.4 Considerations on 4D Printing

The promising results of 3D bioprinting in creating a dynamic microenvironment similar to that of native bone is a well-known reality in the field of bone tissue engineering. In spite of several successes in vitro, maintaining the viability and cellular differentiation potential of artificial constructs overtime and their subsequent preclinical testing in terms of stability, mechanical loading, immune responses, and osteogenic potential still needs to be explored [33]. Advances in 3DP mean to give manufactured constructs the power of changeability, motility and reaction to biochemical, electric or electromagnetic stimuli, possibly with no external intervention. 4D Printing is the new scenario in biomedical sciences, allowing 3DP manufacture to become "intelligent," changing its shape or functionalities with time, in response to changes in pH, temperature or osmolarity, environmental fluctuations of growth factors, and many other external stimuli just like in physiological conditions [44]. The skeletal and vascular systems fit well with this unique opportunity. Methacrylated alginate and hyaluronic acid-composite tubes mimicking small blood vessels or stents with self-folding or shape-changing features in response to blood pressure, physical stress, or blood flow have been developed [45], as well as thermo-responsive PCL micro-particles or shape memory polymers that behold mechanical properties comparable to cancellous human bone [46–48]. Another amazing potential could be smart advanced medications and bandages with lattice-based devices able to release oxygen or even antibiotics at the wound site in trauma injuries or after surgery to hasten healing and reduce the risk of infection [3].

16.5 3D Graphy Banking: To Go Over the Patient's Specific Bio-Modeling

Time and costs of production still limit the widespread diffusion of 3DP in the clinical setting. The available literature reports that the overall time to complete the printing process, from image elaboration to the final output, can range between about half a day to several weeks. At this stage, 3DP remains, therefore, only suitable for elective surgery [11]. The impact of 3DP has to be fully assessed in its capability to print large volumes of materials (economically), material durability must be established, and long-term safety of implantation has to be ascertained. The research on creating computer designs involved in the production of soft and rigid polymers that serve as manufacturing material for 3D printers is ongoing [3]. Developing the capability to print multiple manufactured materials (or composites) from the same printer is a precious opportunity for future medical practice. While this technology has yet to be fully realized, future soft tissue and bone surgery will be ever more highly demanding and patient-specific. No procedure of resection, osteosynthesis, reconstruction, graft or joint replacement fits all. Theoretically, a 3D synthetic bone or a composite from the combination of two synthetic polymers—soft collagen protein and rigid HA mineral—not only could have a structure similar to bone, but could even show a greater resistance to fracture than natural bone tissue. Advances in sterilizable biomaterials could make 3DP replicas and hundreds of different templates readily accessible for surgical planning or even intraoperative use in urgent cases. Postoperatively, these patient-specific physical models and their electronic files could be kept to build a library of various types of fractures, osteochondral and bone defects and tumors so that the models can be 3D-printed again when necessary [25]. Such a collection of 3DP templates could be precious for educational surgical training as well as for discussions of complex clinical cases among specialists of different disciplines and for better adherence of patients and their families to the treatment decision-making process.

16.6 Conclusions

Goals presently achieved in RP consist in manufacturing products that are either highly complex, highly customized or where the quantity needed is small and other production techniques are cost-effective [3, 12]. In terms of further technological development and research, the issue will be to overcome current limitations as biocompatibility and biodegradability, the compatibility of stem cells and growth factors and their endurance to thermal or chemical treatments. Commercialization of 3DP systems and their high price for biomedical use is still a concern among certain research groups and institutions. There is also a lack of information on the survival of manufactured prostheses, the functional outcomes and the complications, limited by the short-term follow-up and lack of control for comparison purposes between different reconstruction methods [15]. The lack of large-scale data sets and subjective assessments of many qualitative studies pose the issue of bias and make standardization in terms of reliability and validity difficult, thus quantitative studies including large sample sizes for a more accurate analysis are recommended. Further developments of 3D printed bone implants should be implemented and optimize standard practice. This goes through sharing multicenter data collections to encourage an honest discussion from different hospitals and from different countries on current limitations yet to be overcome. Anyway, talking about the exponential development of 3DP in bone surgery means assessing that the future of Orthopedics and Traumatology is now. And today the greatest challenge is that availability of 3DP and its bony in-growth potential is "within everyone's reach."

References

1. Banks J. Adding value in additive manufacturing: researchers in the United Kingdom and Europe look to 3D printing for customization. IEEE Pulse. 2013;4(6):22–6. https://doi.org/10.1109/MPUL.2013.2279617.
2. Mills DK. Future medicine: the impact of 3D printing. J Nanomater Mol Nanotechnol. 2015;4:3. https://doi.org/10.4172/2324-8777.1000163.
3. Zamborsky R, Kilian M, Jacko P, Bernadic M, Hudak R. Perspectives of 3D printing technology in orthopaedic surgery. Bratisl Lek Listy. 2019;120(7):498–504. https://doi.org/10.4149/BLL_2019_079.
4. Woo SH, Sung MJ, Park KS, Yoon TR. Three-dimensional-printing Technology in hip and Pelvic Surgery: current landscape. Hip Pelvis. 2020;32(1):1–10. https://doi.org/10.5371/hp.2020.32.1.1.
5. Park JW, Kang HG, Lim KM, Park DW, Kim JH, Kim HS. Bone tumor resection guide using three-dimensional printing for limb salvage surgery. J Surg Oncol. 2018;118(6):898–905. https://doi.org/10.1002/jso.25236.
6. Park JW, Kang HG, Lim KM, Kim JH, Kim HS. Three-dimensionally printed personalized

implant design and reconstructive surgery for a bone tumor of the calcaneus: a case report. JBJS Case Connect. 2018;8(2):e25. https://doi.org/10.2106/JBJS.CC.17.00212.
7. Liu X, Liu Y, Lu W, Liao S, Du Q, Deng Z, et al. Combined application of modified three-dimensional printed anatomic templates and customized cutting blocks in pelvic reconstruction after pelvic tumor resection. J Arthroplast. 2019;34(2):338–345.e1. https://doi.org/10.1016/j.arth.2018.10.001.
8. Angelini A, Trovarelli G, Berizzi A, Pala E, Breda A, Ruggieri P. Three-dimension-printed custom-made prosthetic reconstructions: from revision surgery to oncologic reconstructions. Int Orthop. 2019;43(1):123–32. https://doi.org/10.1007/s00264-018-4232-0.
9. Lador R, Regev G, Salame K, Khashan M, Lidar Z. Use of 3-dimensional printing Technology in Complex Spine Surgeries. World Neurosurg. 2020;133:e327–41. https://doi.org/10.1016/j.wneu.2019.09.002.
10. Park JW, Kang HG, Kim JH, Kim HS. The application of 3D-printing technology in pelvic bone tumor surgery [published online ahead of print, 2020 Apr 1]. J Orthop Sci. 2020.;S0949-2658(20)30075-0; https://doi.org/10.1016/j.jos.2020.03.004.
11. Pugliese L, Marconi S, Negrello E, et al. The clinical use of 3D printing in surgery. Updat Surg. 2018;70(3):381–8. https://doi.org/10.1007/s13304-018-0586-5.
12. Bagaria V, Bhansali R, Pawar P. 3D printing- creating a blueprint for the future of orthopedics: current concept review and the road ahead! J Clin Orthop Trauma. 2018;9(3):207–12. https://doi.org/10.1016/j.jcot.2018.07.007.
13. Shilo D, Emodi O, Blanc O, Noy D, Rachmiel A. Printing the Future-Updates in 3D Printing for Surgical Applications. Rambam Maimonides Med J. 2018;9(3):e0020. https://doi.org/10.5041/RMMJ.10343.
14. Rengier F, Mehndiratta A, von Tengg-Kobligk H, Zechmann CM, Unterhinninghofen R, Kauczor HU, et al. 3D printing based on imaging data: review of medical applications. Int J Comput Assist Radiol Surg. 2010;5:335–41. https://doi.org/10.1007/s11548-010-0476-x.
15. Fan H, Fu J, Li X, et al. Implantation of customized 3-D printed titanium prosthesis in limb salvage surgery: a case series and review of the literature. World J Surg Oncol. 2015;13:308. https://doi.org/10.1186/s12957-015-0723-2.
16. Horn TJ, Harrysson OL. Overview of current additive manufacturing technologies and selected applications. Sci Prog. 2012;95(Pt 3):255–82. https://doi.org/10.3184/003685012X13420984463047.
17. Harrysson O, Cansizoglu O, Marcellin-Little DJ, Cormier DR, West HA II. Direct metal fabrication of titanium implants with tailored materials and mechanical properties using electron beam melting technology. Mat Sci Eng C. 2008;28:366–73.
18. Ponader S, von Wilmowsky C, Widenmayer M, Lutz R, Heinl P, Körner C, et al. In vivo performance of selective electron beam-melted Ti-6Al-4V structures. J Biomed Mater Res A. 2010;92:56–62.
19. Cui H, Zhu W, Nowicki M, Zhou X, Khademhosseini A, Zhang LG. Hierarchical fabrication of engineered vascularized bone biphasic constructs via dual 3D bioprinting: integrating regional bioactive factors into architectural design. Adv Healthc Mater. 2016;5(17):2174–81. https://doi.org/10.1002/adhm.201600505.
20. Li CS, Vannabouathong C, Sprague S, Bhandari M. The use of carbon-fiber-reinforced (CFR) PEEK material in orthopedic implants: a systematic review. Clin Med Insights Arthritis Musculoskelet Disord. 2015;8:33–45. https://doi.org/10.4137/CMAMD.S20354.
21. Kersten RF, van Gaalen SM, de Gast A, Öner FC. Polyetheretherketone (PEEK) cages in cervical applications: a systematic review. Spine J. 2015;15(6):1446–60. https://doi.org/10.1016/j.spinee.2013.08.030.
22. Piccioli A, Piana R, Lisanti M, et al. Carbon-fiber reinforced intramedullary nailing in musculoskeletal tumor surgery: a national multicentric experience of the Italian Orthopaedic society (SIOT) bone metastasis study group. Injury. 2017;48(Suppl 3):S55–9. https://doi.org/10.1016/S0020-1383(17)30659-9.
23. Honigmann P, Sharma N, Okolo B, Popp U, Msallem B, Thieringer FM. Patient-specific surgical implants made of 3D printed PEEK: material, technology, and scope of surgical application. Biomed Res Int. 2018;2018:4520636. https://doi.org/10.1155/2018/4520636.
24. Vaezi M, Black C, Gibbs DM, et al. Characterization of new PEEK/HA composites with 3D HA network fabricated by extrusion Freeforming. Molecules. 2016;21(6):687. https://doi.org/10.3390/molecules21060687.
25. Wong KC. 3D-printed patient-specific applications in orthopedics. Orthop Res Rev. 2016;8:57–66. https://doi.org/10.2147/ORR.S99614.
26. Biazzo A, De Paolis M, Donati DM. Scapular reconstructions after resection for bone tumors: a single-institution experience and review of the literature. Acta Biomed. 2018;89(3):415–22. https://doi.org/10.23750/abm.v89i3.5655.
27. Angelini A, Kotrych D, Trovarelli G, Szafrański A, Bohatyrewicz A, Ruggieri P. Analysis of principles inspiring design of three-dimensional-printed custom-made prostheses in two referral centres. Int Orthop. 2020;44(5):829–37. https://doi.org/10.1007/s00264-020-04523-y.
28. Baauw M, van Hellemondt GG, van Hooff ML, Spruit M. The accuracy of positioning of a custom-made implant within a large acetabular defect at revision arthroplasty of the hip. Bone Joint J. 2015;97-B(6):780–5. https://doi.org/10.1302/0301-620X.97B6.35129.
29. Heinl P, Müller L, Körner C, Singer RF, Müller FA. Cellular Ti-6Al-4V structures with interconnected macro porosity for bone implants fabricated

by selective electron beam melting. Acta Biomater. 2008;4(5):1536–44. https://doi.org/10.1016/j.actbio.2008.03.013.

30. Ma L, Zhou Y, Zhu Y, et al. 3D-printed guiding templates for improved osteosarcoma resection. Sci Rep. 2016;6:23335. https://doi.org/10.1038/srep23335.
31. Murphy SV, Atala A. 3D bioprinting of tissues and organs. Nat Biotechnol. 2014;32(8):773–85. https://doi.org/10.1038/nbt.2958.
32. You F, Eames BF, Chen X. Application of Extrusion-Based Hydrogel Bioprinting for Cartilage Tissue Engineering. Int J Mol Sci. 2017;18(7):1597. https://doi.org/10.3390/ijms18071597.
33. Midha S, Dalela M, Sybil D, Patra P, Mohanty S. Advances in three-dimensional bioprinting of bone: Progress and challenges. J Tissue Eng Regen Med. 2019;13(6):925–45. https://doi.org/10.1002/term.2847.
34. Daly AC, Cunniffe GM, Sathy BN, Jeon O, Alsberg E, Kelly DJ. 3D bioprinting of developmentally inspired templates for whole bone organ engineering. Adv Healthc Mater. 2016;5(18):2353–62. https://doi.org/10.1002/adhm.201600182.
35. Levato R, Webb WR, Otto IA, et al. The bio in the ink: cartilage regeneration with bioprintable hydrogels and articular cartilage-derived progenitor cells. Acta Biomater. 2017 Oct 1;61:41e53. https://doi.org/10.1016/j.actbio.2017.08.005.
36. Araujo Borges R (2017) 3D printed PCU/UHMWPE polymeric blends for artificial knee meniscus. Theses and Dissertations Retrieved from https://scholarworks.uark.edu/etd/2653.
37. Zhang Y, Xia L, Zhai D, et al. Mesoporous bioactive glass nanolayer-functionalized 3D-printed scaffolds for accelerating osteogenesis and angiogenesis. Nanoscale. 2015;7(45):19207–21. https://doi.org/10.1039/c5nr05421d.
38. Weisman JA, Nicholson JC, Tappa K, Jammalamadaka U, Wilson CG, Mills DK. Antibiotic and chemotherapeutic enhanced three-dimensional printer filaments and constructs for biomedical applications. Int J Nanomedicine. 2015;10:357–70. https://doi.org/10.2147/IJN.S74811.
39. Lee JH, Baik JM, Yu YS, et al. Development of a heat labile antibiotic eluting 3D printed scaffold for the treatment of osteomyelitis. Sci Rep. 2020;10(1):7554. Published 2020 May 5. https://doi.org/10.1038/s41598-020-64573-5.
40. Dong J, Zhang S, Liu H, Li X, Liu Y, Du Y. Novel alternative therapy for spinal tuberculosis during surgery: reconstructing with anti-tuberculosis bioactivity implants. Expert Opin Drug Deliv. 2014;11(3):299–305. https://doi.org/10.1517/17425247.2014.872625.
41. Zhang Y, Zhai D, Xu M, Yao Q, Chang J, Wu C. 3D-printed bioceramic scaffolds with a Fe3O4/graphene oxide nanocomposite interface for hyperthermia therapy of bone tumor cells. J Mater Chem B. 2016;4(17):2874–86. https://doi.org/10.1039/c6tb00390g.
42. Zhang Y, Zhai D, Xu M, et al. 3D-printed bioceramic scaffolds with antibacterial and osteogenic activity. Biofabrication. 2017;9(2):025037. https://doi.org/10.1088/1758-5090/aa6ed6.
43. Byambaa B, Annabi N, Yue K, et al. Bioprinted osteogenic and Vasculogenic patterns for engineering 3D bone tissue. Adv Healthc Mater. 2017;6(16) https://doi.org/10.1002/adhm.201700015.
44. Yang GH, Yeo M, Koo YW, Kim GH. 4D bioprinting: technological advances in biofabrication. Macromol Biosci. 2019;19(5):e1800441. https://doi.org/10.1002/mabi.201800441.
45. Kirillova A, Maxson R, Stoychev G, Gomillion CT, Ionov L. 4D biofabrication using shape-morphing hydrogels. Adv Mater. 2017;29(46) https://doi.org/10.1002/adma.201703443, https://doi.org/10.1002/adma.201703443.
46. Sawkins MJ, Mistry P, Brown BN, Shakesheff KM, Bonassar LJ, Yang J. Cell and protein compatible 3D bioprinting of mechanically strong constructs for bone repair. Biofabrication. 2015;7(3):035004. https://doi.org/10.1088/1758-5090/7/3/035004.
47. Morouço P, Lattanzi W, Alves N. Four-dimensional bioprinting as a new era for tissue engineering and regenerative medicine. Front Bioeng Biotechnol. 2017;5:61. https://doi.org/10.3389/fbioe.2017.00061.
48. Rychter P, Pamula E, Orchel A, et al. Scaffolds with shape memory behavior for the treatment of large bone defects. J Biomed Mater Res A. 2015;103(11):3503–15. https://doi.org/10.1002/jbm.a.35500.

GPSR Compliance

The European Union's (EU) General Product Safety Regulation (GPSR) is a set of rules that requires consumer products to be safe and our obligations to ensure this.

If you have any concerns about our products, you can contact us on ProductSafety@springernature.com

In case Publisher is established outside the EU, the EU authorized representative is:

Springer Nature Customer Service Center GmbH
Europaplatz 3
69115 Heidelberg, Germany

Batch number: 10731385

Printed by Printforce, the Netherlands